HEALTHY BODY IMAGE

Teaching Kids to Eat and Love Their Bodies Too!

Second Edition

Promoting healthy body image, eating, fitness, nutrition, and weight

❖

A comprehensive resource manual and lesson guide with scripted-lessons and activities for grades four, five, or six

KATHY J. KATER

Healthy Body Image

Teaching Kids to Eat and Love Their Bodies Too!

Second Edition

Published in the United States by the National Eating Disorders Association

603 Stewart Street, Suite 803

Seattle, WA 98101

www.NationalEatingDisorders.org

206-382-3587

Cover art by Erik Brooks

This is a trade paperback, second edition of a three-ring-binder curriculum guide first published by Eating Disorders Awareness and Prevention, Inc. (currently the National Eating Disorders Association) in 1998. In this 2005 edition, the author has updated and revised the entire text.

ISBN 0-9772861-0-X

Disclaimer

The information contained in this book is not intended as a substitute for medical or mental health treatment. Information is offered to inform education related to health, eating, physical activity, and healthy weight. Readers and students of this guide are advised to seek care from a doctor or other appropriately trained professional for concerns related to a medical condition.

Actually, I felt pretty good about my body until about sixth grade. But then everyone else hated theirs, so I thought I should, too.

❖

A culture is formed by the stories its children are told.

Healthy Body Image
MISSION STATEMENT

To empower boys and girls
to maintain positive body esteem
based on recognition of what they can
and cannot control in regard to size and shape.

To empower boys and girls
to resist unrealistic and unhealthy
cultural pressures regarding body image,
eating, nutrition, fitness, and weight.

To inspire boys and girls to develop a stake
in wholesome eating and physical fitness.

TABLE OF CONTENTS

ACKNOWLEDGMENTS

This *Healthy Body Image* curriculum would not exist were it not for the ongoing efforts of literally hundreds of colleagues around the world who have dedicated their time to research, treatment, education, publication, and a joint effort to prevent the full spectrum of body image, eating, nutrition, fitness, and weight problems. However, I am particularly grateful to Michael Levine and Margo Maine for taking precious time away from their already overloaded schedules to provide meticulous and judicious feedback on the revised manuscript for this edition. The exceptional contributions that each of these two individuals has made to the field of eating disorder treatment, prevention, and research seems incalculable, but their warm collegiality, generous leadership, humor, and perseverance are beyond measure as well.

In no particular order, additional individuals whose work has inspired and supported my own include Linda Smolak, Glen Gaesser, Catherine Steiner-Adair, Karin Kratina, Frances Berg, Leigh Kohn, Dianne Neumark-Sztainer, Walter Kaye, Cynthia Bulik, Joe Kelly, Niva Piran, and the late Lori Irving and Ansel Keys. In addition, teachers across the country who have made these lessons come alive in their classrooms have provided invaluable feedback to make this guide better than ever.

I am indebted to the vision and commitment of the board and staff of the National Eating Disorders Association (NEDA), who believed in and piloted the production of both the original publication of *Healthy Body Image* in 1998 and this revised edition. At the NEDA central office Tracy Kahlo, Tonia Brown, and Kari Augustyn in particular committed time and skill to the endless details, decisions and arrangements that turn a manuscript into a publication.

As was true for the original manual, it is my clients, young and old, whose struggles drive my search for effective ways to challenge the destructive, cultural forces that they and we all face. I am ever grateful to them for trusting me with their stories of feeling too long at odds with bodies that were perfect from the start.

Finally, I am unspeakably thankful to my family—Lincoln, Adam and Anya—for their enthusiastic support of my work and willingness to take over many of my chores during the final phase of editing.

PREFACE TO THE REVISED *HEALTHY BODY IMAGE* CURRICULUM

Beyond Prevention of Eating Disorders

Many will assume this curriculum was designed to prevent eating disorders and/or stem the rising tide of obesity in young students, but this would miss a much bigger picture. While too many children will suffer a diagnosable eating or weight disorder, almost *all* children growing up today—particularly the vast majority of girls—will become anxious and/or dissatisfied with their body size and shape and will learn to make unhealthy, nutritionally inadequate, counterproductive, and even dangerous lifestyle choices as a result. Primary prevention efforts are therefore needed to target the seedbed within which the full spectrum of body image, eating, nutrition, fitness, and weight problems take root and grow. In response, the *Healthy Body Image* curriculum was developed to prevent or reduce the influence of insidious risk factors that diminish the body esteem, well-being, and health of the vast majority of children today, regardless of size.

First, Do No Harm

While most body image, eating, nutrition, fitness, and weight disorders are cultivated in the same, increasingly "toxic," cultural environment, these problems have generally been regarded separately when it comes to prevention and intervention. It has become progressively clear that this approach is counterproductive, resulting in recommendations that are frequently contradictory, and thereby contribute to long-term problems. The end result is an *increase* in body image, eating, nutrition, fitness, and weight problems that affect ever-younger children. With an upsurge of headlines announcing a "war on obesity," and an increase in generalized advice to the American population to "lose weight," a reminder about the directive to "first, do no harm" has never been more urgent. This *Healthy Body Image* curriculum is specifically designed to take into account all known factors contributing to the full spectrum of body image, eating, nutrition, fitness, and weight concerns, and to pro-actively teach children a model for long-term health that is realistic, non-contradictory and non-discriminatory. The model upon which the curriculum lessons are based provides both goals and the means to reach them—healthy body image attitudes and healthy lifestyle choices—that are equally attainable by all, regardless of size, shape, cultural and socio-economic background, genetic predisposition, or gender.

Teachers should carefully read the introductory chapter, entitled *Background for Educators,* in order to become very well acquainted with the new paradigm these lessons teach and why a new approach is critical to avoid causing new problems with short-sighted solutions. In fact, schools and organizations are advised to make this background section available to all teachers and staff who interact with students in order to encourage a consistent set of messages about body image, eating, nutrition, fitness, and weight in students' educational environments.

Targeting the Risk Factors That Are within Our Power to Change

Several risk factors for body image, eating, nutrition, fitness, and weight problems have been identified in recent years. Most of these fit into one of two fairly distinct categories: 1) those arising out of the cultural context (this includes the wider culture but also family and micro-cultures), and 2) individual factors, including the innate constitution or biological predisposition that a person brings to that context. While studies have shown that social context alone is enough to generate body image, eating, nutrition, fitness, and weight problems, certain genetic factors, such as a tendency for anxiety, perfectionism, obsessive compulsivity, depression, and certain innate appetites appear to increase an individual's vulnerability and susceptibility to this environment. On the other hand, the existence of predisposing factors are not, by themselves, likely to result in body image, eating, nutrition, fitness, or weight problems without exposure to particular environmental risk factors, or triggers. This is illustrated in the following graph:

Presence of cultural risk factors for body image, eating, nutrition, fitness, and weight problems		⇒	⇒	*Good likelihood* that body image, eating, nutrition, fitness, and weight problems will develop.
Presence of cultural risk factors for body image, eating, nutrition, fitness, and weight problems	+	Presence of innate vulnerabilities	⇒	*Greater likelihood* that serious body image, eating, nutrition, fitness, and weight problems.
No or few cultural risk factors for body image, eating, nutrition, fitness, and weight problems	+	Presence of innate vulnerabilities	⇒	*Not likely* that body image, eating, nutrition, fitness, and weight problems will occur. (Vulnerabilities may be expressed in other ways.)

While it is important to recognize and respond to innate vulnerabilities, these are not within our power to *prevent*, nor should prevention necessarily be a goal, since their existence enhances the rich diversity of our humanity. In contrast, risk factors arising from the cultural context offer tremendous opportunities for prevention. Challenging a set of unhealthy norms that promote significant body image, lifestyle, and health problems for nearly everyone is the goal of this curriculum. Although this task can seem daunting, creating micro-environments (classrooms or schools) that support new and positive attitudes and behaviors should not be underestimated as a change agent.

> ***Never doubt that a small group of thoughtful, committed people can change the world: indeed it's the only thing that ever has!***
>
> **Margaret Mead**

The goals of the *Healthy Body Image* curriculum have been actualized in the past several years by many teachers across the country, demonstrating that teachers and students together can create an environment that contrasts positively with the wider culture. Outcome studies, conversations with veteran teachers and their students, and observations of classroom settings reveal how this is working. Students who have learned the *Body Image Building Blocks* talk openly and non-judgmentally among themselves about size diversity (taller/shorter, fatter/thinner), and matter-of-factly discuss the value of attention to deeper qualities (versus placing undue emphasis on looks). They are savvy about cultural messages that push the *thin-ideal* as "the way to look," as well as high calorie/low-nutrient treats as "the way to eat." They can tell you why it's good that the Ugly Duckling didn't stay with the ducks, and how she thereby avoided what occurs for so many in our culture: people comparing themselves year after year to a standard that was never realistic for them and feeling ugly or at least unattractive and undesirable as a result. Posters in these classrooms reflect diversity. Projects such as the *Identity Mobile* (from Lesson 2) hang from the ceiling, and books are displayed that reflect acceptance of a variety of healthy sizes and shapes, body esteem, and the value of nutrition and fitness for every body. The result is as follows:

Presentation of concepts presented by the *Body Image Building Blocks*	+	Presence or no presence of innate vulnerabilities	⇨	*Less* likelihood of body image, eating, fitness, nutrition and weight problems; greater likelihood of empowerment through having a "voice" with which to resist destructive norms.

The normative "voice" of their classroom is educational and empowering to students, despite their awareness that outside of their classroom, even in their school and in their homes, many have not had these lessons and thus have different perspectives. The general response is one of understanding and acceptance that peers and adults have not all had the same educational opportunity as they have had. This is not dissimilar from the experience of the 1970s, when education regarding the dangers of smoking was taught in classrooms even as students walked daily past smoke-filled teachers' lounges and went home to smoking parents.

Students of these lessons are not naïve. They know they may be vulnerable to negative cultural pressures about looks as they move into their teen years. Still, they state their belief that these *Healthy Body Image* lessons will help them along the way. A video of fifth-grade children talking about their experiences with the *Healthy Body Image* curriculum is available at cost from the author for limited viewing. (See the Appendix for contact information.)

The Primary Cultural Risk Factors for Body Image, Eating, Fitness, Nutrition, and Health Problems

The cultural risk factors known to contribute to body image, eating, fitness, nutrition, and weight problems include the following set of pervasive values, beliefs, and responses:

- **Image is valued over substance:** *"How I look" is more important than "who I am." An essential criterion for the "right look" is a thin or lean body.*
- **Denial of biological diversity:** *Anyone can be slim if he or she works at it. Fatter people inevitably eat too much and/or are inactive. Fat is bad/wrong.*
- **Denial of the universal effects of externally prescribed hunger regulation:** *Dieting is an effective weight-loss strategy.*

- **Discounting the value of health; complacency about healthy lifestyle choices that do not result in the desired look:** *"Eat, drink, and be merry." Healthy choices (for health's sake) are too much work.*

Students growing up today are exposed from an early age to these risk factors through multiple interpersonal and media channels. In fact, children and adults today are so universally bombarded with messages promoting body image, eating, fitness, and nutrition problems that few escape the effect. It is important to note that all of these now normative values or beliefs directly conflict with basic biological facts and/or principles that support healthy body image and health in general. The result is a population who, by and large, worry more about size and the drive to be thin than wellness and vitality while paradoxically growing fatter by the decade.

The majority of females of all ages and sizes in Western cultures learn to incorporate this negative set of attitudes, beliefs, and behaviors into their daily lives, even those who intellectually "know better," i.e., reject the premise as invalid, unrealistic, unhealthy, and unhelpful. Males, many of whom have learned to tolerate, endorse, or push unrealistic expectations of females based on this set of beliefs, are now applying similar standards to themselves.

Reclaiming health as a goal.

As the thin-ideal and the drive to be thin have become normative values, the concept of "health" as a core value has been gradually lost or re-constructed. Instead of strength, stamina, flexibility, vitality, and vigor (including metabolic fitness and nutritional soundness), a more slender or lean appearance is routinely the primary objective. This value shift has been accepted even if the means to achieve a reduced size defy principles of health, biological diversity, and internal hunger regulation. The disappearance of hardiness and heartiness as key values undermines the welfare and well-being of our population. The *Healthy Body Image* curriculum teaches 1) that health is a primary goal that should not be sacrificed for the sake of appearance, and 2) the lifestyle choices and attitudes conducive to achieving it.

Fortunately, since all of these risk factors are imbedded in the culture, change, while difficult, is possible. Lessons designed to counteract their influence through promoting positive, healthy attitudes and choices can help the next generation. Students can learn to maintain innate body esteem and body integrity, develop realistic body image attitudes and perspectives, and cultivate a lifelong habit of competent eating and fitness choices even in the face of toxic cultural pressures. The *Healthy Body Image* curriculum is designed as a tool for this purpose.

Changes in This Revised *Healthy Body Image* Curriculum

Those who are familiar with the first edition of this curriculum will find this revision to be familiar. The *Model for Healthy Body Image* upon which it is based is unchanged, and lessons include most of the same activities. There are three major differences: 1) The *Background for Educators* has been expanded to address the health concerns resulting from inactivity and excessive high-calorie/low-nutrient eating that have increased exponentially in recent years. *Healthy Body Image* lessons have always targeted prevention of unhealthy weight gain, inadequate nutrition, and poor fitness habits as well as prevention of body image problems and unhealthy dieting behaviors. That comprehensive purpose is now more clearly and explicitly expressed. 2) While feedback from teachers of the *Healthy Body Image* curriculum has been positive, suggestions for minor changes from those experienced in teaching the lessons have been incorporated. 3) The overall formatting and presentation of the curriculum has been simplified and reorganized. Several auxiliary pages that were previously found in the front of the manual have been moved to the Appendix. In addition, rather than a three-ring binder, a bound book with perforated handouts and overheads that can be removed for photocopying protects the physical integrity of the manual. (Perforated pages may be found in the Appendix.)

Updated Empirical Basis for This Curriculum

For those wanting to examine the scientific basis for the concepts taught in this prevention initiative, an extensive reference section is included in the Appendix. While much remains to be understood, even more has been learned about the risk factors for unhealthy body image, eating, nutrition, fitness, and weight problems since the first edition, pointing the way to promising methods of prevention. Research has demonstrated that it is possible to help children to develop a healthy body image and positive lifestyle habits at an early age, in addition to helping them to resist conflicting socio-cultural messages as they progress through middle school. In turn, the primary purpose of eating and movement for health, energy, and satisfaction can be protected. Curricular interventions using a combination of cognitive and experiential education methods are most effective. That said, studies further show that a systematic, *whole-school*, family, and community education effort will result in the best outcome (for more information about a *whole-school* approach, see the Appendix.)

Outcome Data

Outcome studies using this curriculum have been promising, measuring significant positive change in student attitudes, behaviors, and knowledge. Information about two published reports can be found in the *Background for Educators* as well as in the Appendix.

Anecdotal Basis for This Curriculum—Beyond the Numbers

The *Background for Educators* presents the empirical need for lessons included in this curriculum. The following quotes more personally illustrate the problems this curriculum is designed to prevent.

> *Why should I eat healthy if it won't make me thin?*
>
> —Fourteen year-old girl

> *I exercised five times a week for three months, but I didn't lose any weight.*
> *What's the point?*
>
> —Mother of three elementary school girls

If I eat healthy, I feel like I'm on a diet and I can't wait to eat some junk food.

—Sixteen year-old girl

I played soccer four or five times a week all year, and I ate better than almost anyone I know. But then my coach said I would play better if I lost weight. At first it made me mad, since I'm one of the best players on the team. But after a while it got to me, and I thought maybe I should go on a diet. At first it was hard, but then the more I didn't eat, the easier it was. I lost 45 pounds in about six months. Then one day, something snapped. I started bingeing in the evening. Every day it got worse. All day I would try to eat as little as possible to make up for the last night's binge, but after school when I was home alone, I just couldn't control myself. Now I'm terrified to eat, because once I do. . . Well, there's no end until I'm stuffed.

— High School All-State athlete who developed bulimia

You won't believe this, but in my school, how you look is everything. If I don't lose 10 pounds by next fall, I might as well not even go to high school.

— Beautiful and slim-by-any-standard eighth-grade girl

When I was in second grade the school nurse told my mother she should put me on a diet or my chubby little body might get too fat. At first I was excited because I felt special that I got to go through the teacher's lunch line where they had salad and other low-cal foods that weren't offered to the kids. But it didn't take long before I realized this was no great deal. Mainly, I remember I was starving all the time. In the morning, I spent my time waiting for lunch. But what they gave me was never enough, and so all afternoon I would wait to go home and eat. My mom tried to limit my snacks, but I would find ways to get food and hide it in my room, or go to the corner store and stock up. I couldn't figure out why I had to be hungry all the time just because I was fat. That was when my resentment started to grow. I was determined not to let them succeed in their plan to slim me down. I began to eat whatever treats I could get my hands on whenever I could. They couldn't figure out why I didn't lose weight! By the time I was in high school I was very obese. But I was never a wallflower. I had a lot of friends because I'm outgoing and always had fun ideas about things to do. I still love to go to restaurants, order a lot of greasy food, and then watch the waitress squirm when I look her in the eye and say, "Bring a little extra butter on the side with that, would you, dear? Oh, and a slice of that double-Dutch cake for dessert, please."

—Thirty-four year-old clinically obese registered nurse in psychotherapy for depression

I heard my aunt tell my mom that I have the Anderson body. I really hate my legs because I know they are like my mother's and she has big thighs. A couple of times my mom stayed home because she said she looked so fat, and she went in her room and cried. I feel like my legs are really big and fat, and I have to eat as little as possible to keep them from growing.

—Nine-year-old girl, five feet tall, weighing 71 pounds, diagnosed with anorexia

All anyone ever talks about at lunch is how fat and ugly they are and how they can't eat this and can't eat that. It makes me so mad! I used to feel fine about my body, but how can you feel ok when the skinniest girls in the school go on and on about how they need to lose weight. It wears you down. Now I worry just like they do about being fat, and wonder what other people think about me. How can I eat lunch when that's what's going on? What if people think you are fat, and there you are, eating right in front of them?

—Normal-weight thirteen-year-old girl

I hate my body. Really. I just hate it. I have ever since I was in fourth grade. I feel it every minute of every day.

—Thirty-four year-old mother of three daughters

Actually, I felt pretty good about my body until 6th grade. But then everyone else hated theirs, so I thought I should too.

—Twenty-two year-old women in treatment for her bulimia

BACKGROUND FOR EDUCATORS

Body image, eating, fitness, nutrition, and weight problems are pervasive in our culture and affect children at increasingly young ages. At a time when they should feel secure in their body's growth, most children today learn to worry about size, shape, and weight and to make choices that cause the very problems they wish to avoid. The results diminish the self esteem and integrity of growing bodies and egos, as well as consuming attention and energy that should be available for other important developmental tasks. Ironically, as the drive to be thin and dieting for weight loss have consumed our population, America has become the fattest nation on earth. In four decades, the thinner we have tried to be, the fatter we have become. Clearly something is wrong with our approach.

Headlines draw our attention to debilitating eating disorders and the rapid rise in obesity. But underlying these extremes are the culturally propagated seeds for body image, eating, nutrition, fitness, and weight problems that negatively affect virtually *all* children today. It is these environmental risk factors that must be the focus of our educational efforts. It is important to note that students would not need a curriculum such as this one in an setting in which body esteem, respect for size diversity, internal hunger regulation, wholesome eating and physical fitness were well supported. Unfortunately, the context in which today's children grow up, instead, presents them, from an early age, with multiple, conflicting messages that specifically promote unhealthy perspectives and behaviors. These messages have an especially negative effect as children experience the natural reshaping of their bodies that comes with puberty.

Body-angst, eating, fitness, and weight problems are extremely difficult to reverse once they are established. We now know enough about the toxic cultural risk factors that give rise to these concerns to prevent much of the trouble *before* it starts. Children can and should be taught from an early age to recognize and resist unhealthy pressures, to maintain body integrity, and to make competent choices that will enhance their health and well-being. This *Healthy Body Image* curriculum is designed to positively and proactively support that objective.

These introductory pages provide the background that is necessary to teach this *Healthy Body Image* curriculum. Teachers should read the *Background for Educators* in its entirety before proceeding with lesson plans. This material is organized as follows:

Part I: Introduces the full spectrum of body image, eating, fitness, nutrition, and weight problems that routinely affect students.

Part II: Describes the cultural risk factors that encourage body image, eating, nutrition, fitness, and weight problems and presents the *Model for Healthy Body Image* that was developed to challenge these risk factors. This model provides the foundation for the *Body Image Building Blocks* presented in the *Healthy Body Image* lessons.

Part III: Further orients teachers as they prepare to teach the lessons.

PART I: THE SPECTRUM OF PROBLEMS

The following interrelated topics will be addressed in this section:

A. Negative body image and the drive to be thin
B. The rising rate of overweight and obesity
C. Poor nutrition and lack of fitness at every size
D. The purpose of this *Healthy Body Image* curriculum in addressing this spectrum of problems

A. Negative body image and the drive to be thin

The effect on females

It is rare for adolescent girls to feel content with their natural bodies. Between 70% to 80% report unhappiness with their shape and say they "feel fat," a disparaging self-judgment that may or may not have anything to do with *being* fat. While people have always been interested in appearance, the current emphasis on physical beauty for women and the pressure to be thin in order to achieve it is unprecedented. In response, attempts at weight control through various methods of restrictive eating have become the norm. Up to 70% of teenage females report they have engaged in restrictive eating practices to attempt control or loss of weight. By comparison, in the early 1960s similar attitudes and behaviors were measured in the 30% to 35% range.

Body image, eating, and weight concerns have proliferated in a social context that equates desirability in females with appearance, and the "right look" with a lean body that is unrealistic for most. Given this environment, we cannot be surprised at the prevalence of negative body image among girls. In light of cultural norms, it is *adaptive* for them to become anxious about and dissatisfied with their naturally developing, fuller shapes. Studies have documented the following statistically normal developmental sequence for this adaptive process. The sequence:

→ begins with internalization of Western culture's unrealistic thin-ideal.

→ progresses to body dissatisfaction, "feeling fat" or fear of becoming fat.

→ leads to dietary restraint for weight loss (or in hopes of preventing weight gain).

→ results in the expected and predictable consequences of dieting for weight loss: preoccupation with food, compulsive- or binge-eating problems, and regaining of weight.

→ focuses attention on feelings of failure and/or heightened fear of fat.

→ begins again.

In today's culture it is normative for females of all sizes to learn to feel dissatisfied with their natural size, weight, and shape and to fear that their hunger will make them unattractive (fat). This attitude is reflected by this statement from a 22-year-old victim of bulimia:

Actually, I felt pretty good about my body until about sixth grade.
But everyone else hated theirs, so I thought I should, too.

It should be clarified that most girls and women in our culture, not just those who are visibly fatter, either "feel fat" and develop the accompanying self-condemnation, or they fear becoming fat. In fact, there is indication that some relatively slender girls who see "perfection" as only a few pounds away may be more likely to use manipulative eating practices to achieve the cultural ideal than those for whom this possibility is more distant. While fatter girls may not feel better about themselves, they may at least be more realistic!

Younger children are affected

Once considered to be a problem of college-age, and then high school females, now the vast majority of third- to sixth-grade girls, biologically primed for their pubescent growth spurt, say they are "very afraid of gaining weight." Almost half, regardless of size, say they would "like to lose weight," and one-third of girls this age acknowledge they have already tried restrictive dieting. Even kindergarten teachers say they hear their young students mimicking the fat-talk of their elders. Whether or not such young children fully understand their own words, clearly they are learning the language of fat-phobia. These children are not learning to feel integrity in their bodies, to trust inner cues about what they need, or that we want them to eat well for health and well-being. Instead, from a very early age, they are learning to feel insecure and self-conscious, to mistrust their hunger, to think of themselves as "good" or "bad" based on the size of their stomachs, and to set themselves on a course in which weight loss and gain are a central focus of their lives.

Boys are not exempt

Body scrutiny for boys in our culture is gradually following the path previously prescribed for females. Still, surveys show that important differences between boys and girls remain: fewer boys feel bad, and those who do begin at a later age. Experts suggest this may be because fewer comments are made to boys about their appearance, and the standards for an acceptable male physique are broader. As a result, the risk of harsh judgments seems to be generally less for males than for females in our culture. While surveys show that boys increasingly have an aversion to becoming fat, unlike girls they rarely describe themselves as being or feeling fat unless there is visible, objective evidence to support that description.

Coping styles for boys are also different. Studies show that boys are not as likely as girls to take it out on themselves if they feel their appearances are not ideal or are merely "Ok." In particular, this perception is less likely to affect overall self esteem, activities they pursue, or to interfere with healthy behaviors. Boys tend to seek other outlets (hobbies, sports) rather than trying to make themselves over at any cost.

While few studies exist, there is consensus that males have been significantly affected by a rise in the number of images of "ideal" pumped-up men in today's mass media. Despite different coping styles, as they are increasingly surrounded by images of "ideally handsome" men with the "chiseled body" look, studies show males succumb to comparisons, and feel deficient as a result. It is the desire for a "ripped" (muscular) look that seems to occur most frequently. When the lean-but-buff-body look is presented as if it were normal, more men and boys feel their body build is lacking. For example, in 1972, only 18% of males said they "disliked their upper torso," but by 1996 the percentage had more than doubled to 38%, and has risen to nearly 50% today. Compulsive weightlifting and consumption of expensive bulking-up substances has increased with these changes. Most alarming is the use of anabolic steroids to build muscles and exaggerate male sexual characteristics. While these drugs are not legal without a prescription, abusers find ways to obtain them, and advice about their use is readily available on the Internet. The effectiveness of these drugs makes them extremely seductive, and most users are either not aware of or deny the serious medical complications that are inevitable with long-term use.

Finally, boys are vulnerable and at risk for adopting unrealistic and distorted expectations of girls when only unrealistic, idealized images of females are presented as acceptable and desirable. "Image is everything!" and the thin-ideal puts both girls and boys at risk.

Cultural differences

Some cultural and racial groups have fared better in maintaining their acceptance of more realistic and diverse body types. For example, some studies have shown that African American females are more satisfied with their diverse bodies than White women. Surveys reveal that among these women "looking good" spans a wider range of options and reflects individual style rather than conformity. However, new research suggests that acceptance of diverse sizes is diminishing. As financial conditions improve among minority groups, so apparently does anxiety about weight and identification with the current "ideal" female role model: five-feet seven-inches tall and 110 pounds. Certainly the process of acculturation—the identification of a small group with the values of the larger group—has taken a toll on many ethnic minorities and immigrants to Western cultures. Integration into mainstream society generally includes adoption of the prevailing standard of thinness and perceived pressures to diet.

The idea that the drive to be thin is for White kids only is no longer sound, as messages placing a premium on thinness (and dieting as a means to achieve it) permeate the far corners of the globe. While dieting is not generally associated with developing countries, headlines such as this one suggest a change: *Anorexia Takes Hold in India* (British Broadcasting Company, 2003). Diet disorders have increased exponentially in places like India, Venezuela, the Philippines, and Mexico. So, too, have they increased in the inner cities, rural towns, and ethnic communities across the USA.

To the degree that some groups or individuals have held onto their healthy body image attitudes and behaviors in the face of mainstream counter-pressures, we can learn from their model. This curriculum echoes and affirms that wisdom.

The cost of negative body image and the drive to be thin

Many people believe that, unless body image and eating problems progress to a diagnosable eating or weight-related disorder, there is not so much cause for concern. But how students feel in their own skins is not trivial. Negative body image costs our children, our families, and our society at large in several important ways:

1. Time, attention, energy, self esteem and money drain

   Body dissatisfaction is a significant distraction, consuming a tremendous amount of energy and attention that children need for more important developmental tasks. Self-consciousness feels bad, provoke feelings of shame, erodes self esteem, and makes it difficult to concentrate. Students who routinely worry about their size and shape as they navigate school hallways or sit at their desks are anxious and preoccupied students. Students who fear they are being judged as they eat (or don't eat) in lunchrooms or who worry about how they look in physical education classes would rather be anywhere else. Body self-consciousness hampers children's ability to focus on academic, social, and character development as well as other important skills and events.

2. A crisis of disconnection from the self

   A growing child's inability to feel comfortable in his or her own skin is detrimental to the formation of his or her identity. Children who struggle with body image learn to view themselves from the outside-in, rather than the inside-out. "How I look" becomes more important than "Who I am." As teachers try to guide students to listen to and express their inner voices, our culture's emphasis on superficial appearance teaches children to worry more about how people will judge them.

   Today's students feel pressured at increasingly younger ages to present an exterior appearance that will be favorably received, whether or not that appearance is even remotely possible for them. They feel forced to choose between staying connected to who they are, on the one hand, and trying to "fit in," on the other. For girls this usually begins with objectifying their bodies as they search for external cues to tell them what will be considered desirable instead of role models who encourage expression of their honest selves. This "dissociative crisis" makes many girls willing to risk even their health (deny their hunger, exercise excessively, look good at any cost) in order to have relationships. Rather than *who they are*, it is *who they appear to be* that matters. This perceived need to bury the authentic self takes a tragic toll on the self esteem and health practices of many adolescent girls.

3. Poor nutrition and spiraling fatness

    Negative body image is a primary risk factor for many of the nutrient-deficient eating habits that are now routine for many Americans. Instead of holding good nutrition and health as the highest priority, eating or not eating is done in hopes of achieving a particular body size or shape, or to sooth disappointment when these efforts fail. Eating habits that disregard the primary purpose of eating for nutritional sustenance, energy, and satisfaction of hunger severely test the functioning of the internal weight regulatory system. When adolescents swing from restrictive eating one day to "junk food" overloads the next, they routinely miss important nutrients, frequently add pounds, and lose touch with what it means to eat normally.

4. Eating disorders

    Feeling fat and the dieting behaviors it spawns are the primary triggers for life-threatening and difficult-to-treat eating disorders. New research strongly suggests that eating disorders may be a response to an underlying anxiety disorder, perfectionism, and/or obsessive-compulsive traits, all of which are believed to have a genetic basis. However, a person with this type of predisposition is not as likely to develop an eating disorder without exposure to the thin-ideal and pressures to restrict eating for weight loss.

While only about 6% of adolescent girls and 1% of boys will progress in their body image concerns to a restrictive- or binge-eating disorder, the *vast majority* of young students today will be negatively affected by our culture's thin-ideal. Increasing anxiety about appearance, obsessive inner dialogues about weight and shape, and the consequences of restricted, defiant, or complacent eating are serious problems that interfere with important emotional and health needs for most girls and an increasing number of boys today.

Body image is central to the emerging self as children enter puberty

As students enter puberty, they begin to anticipate the looming judgment of their own physical attractiveness. Looks do matter. In the American social context, almost any degree of visible fatness is considered to be unattractive, whether it is 5 pounds or 200. Since it is normal for developing females to add 20% of their body weight in fat, sometimes as much as 20 pounds or more in a single year between the ages of 10 and 14, the result is frequently devastating to girls' self esteem and confidence. Likewise, boys often round out before shooting upward as they enter puberty. When this development is labeled "getting fat" (negative connotation implied) rather than celebrated as the start of a new stage of growth, self-consciousness, preoccupation, anxiety, and often hunger (from dieting to ward off normal development) begin to consume attention. Just when young students should begin to discover who they are—their preferences, personal style, and their own voices about what is right and just in the world—more and more of them are overwhelmed and silenced by pressures to acquire the "right look." "Good" students of the culture will learn to suppress their individuality, to view themselves as objects, to adopt the drive to be thin and to suffer the negative body esteem this spawns. The long-ranging effects into adulthood are well documented.

B. The rising rate of overweight and obesity

Awareness and concern about negative body image and the drive to be thin in children are growing. But given coinciding trends, a frequent question seems almost to counter this: *Aren't a slender-ideal and a self-critical eye regarding fatness needed to prevent unhealthy weight gain?*

This question is best answered by a second one: Have a pervasive focus on weight, fear of fatness, critical body scrutiny, and the drive to be thin kept us lean? Since the early 1960s, Americans have assumed more personal responsibility for their weight, claimed more weight-loss intentions, and engaged in more weight-loss efforts than ever before. On any given day, 46% of the population is actively on a weight-loss diet, and many more are planning to begin (or resume) dieting soon. Roughly 70% of females routinely cycle on and off of various weight-loss plans, and they are being joined by a growing number of men who diet and exercise in an effort to shed fat. Yet, Americans as a group are fatter now than any population has ever been.

Since the drive to be thin and efforts to lose weight have become pervasive, the incidence of overweight and obesity has more than doubled. When adjusted for changing standards, the number of Americans considered overweight has risen from somewhere around 14% in the 1960s to over 50 % today. At this rate of increase, statisticians tell us the nation will be 100% overweight by 2030. *Clearly weight loss or even weight control as a goal has failed and continues to fail.* It is critical to understand the complex set of factors that hinders this objective in order to avoid inadvertently contributing to the problem.

Dieting as a solution

There is widespread agreement that, for those who want to lose weight, dieting (eating according to a prescribed plan to limit food intake with the goal of weight loss) should be part of the formula. As previously noted, dieting has become a normative eating style in the United States.

The diet mentality remains strong despite significant empirical data and clinical outcomes showing that restricting calories or food groups for the purpose of weight loss is counterproductive for weight loss in the long run. In fact, for mentally well individuals, dieting for weight loss reliably produces results that are not only contrary to sustained weight loss but frequently result in weight gain. Studies show that dieting behaviors consistently and reliably lead to:

- An increased preoccupation with food and difficulty concentrating on anything else.
- A dramatic increase in food cravings, especially for calorie-dense foods, such as sugars and fats.
- Irritability and depression.
- Decreased metabolic rate.

- A ravenous hunger when restraints on eating are removed.
- Compulsive or binge rebound-eating that may persist for some time once the diet is ended.
- Disruption of the normal internal hunger regulatory system if dieting is sustained or repeated over time.
- Regain of weight that was lost, often with added pounds.

Dieting is very seductive. Short-term results are almost always promising. However, given the normal, expected response to dieting over time, weight that is lost is predictably regained. Conservative estimates suggest that at least 90% of weight that is lost through any type of weight reduction plan is ultimately regained and often with added pounds. Even so, since dieting is generally viewed as part of the "solution" for weight loss, most dieters resume their efforts again and again. Over time, diet cycling results in significant weight gain over and above the starting weight for many chronic dieters. Efforts to lose weight through dieting are therefore not merely ineffective but are actually harmful, contributing to long-term problems for a significant number of people.

Because restricting calories (by any means—restricting overall intake or selected food groups, such as carbohydrates) works at first, there is a reluctance to acknowledge its dismal long-term record and negative side-effects. Most dieters incorrectly accept a sense of personal failure for their futile efforts and blame themselves for the compensatory eating that routinely follows. Even many health-care-providers remain uninformed or discount the evidence against dieting as a weight-loss strategy. For example, a study published in *Pediatrics* (2003) followed 15,000 dieting and non-dieting boys and girls, ages 9 to 14, for three years. In the end, dieting children gained significantly *more* weight than non-dieters and were more likely than non-dieters to report binge or compulsive-overeating behaviors. The more often dieting occurred, the more weight was gained. Despite such warnings, prescription of diets for weight loss continues, even for children.

With headlines stressing a correlation between weight gain and health problems, worried physicians and parents often do not know what else to do as more and more chubby children test positive for type-two diabetes, high blood pressure, cholesterol, and other ailments. But a careful history of obese adults reveals that many can trace a pattern of disordered eating to diets that were urged on them by well-meaning adults when they were children. Prescribing a diet for weight loss teaches children that they cannot trust and should not listen to the internal cues that regulate their hunger and weight, and that they must rely on external rules in order to be both healthy and acceptable in the eyes of others. Such a plan is a set-up for failure. Teaching children of any size that weight loss should be their goal and that a diet plan is the means to achieving it is a dangerous, reactionary response, swinging the pendulum to a dysfunctional alternative that is not benign. Following the maxim, "do no harm," a more effective approach is imperative.

What to say to students who are on weight loss diets prescribed by health-care providers: Lessons in this curriculum teach students that, instead of dieting for weight loss, a more realistic, effective, and no-risk method is 1) to satisfy hunger fully with a variety of wholesome foods, 2) to be physically active for strength and fitness, and 3) to trust that the resulting size and weight is right for them. Lesson 8 specifically demonstrates to children why dieting for weight loss is not generally successful in the long run and may actually cause problems. This will pose a conflict for students who have been advised to lose weight through calorie restriction by their medical-provider. It is probably best to address this discrepancy directly. Teachers then might say, "Your health-care-provider and parents want only the best for you. It's possible they may not be aware of the problems that can be caused by dieting for weight loss." The Recommended Reading list in the Appendix includes books for parents and/or physicians requesting more information.

The "obesigenic environment"

Many things have changed in the four decades during which the drive to be thin and dieting for weight loss became normative. Alongside marketing of the thin/buff-ideal and the various means to achieve it, the introduction and mass marketing of low-nutrient/calorie-dense, taste-stimulating foods have competed for a bigger and bigger share of the American food market. Simultaneously, new sedentary work and entertainment options have come to occupy more daily hours than ever previously imagined. Without a doubt, the explosion of fast-food, entertainment-food, and ready-made or easy-to-prepare processed-food markets has resulted in very real changes in the eating style and quality of food eaten by the average American. This environmental change certainly supports less wholesome lifestyle choices that may result in unhealthy fatness for many, and diminished health for most.

There is little argument that the availability, portability, attractive packaging, great taste, and a cheap price have made an abundance of generally calorie-dense/nutrient-deficient, ready-to-eat foods widely and wildly appealing to children as well as to most adults. By comparison, most whole, unprocessed groceries and fresh produce and meats are usually available only at higher cost at grocery stores or markets situated in locations that are often not within easy walking distance of homes, schools, work, or recreational sites. Once purchased, whole foods may need at least some preparation before they are ready to eat. All in all, satisfying hunger with a variety of nutrient-dense foods requires more planning, effort, and expense than with many "convenience" or fast foods.

Coupled with a host of other lifestyle changes—fewer stay-at-home parents, busier schedules, fewer family meals, more disposable income, and especially the rise in sedentary work and leisure options—and the resulting environment can easily be blamed for a sharp drop in wholesome eating and physical activity. That said, a dangerous perspective emerges when concern about *lifestyle choices* is redirected and *fatness* is instead identified as the problem. Not only does this add fuel to fat-phobia and encourage weight loss as the goal; it implies that weight (which is not a behavior) can be chosen or controlled and that health is dependent on size.

Belief that weight is a choice

American children as young as five believe that, if an individual is fat, he or she eats too much and exercises too little. The belief that fatter people are inevitably doing something wrong and that they should lose weight is normative in our population. However, this assumption discounts our knowledge of biological size diversity and the fact that well over 50% of the influence for size and shape, including fatness and thinness, is genetically predisposed. This includes not only bone structure but also fat-to-lean body-tissue composition, the location of fat stores, and metabolic rate. This does not mean that weight cannot be *influenced* by lifestyle choices—clearly the increasing rate of fatness across the population is not due to a change in genetic predisposition. What it means is that, given equal, optimal lifestyle habits of healthy eating and fitness across the population, bodies will still be diverse, ranging from very thin to very fat, with most people somewhere in the middle. It further means that assumptions cannot be made about a person's lifestyle habits by merely observing that they are fat or thin, or by measuring body mass index (BMI). Despite the abundance of messages implying that weight is a matter of choice, *that concept is not accurate.* Choices may be made about behaviors: how one will eat and how much one will move. Such choices frequently influence weight, but they cannot be counted on to result in a particular, prescribed weight or recommended BMI. Instead, even when optimal choices are made, the expected outcome is improved health in individuals who will maintain diverse sizes, ranging from fat to thin.

Belief that health is dependent on size

An excess of high-calorie/low-nutrient food and a too-sedentary lifestyle pose a very real health risk. One common outcome is increased fatness. But before pointing to fatness as a risk factor for health problems, we must step back and consider the facts. Major studies, including one that carefully followed 21,925 men over eight years, have documented that fatter people who are physically fit are actually at lower risk for health-related problems than thinner people who are not fit. This challenges our basic assumption and raises an important new question: *Is fatness or lack of fitness the causal factor when it comes to health concerns?* Many fatter people are not fit (perhaps in part because of the stigma associated with fatness), but when fitness improves, even with minimal weight loss, vital measures of health improve, as well. In light of this, a focus on *fitness*—which is an achievable goal, regardless of size, rather than reduced fatness, which may or may not be achievable—is both non-discriminatory and likely to improve health.

Defining a more realistic goal

It should be clear that the identification of *fatness* as the problem and resulting emphasis on *weight loss* as the solution has done little to address the health concerns of the next generation of children and, in fact, is making matters worse. This paradigm encourages the drive to be thin and diet mentality, while having little positive effect on the eating, fitness, or weight of the average adult or child. When we instead shift the focus from fat and weight to choices leading to nutritional health and metabolic fitness we sacrifice nothing while gaining an approach that enhances the well-being of all.

C. Complacency about nutrition and fitness

Complacency about nutrition and physical activity is epidemic in the American population among people of all sizes and shapes. Surveys show that the primary motive for being physically active and eating a variety of fruits, vegetables, whole grains, low-fat milk, and protein-rich foods today is to lose or control weight. When healthy choices do not always result in the desired weight, the temptations of today's *obesigenic* (fat inducing) environment become an all too appealing alternative. Health as a goal is considered to be a poor and uninspiring second choice, if not irrelevant, especially for the young.

> *Why should I eat healthy if it won't make me thin?*
>
> –Fourteen year-old girl

> *I exercised five times a week for three months and didn't lose any weight. What's the point?*
>
> – Twenty-seven year-old mother of two preschool children

A dangerous perspective arises when weight loss is presented as the reward for healthy lifestyle habits, leading too many people to abandon good nutrition and fitness if these "only" result in improved health versus a lean physique. This skewed perspective has contributed to the rising rates of overweight and obesity in the American population. In addition, when weight loss is the much touted objective of a wholesome lifestyle, complacency is inadvertently encouraged among those who do not perceive a need to lose weight:

> *It doesn't matter what I eat. I've never been fat!*
>
> – Fifteen year-old boy

> *I eat every day at some fast-food place, just like in that movie* Supersize Me. *The difference is, somehow I stay slim! So who cares?*
>
> – Twenty-eight year-old office worker

> *My friends hate me because I eat junk all the time, I never exercise, and I'm still skinny!*
>
> – Eighth-grade girl

Do we really want to convey that the nutritional and fitness needs of slim students are less important than those of their rounder peers? The number of children *of all sizes* today who lack balanced nutrition and are inactive is alarming. Sometimes the basis for this is economic, and food is scarce. But when children of adequate means eat a disproportion of high-calorie/low nutrient foods or, alternatively, restrict calories for the purpose of weight loss or because of a misguided sense of "being in control," a *disconnect* from the primary purpose of eating well for self-care—for health, vitality, well-being, and enjoyment—is evident. When poor nutritional habits are accepted *or supported* by adults, either through the foods that are offered, through turning a blind-eye, or through modeling, then a normative complacency about the relationship between health, nutrition, and fitness as a value in its own right can be expected in the next generation.

Eating well and physical fitness require some time and effort. When bodies are already naturally slim, when wholesome choices do not pay off in the "right" (slim) look, or when restricting calories solicits in admiration for "willpower" or a slimmer physique, "who cares about nutrition" is an all too common response. Children today need *new incentives* to eat a balanced, wholesome variety of food and to seek out activities that promote their physical fitness. *When health replaces size or appearance as the primary enticement, then students of every size will have measurably better health.*

Pseudo-control versus real control

In cultures where food is plentiful, the freedom to choose what and how much to eat has become an arena in which a misguided sense of being in control is played out. On the one hand, in times of plenty, we have come to admire restrictiveness and view the willpower to cut calories (skip lunch, say "no" to dessert, count carbs, *be anorexic*, etc.) and ultimately *to be slim* as a signs of being "in control." This is a strange anomaly of our time. At the same time, free will is viewed as a privilege of an autonomous self; and an excess of eating "whatever/whenever" or an escape into sedentary entertainment is sometimes considered a defiant right of passage (often carried into adulthood)—perhaps especially for those who have been pressured at an early age to restrict eating or to exercise to reduce chubbiness or fatness. In contrast, the *Healthy Body Image* curriculum presents competency about nutrition, fitness, body esteem, and resistance to unrealistic norms as a model for students who aspire to be independent and "in control."

D. The Purpose of this Updated *Healthy Body Image* Curriculum

In May 1996, the U.S. Department of Health Task Force on Eating Disorders published a report calling for curricula to be developed targeting the known risk factors for eating disorders for students in upper elementary school grades. The report stated that topics should cover pubescent development, *weightism* (prejudice regarding size diversity) gender-specific pressures, and body esteem. Emphasis should be placed not on external weight prescriptions, but rather on discovery of individual best weights through natural eating responses to internal cues of hunger and satiety, and through enjoyable physical activity. Such a curriculum must also include complementary materials for parents. In response to this call, the first edition of *Healthy Body Image: Teaching*

Kids to Eat and Love Their Bodies Too! was developed and pilot-tested over a two-year period of time before its publication by the National Eating Disorder Association in 1998.

Since its publication, this curriculum has been recommended by the USDA Department of Women's Health in their *Bodywise Packet for Middle School Educators.* It is used in hundreds of schools across the United States and has been adapted for special populations, such as those served by the New York City Board of Jewish Education. A companion book for parents and other non-educators has been written, entitled *Real Kids Come in All Sizes: Ten Essential Lessons to Build Your Child's Body Esteem* (Broadway Books/Random House, 2004). In addition, while this manual is designed to be self-instructive for teacher use, the author is available on a limited basis for in-service training and community education presentation (see the Appendix for contact information).

This updated *Healthy Body Image* edition incorporates new research in the field of eating disorders, health, nutrition, and fitness standards, as well as feedback from a host of teachers and parents. It also responds to clear trends in the popular press. The purpose remains the same as in the original guide, published in 1998: to inoculate children with information, perspectives, values, and behavioral competencies that will help them resist the primary risk factors for the full spectrum of body image, eating, nutrition, fitness, and weight problems. Classrooms should provide a micro-environment that surrounds students with new norms and standards to draw upon. The common goal is to raise a generation of students with healthy, realistic body images who eat well and value physical fitness for the health, strength, and well-being these afford.

PART II: DEVELOPING A NEW MODEL FOR HEALTHY BODY IMAGE

Learning from prior prevention efforts

Several initiatives to prevent eating and weight problems have been tested in the last decade. It is important to examine what has worked and not worked as we move ahead. Prior to the 1998 publication of this curriculum, available lesson plans targeted only middle- or upper-school students—an age when body image problems are already prevalent and primary prevention is too late. Since it is extremely difficult to reverse negative body image attitudes once they are established, students should have the benefit of lessons at an earlier age that are designed to help them maintain (rather than regain) body esteem.

Some curricula for middle and upper school aim to deter students from problems by informing them about eating disorders and the damage they cause. There is some evidence that this approach may backfire, teaching eating-disorder behaviors to already fat-phobic adolescents. The *Healthy Body Image* curriculum takes a different approach, teaching students *what to do* versus *what not to do.*

Curricula that are exclusively didactic and that do not involve children experientially may transmit knowledge but without the desired attitudinal or behavioral changes. Better results occur when concepts are presented through engaging activities, stories, and discussions. Additionally, since a positive body image and a focus on wholesome eating and fitness for health (versus size) are not culturally normative today, development of a *whole-classroom micro-culture* that consistently normalizes and values these concepts is very important. Posters, books, art, and music that reinforce size diversity, appreciation of deeper qualities (beyond superficial appearances), eating well, and fitness make healthy norms the *status quo* in contrast to the wider culture in which children live.

Last, but not least, approaches that educate and foster change in the wider community within which children grow hold even more promise. Changing a classroom environment is potent, but when the wider school culture, including administration, staff, and parents, embrace a *whole-school approach* (see the Appendix for more information about a *whole-school approach*) this larger micro-culture clearly reinforces students' responses as they move through higher grades.

The *Healthy Body Image* curriculum is scripted with activities for grades four through six. However, the concepts taught by the *Model for Healthy Body Image*, upon which lessons are based, are *not* grade-specific. Many schools have adapted lessons to reinforce concepts as students progress through high school. While long-term studies are needed, anecdotal evidence and observations suggest that the creation of a whole-school culture that values health over size or appearance is both possible and desirable.

Criteria for a new model: *First, do no harm.*

To be effective in preventing or reversing culturally induced body image, eating, nutrition, fitness, and weight problems, it is essential that new models correct a serious flaw of most current prevention initiatives regarding weight. When we examine these initiatives, we too often find one approach designed to stop the rising rate of fatness, a contrasting approach to prevent or reverse eating disorders, and a third approach to encourage body esteem and to battle prejudicial, weightist attitudes. When these contrasting approaches recommend solutions that are contradictory, which they frequently do, or when they encourage short-term solutions that are counterproductive in the long run, confusion and failure prevail. In this light, we cannot be surprised when the general public is frustrated and, in many cases, complacent about healthy eating and fitness choices. Prevention experts agree that a new approach is needed that is capable of targeting: 1) the unrealistic drive to be thin and the restrictive eating that accompanies it, 2) the rise in unhealthy fatness, 3) poor nutrition and fitness in children of all sizes, and 4) weightist attitudes that deny the integrity of size diversity—*simultaneously and without discrimination or contradiction.*

In creating a new model, we must start by recognizing that the pervasive thin-ideal, the diet mentality, poor nutrition and fitness habits, and weightism are not separate concerns but are interrelated: They are part of one dynamic, whole problem. Therefore, any non-discriminatory approach must reject methods that may appear to solve one problem at the expense of another and must also vigorously avoid recommendations for short-term-only solutions. Both the goals—healthy body image attitudes and healthy lifestyle choices—and the opportunity to reach them should be equally attainable for all students, *regardless of size, shape, weight, age, gender, socio-economic status, or cultural milieu.*

To avoid "solutions" that cause problems, new models must address all of the various documented, culturally-induced risk factors that promote most body image, eating, nutrition, fitness, and weight problems simultaneously, and must make recommendations that are not at cross purposes. Four toxic myths are known to provide the seedbed for the majority of problems. The diagram below illustrates the dynamic flow of these myths.

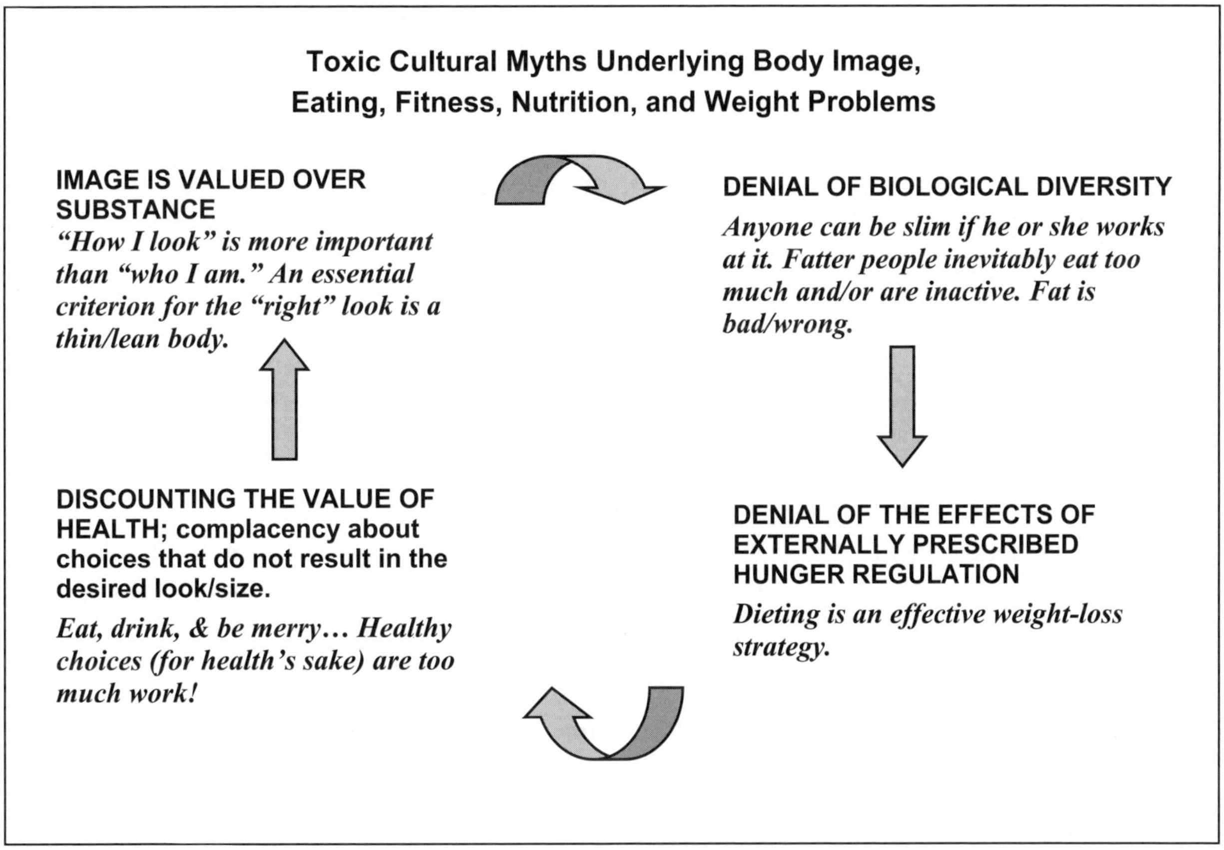

The *Model for Healthy Body Image*

The *Model for Healthy Body Image* (see page xxxviii) was designed as a response to the four interrelated cultural-risk factors that underlie most body image, eating, nutrition, fitness, and weight problems today. By keeping all four toxic myth clusters in mind at all times, the model successfully avoids short-term "solutions" that may conflict or boomerang. The health principles in the *Model for Healthy Body Image* provide the framework for the *Healthy Body Image* curriculum, and have also been translated into a set of *Body Image Building Blocks* for children (see page xxxix). Each *Healthy Body Image* lesson teaches a concept represented by one (or, in one case, two) of the *Building Blocks*.

Rather than warning children about what to avoid, the *Model for Healthy Body Image* teaches students what to embrace to maintain health and integrity in the face of unhealthy pressures. More specifically, each of the *Body Image Building Blocks* serves as an *antidote* to help children resist one of the four toxic myths. Teachers (who are themselves students of the culture) should be well-versed about the toxic myths and their antidotes before beginning to teach any of the *Healthy Body Image* lessons. A summary follows:

Myth 1: Image over substance. *"How I look" is more important than "who I am." An essential criterion for the "right" look is a thin/lean body.*

Children routinely learn that *beauty is only skin deep,* and *you can't judge a book by its cover.* But today's students must be prepared to defend themselves in light of another adage: *One picture is worth a thousand words.* Since the explosion of visual media in the late 1950s, people no longer assume that other ordinary-looking people should be the basis for comparing their looks. Instead, millions of images of extraordinarily photogenic models all chosen for a particular "look" have revolutionized the value placed on appearances in general and have created a mandate for a *slim* or *lean* appearance in particular.

As children enter puberty, it is developmentally normal for them to begin to identify less with parents regarding certain issues and more with friends, especially regarding what looks good and is considered "cool" or socially desirable. Belonging means *fitting in*, and whatever is perceived as normal carries tremendous value. Playing on this human need for inclusion, intensive marketing of a generally unattainable, slim/lean beauty ideal *as if* this look was normal, especially for females, has been very effective in creating tremendous anxiety about appearance.

Most people are not aware that the *manufacturing of anxiety* about social acceptability is a purposeful marketing strategy. Insecurity about looks is a desired outcome for advertisers, who then offer products that promise to correct the perceived deficiency. Because the thin-ideal is unrealistic for most females (fewer than 3% of females have the natural physique of most fashion models, just as a sculpted, muscular physique is not common to most males), the prevalence of such images in advertising has been especially successful in generating appearance anxiety. As a result, excessive preoccupation with the "right" look, and the belief that slimness is an essential criterion for it have become normative.

***Building Blocks for Healthy Body Image* (Lessons)**

Teach students to understand and resist objectification:

Lesson 1: Acquire historical perspective on today's body image attitudes. Understand that an emphasis on an "ideal look" is a formula for unhappiness.

Lesson 2: Develop a strong sense of identity based on a balance of *inner* qualities rather than on appearance.

Lesson 6: Become media literate and recognize advertising strategies. Think critically about media messages that encourage unrealistic, unhealthy body image attitudes and low nutrient, sedentary lifestyle choices.

Myth 2: Denial of biological diversity: *Anyone can be slim if he or she works at it. Fatter people inevitably eat too much and/or are inactive. Fat is bad/wrong.*

For the thin-ideal to be widely embraced, facts pertaining to biological diversity of body size and shape must be dismissed, discounted, or denied. In its place, we have learned to mistrust the body's ability to regulate weight and to believe that fatter people must inevitably be doing something wrong. With the assumption that fatness of any degree is bad, prejudicial assumptions regarding fat freely develop. As a result, weightism has become normative, and anxiety about weight is rampant.

Weight may, of course, be influenced by lifestyle choices, but the idea that weight can be "controlled" through healthy means over the long term is flawed. In fact, weight is not a behavior. It is an outcome of highly complex variables, many of which are not in our control. Because of this complexity, long-term efforts to manipulate weight frequently backfire, resulting in a greater loss of control. Healthy weight is best determined by taking charge of variables that are in our control: by observing the outcome of stable, healthy eating and a physically active lifestyle over time. In this light, we see that "overweight" cannot be determined by appearance alone or by comparison to an external standard, even when we see that someone is fat. Individuals who eat well and are active and fit will have normal weights and BMIs that are diverse, showing a natural distribution ranging from quite fat to quite thin.

***Building Blocks for Healthy Body Image* (Lessons)**

Teach students the biological principals of size diversity:

Lesson 3: Understand the normal, expected addition of body fat that is common during puberty and other developmental stages of life.

Lesson 4: Respect and appreciate the genetic diversity of body shapes and sizes.

Lesson 5: Understand how the internal weight regulatory system *limits* the extent of long-term control that is possible over weight.

Myth 3: Denial of the universal effects of externally prescribed hunger regulation: *Dieting is an effective weight-loss strategy.*

When slimness is culturally mandated, a means to attain it is needed. Because restrictive eating results in weight loss in the short run for most people, this instant reward is routinely used as evidence for the belief that anyone could be slim(mer) if he or she worked at it through diet and exercise. Denial of the long-term, counterproductive effects of dieting for weight loss is essential to support the drive to be thin. Most people, including many medical providers, continue to blame a dieter's lack of willpower rather than accept that the method is intrinsically flawed. Erroneous beliefs about the effectiveness of dieting are boldly transmitted without qualifiers side by side with the thinness schema, creating dual pressures for an unsuspecting public who have not been educated about the expected outcomes.

Long-term efforts to "control" hunger by overriding internal hunger cues are counterproductive. Hunger demands to be fed and will subside naturally when it is satisfied.

***Building Block for Healthy Body Image* (Lesson)**

Teach children the facts about dieting for weight loss:

Lesson 7: Recognize that there are predictable, counterproductive results when hunger is restricted according to an external plan. At least 90% percent of weight lost through dieting is predictably regained, usually with added pounds.

Myth 4: Devaluing health; complacency about lifestyle choices that do not result in the desired look: *Eat, drink, and be merry! Healthy choices (for health's sake) are too much work.*

In a social context in which appearances, the drive to be thin, denial of size diversity, and the diet mentality dominate, the primary purpose of eating and fitness for health and well-being has become lost for a significant portion of the population. Too many children today grow up to believe the only reason to eat well and be physically active is to lose or control weight. But the American promise of weight loss or slimness as the reward for a healthy lifestyle has backfired. When frustrated that diet and exercise do not provide them with the promised lean look, a majority of individuals of varying sizes and shapes understandably throw-up their hands and throw-out wholesome choices. "Why bother?" is the understandable response.

An additional problem arises when weight loss is promoted as a goal of healthy nutrition. This presentation inadvertently sends a message that balanced nutrition and exercise are only important for people who are fat. This conclusion leaves normal weight or slim individuals more vulnerable to seduction by an ever expanding array of low-nutrient entertainment foods as the foundation of their eating. Promoting good nutrition and fitness as a means to weight loss contributes to poor nutrition for people of all sizes.

Eating well and maintaining an active lifestyle require some effort. If the primary objective is to manipulate weight we can expect the current outcome: a nation growing less healthy and in many cases fatter on feelings of failure or complacency. Alternatively, students can be taught that *health*—not size or shape—is a more reliable reward for healthy choices. With this non-discriminatory goal, self-respect and body esteem, as well as nutritional health and physical fitness are achievable for every student at every size.

Building Blocks for Healthy Body Image **(Lessons):**

Teach children of every size to value health:

Lesson 8: Eat well. Satisfy hunger completely with a balanced variety of wholesome foods that provides all the nutrients and energy your body needs. Enjoy entertainment eating in limited doses that do not interfere with nutritional needs or ignore hunger satiation.

Lesson 9: Make movement a priority. Spend enough time and energy engaged in physical activity to maintain your body's fitness level throughout the life cycle. Enjoy sedentary entertainment in limited doses that do not interfere with physical endurance, strength, and agility.

Lesson 10: Accept the diverse sizes that result from healthy choices. Look for realistic role models that help you to feel good about who you are. Resist unhealthy and unrealistic pressures about prescribed weight standards, dieting, low-nutrient food choices, and sedentary entertainment.

The Model for Healthy Body Image

Conceptual Building Blocks	Foundation	Desired Outcome	Goal
Developmental change is inevitable. Normal changes of puberty include weight gain and temporary out-of-proportion growth; fat does not by itself define "overweight." Genetics and other internal weight regulators strictly limit the degree to which shape, weight & Body Mass Index (BMI) can be manipulated through healthy means. Restricted or restrained hunger (dieting) results in predictable consequences that are *counterproductive* to weight loss and interfere with normal hunger regulation.	Recognize and respect basic biology; understand what is *not* in our control regarding size, shape, weight, and hunger.	**Accept the innate body: "This is the body I was born to have."**	**Healthy Body Image**
Balance attention to *many* aspects of identity. Looks are only one part. Consistently satisfy hunger with *enough* varied, wholesome food in a stable, predictable manner. Limit sedentary choices to promote a physically active lifestyle at all ages. Choose role models who reflect a realistic standard.	Emphasize what *can* be influenced or chosen.	**Enjoy eating for health, energy, and hunger satisfaction. Create a physically active lifestyle for fitness, endurance, fun, relaxation and stress relief.**	**Prevention of Unhealthy and Disordered Eating**
Promote historical perspective on today's cultural attitudes related to body image. Teach critical thinking about media messages that influence body image. Support each other in resisting unhealthy norms about weight, dieting, low nutrient food choices, eating for entertainment, and a too sedentary lifestyle.	Develop social and cultural resiliency.	**Develop autonomy, self esteem, confidence, and the ability for critical thinking.**	

The organizational structure of the *Model for Healthy Body Image*

Teachers will notice that concepts in the *Model for Healthy Body Image* are organized into three tiers:

Tier 1: Biological factors influencing size and weight that are not in our control.

Tier 2: Behavioral choices that positively influence health and self esteem.

Tier 3: Competencies to help students resist unhealthy cultural pressures.

This same three-tier framework is used when the *Model for Healthy Body Image* is transposed into the child-friendly *Body Image Building Blocks* shown below.

BODY IMAGE BUILDING BLOCKS

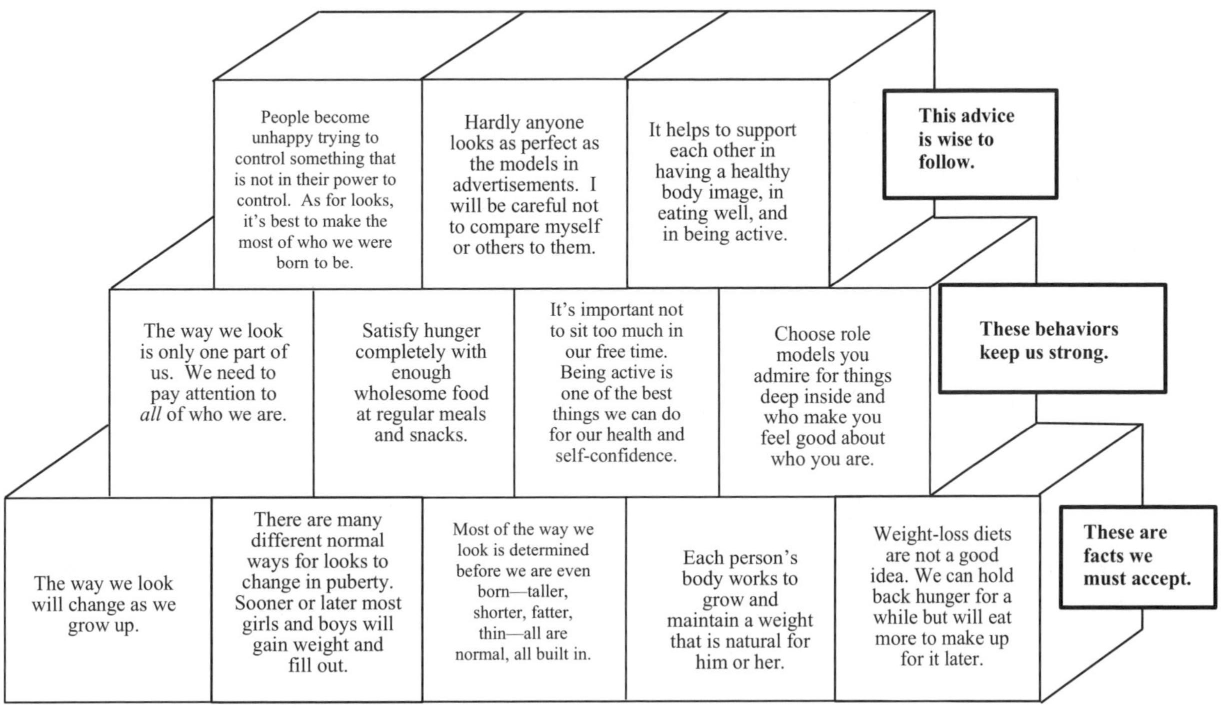

Printable versions of the Model for Healthy Body Image and the Body Image Building Blocks are available in the Supplemental Handouts section of the Appendix.

OUTCOME STUDIES USING THIS CURRICULUM

Outcome studies confirm that a focused body image curriculum such as this one, when presented early in children's development, can make a significant positive difference. Two published studies report measured outcomes of this curriculum:

Kater, K., Rohwer, J., and Londre, K. (2002). *Evaluation of an Upper Elementary School Program to Prevent Body Image, Eating and Weight Concerns,* Journal of School Health; Vol. 72, No. 5: 199-204.

Kater, K., Rohwer, J., and Levine, M.P. (2000). *An Elementary School Project for Developing Healthy Body Image and Reducing Risk Factors for Unhealthy and Disordered Eating,* Eating Disorders: Journal of Treatment and Prevention; Vol. 8, No. 1: 3-16.

These reports document significant positive changes in student knowledge about factors influencing body size and shape, dieting for weight loss, and critical thinking regarding media images. Student attitudes about body-size prejudice, as well as student eating and fitness intentions, were also improved. Teachers interested in reading the abstracts for these studies will find them in the Appendix.

As a follow-up to our initial pilots, students were asked about their response to the *Healthy Body Image* curriculum. In a group of 222 fourth-and sixth-grade boys and girls, 72% of the students said that they liked the lessons and 79% agreed the lessons were being helpful. More than half of the respondents talked about the body image lessons with a parent or guardian at home.

Comments from students included:

- "I learned to feel good about who I am and not worry about what I look like."
- "I liked it all, but the best was you don't have to be thin to be cool."
- "No one is the same, and there's no such thing as a 'perfect' weight."
- "You can't really change how you look. Just eat a lot of good food and don't watch so much TV and your family geens [sic] will tell your body how to turn out right for you."
- "I know that I could never look like those models, and it's good to learn about body image."
- "My dream was to be a model, but now my mind may have a different idea to feed on."

Feedback from teachers participating in the initial pilot included the following remarks:

- "I believe my own life would have been different if I had (this material) in the fourth grade."
- "Everyday the kids asked if they got to have health. That has never happened with a health unit."
- "I wish you could have seen how this material produced magical moments in the classroom."
- "I questioned the need for this (at this age) until I overheard two of my (fourth grade) girls talking about feeling fat."
- "One of my students who is quite fat came up after class and said, 'Thank you.' No one else had ever told her that her fatness might be at least partly genetic."

PART III: HOW TO APPROACH THIS CURRICULUM

This curriculum is based on widely agreed-upon prevention principles recognized by authorities in the fields of eating disorders, biological science, dietary science, pediatrics, and other health specialties. In spite of this, teachers should be aware that in today's world, several of these healthy body image, eating, nutrition, fitness, and weight principals are, in effect, countercultural. This is a reflection that what we *know* to be factual and right does not always shape what we *believe*, how we *feel*, and what we actually *do*. Such is the confusing world today's students face.

Most men and women have been both victims of and participants in perpetuating today's unrealistic beauty standard, weight prejudice, and various ineffective, counterproductive or dangerous eating, dieting, or lifestyle behaviors. As a statistically normal group, many teachers will therefore have to face their own internal dragons to teach these lessons. Do not feel bad if you struggle with these curricula lessons personally. Many of your colleagues will, too. If they do not, try to learn what has helped them to maintain their integrity regarding their diverse body sizes. In the end, if you can embrace these lessons for yourself, do it! If you cannot, then take heart in helping students so they will not have to carry such a burden of judgment when they look in the mirror or at others.

APPROACHING THE LESSONS

You will find perforated versions of all handouts and overheads referred to in the lessons in the Appendix. These may be removed from this book to photocopy for student, classroom, and take-home use. Once removed, store these in a folder or three-ring binder. You will also find supplemental handouts and overheads that may be used for a parent or community education event in this section of the Appendix.

The following points should be considered in approaching this curriculum.

- **Because this *Healthy Body Image* curriculum challenges prevalent cultural beliefs about body image, eating, and weight, the approach needed is somewhat different from that used with other new curricula.** Given the many loaded issues and myths about weight, fat, and bodies in our culture, it is likely you will be faced with your own, your students', and their parent prejudices and questions. To prepare for this, you will need a working knowledge of the new paradigm that is presented and all the concepts that are included before you begin. Since teachers are themselves students of the culture, it is not safe to assume that they are familiar or comfortable with the essential concepts.

  ✓ **Teachers should read the entire manual and be well acquainted with the model, plus the objectives and rationale for *all* lessons in this curriculum prior to presenting any of the lessons to students or prior to selecting portions to integrate into existing classroom curricula.**

- **Plan to teach *all* of the concepts.** Culturally supported attitudes are resistant to change, and education for the purpose of changing unhealthy but entrenched attitudes has unique requirements. Most importantly, presentation of a healthier perspective and approach must be *comprehensive*, covering the topic from all angles to include all of the concepts that support the whole, new model. While the material from each lesson in this curriculum can theoretically stand alone, if some lessons are taught while others are skipped, students and their families will be at risk for yet another distorted "big picture" regarding body image, eating, nutrition, fitness, and weight.

  For example, lessons arising from the *Model for Healthy Body Image* teach students the biological basis for size and weight. But size acceptance does not mean complacency about healthy lifestyle choices. It is therefore of equal importance to teach student's about the means to health at any size through wholesome eating and fitness. In addition, students will need tools to help them resist falling victim to conflicting pressures regarding this topic. All lessons in the curriculum work together to support a whole new perspective. Teachers should understand that concepts presented in later lessons are not less important to the overall model than earlier lessons but rather are different parts of the overall paradigm.

  ✓ **Despite the time constraints, no core concepts from any lesson should be completely skipped. Some lessons may be successfully combined. If concepts have been covered in previous curricula, they should at least be reviewed didactically in the context of this *Healthy Body Image* unit.**

- **If at all possible, plan for a *whole-school approach* to this curriculum.** Teachers have consistently reported that students embrace these curriculum lessons enthusiastically. However, in the face of prevalent norms and pressures that continue to encourage unhealthy body image, eating, nutrition, fitness and weight problems, students will need additional support to maintain their wisdom. Schools in which administrators, school staff, and teachers as well as parents are on-board with the concepts conveyed in this curriculum will be far more likely to succeed in the long term.

    ✓ **You will find guidance for a *whole-school approach* to promotion of healthy body image, eating, nutrition, fitness, and weight in the Appendix.**

- ***Healthy Body Image* lessons are cross-curricular.** Lessons may be integrated into existing science, social studies, history, literature, family life and consumer science, and health teaching blocks. The Table of Contents identifies the appropriate discipline for each lesson. Teachers should plan to complete all of the lessons within a discrete time to allow students to integrate the concepts into a dynamic whole.

Materials in this curriculum may overlap slightly with lessons already being used in the classroom on puberty, nutrition, fitness, and the impact of mass media. However, it is not safe to assume your existing classroom curriculum covers the key *Healthy Body Image* concepts. Teachers should look closely to determine how concepts differ from or add to existing curricula. The critical difference is in the integration of the new paradigm or understanding what can and cannot be controlled about body size and shape and internal hunger cues. *Healthy Body Image* was developed because existing curricula on these subjects lack vital information and/or, in some cases, provide information that is even counterproductive to promotion of healthy body image and positive eating behaviors.

- **If necessary, change your thinking about the size of your students, fat or slim.** It is not a goal of this curriculum to reinforce slimness or to help fat children lose weight. If you feel this way, you are no doubt well-intentioned. However, the wish to help anyone lose weight is based on an assumption that visible fatness inevitably means overweight rather than diversity, that fat children cannot be healthy, and that a focus on weight loss (versus healthy behaviors) can be effective. Fatness that is a by-product of excessive high-calorie/low-nutrient eating and a too-sedentary lifestyle is a serious concern. However, few teachers are in a position to diagnose this. Instead, teachers are in a wonderful position to help all students, regardless of weight, to:

    - Embrace who they are and stay connected to their authentic selves.
    - Accept and respect their own and each other's genetic diversity.
    - Resist negative cultural pressures.

- Expand their notion of health to include vitality and energy, strength and stamina, flexibility and mobility, and metabolic fitness—that which will empower them to enjoy and be productive in life without regard to size.
- Embrace this new notion of health as a value and develop incentives to make lifestyle choices that support it.
- Learn the behaviors that will enhance their health and help them to feel confident that they are the best they can be.

▪ **Include Home Education:** Send your own letter and/or the *Letter to Parents and Guardians* (see Appendix) to introduce this unit to students' families. Alert parents to watch for and read the take-home materials. Family education on this topic is critical. Ideally, a presentation should be provided for parents, although experience shows that many who need it most may not attend. Because parent education may not be realistic, all the handouts, activities, and worksheets are designed to serve also as family education. Consider using the Home Education slips (see Appendix). These can be sent home to be signed and returned, indicating that the material has been shared with at least one adult. You may wish to add incentives for sharing the material with more than one adult (grandparents, cousins, etc.)

✓ **A companion book by the *Healthy Body Image* author entitled *Real Kids Come in All Sizes: Ten Essential Lessons to Build Your Child's Body Esteem,* is available in bookstores or from www.NationalEatingDisorders.org. This book presents all of the concepts in the *Healthy Body Image* curriculum in an easy-to-read format for parents and others. Recommend this book to the parents of your students, or even encourage a book discussion event. It will be helpful for other teachers and administrators in your school to read *Real Kids Come in All Sizes* as well.**

▪ **You may create an enlargement of the *Body Image Building Blocks* to display for classroom use** (see Appendix). This can be introduced at the close of Lesson 1 when students begin to construct their models to take home. The *Building Block* concepts for each lesson are also printed on the Home Education slips for caregivers. It is hoped that the *Building Block* concepts will become imprinted in the minds of students, who may use them to resist unrealistic cultural contradictions.

▪ **Teach to students' developmental levels and reinforce lessons as students progress through higher grade levels.** Given the developmental level of fourth grade students, teachers experienced with the *Healthy Body Image* curriculum recommend teaching the lessons during the second half of the year but early enough to satisfactorily complete the entire unit. In contrast, sixth graders may be most receptive to lessons presented in the first half of the school year.

As with any prevention model that challenges cultural factors that support disease, an initial inoculation is not sufficient to sustain resiliency.

- ✓ **Schools should plan to reinforce the concepts in the *Model for Healthy Body Image* as students progress through middle school and high school. While no separate guide is available for this purpose, many teachers have successfully adapted these *Healthy Body Image* lessons for use with students through college age.**

- **Some elementary-age students will be savvy about eating disorders. You may even have a student in your class who has been diagnosed with or who has shown signs of an eating disorder.** If students comment about the relationship of these lessons to eating disorders, respond in an honest, nonjudgmental but minimalistic manner that does not describe eating disorders. Unfortunately, descriptions of eating disorders, however well intentioned, have too often planted the seed for these disorders in high-risk children. For example, you could safely say, "Eating disorders are very dangerous problems. These can occur when some people, for various reasons, have trouble following the *Body Image Building Blocks*."

- **Be prepared for some pre-pubescent students to be squeamish when faced with talk about their changing bodies**. This appears to be developmentally normal, at least among American students. The more comfortable *you* can be in speaking confidently and reassuringly, while simultaneously respecting individual differences in modesty, the easier it will be for those students who may otherwise feel embarrassed. Students should never be made to feel embarrassed about feeling embarrassed. Consider your particular class when considering whether to provide for gender-separated discussions for Lesson 3.

- **While some teachers may consider combining these lessons with a Family Life Unit (sexual education), there are reasons *not* to do to do so.** It is likely that students will feel freer to talk about body changes as well as size and shape when this topic is not paired with (and therefore "loaded" by) sexual content. This appears to hold true even for middle school and high school students. Based on results from field tests, students participate more fully when the two topics are kept separate.

- **Consider teacher interest.** While this curriculum teaches a straightforward knowledge base, it also does and should provoke discussion of attitudes and cultural myths. Therefore, teachers who are simply not interested in or comfortable with the subject area should not teach it. Consider creative options. For example, consider dividing the lessons between two or more teachers according to discipline. Teachers interested in science can teach those lessons, while teachers loving literature, social studies, health, etc., can take others. If this is done, time the presentation so that the unit cohesion is maintained.

DISCLAIMER

This curriculum addresses most of the known reasons why medically healthy students develop negative body images and disordered eating behaviors. If a child is not getting basic needs for safety, physical care, positive attention, limit-setting, mentoring, and other essentials of healthy development—including the time and space to be a child—then he or she will be "hungry" in ways that are beyond the scope of these lessons. Some of your students are more "emotionally hungry" than they should have to be. It is not likely that you alone will be able to "fill them up" any more than they could themselves through use of food for "comfort." Nor can you insulate them more than they might attempt for themselves through denial of their hunger. These students will be at risk for other harmful or self-limiting behaviors as well. But do not doubt the power of talking to students about what they wrestle with in their hearts as they are forming their self-images. Naming and correcting cultural myths that reinforce their self-blame will not be all they need, but it may be more helpful than you will know.

LESSON ORGANIZATION

Each *Healthy Body Image* lesson is organized as follows:

1. TITLE AND *BODY IMAGE BUILDING BLOCK*
2. BACKGROUND INFORMATION FOR EDUCATORS
    - Lesson objective
    - Background
    - Desired outcomes for students
    - Concepts needed to teach this lesson
    - Critical concepts
    - Vocabulary
    - Materials needed
    - Lesson summary
3. SUGGESTED LESSON SCRIPT
4. HANDOUTS AND OVERHEADS (see Appendix for perforated versions to copy)

HEALTHY BODY IMAGE LESSONS

UNIT INTRODUCTION

GROWTH AND CHANGE IN APPEARANCE

Body Image Building Block:

The way we look will change as we grow up.

LESSON OBJECTIVES

This lesson sets the stage for the *Healthy Body Image* (HBI) Unit and defines ground rules for classroom discussion of sensitive topics. The children will learn the following:

- They are about to begin, or have begun, a new stage of physical development that will result in qualitatively different changes in their external appearance.
- The purpose of this unit is to help them to be confident, comfortable, and capable of maintaining healthy attitudes and behaviors as this transition occurs.
- Tools for coping with change.
- Reasons to be interested in this unit.
- Ground rules for emotional safety in discussion of body development and differences.

Depending on your plan, you may want to reassure students that gender-sensitive material (Lesson 3) will be discussed in gender-specific classes.

BACKGROUND

Children notice changes in their own and each other's outward appearance. If adults do not acknowledge obvious changes out loud, children are likely to interpret this silence as a "no-talk" taboo. In turn, they may worry whether their development is normal or something to be ashamed of. In addition, "taboo" talk is often the fodder for playground teasing.

Many girls are beginning the developmental changes of puberty by the fourth grade. Others may not show much outward change for three to four years. Boys lag behind girls in their growth spurts and may not know this is normal. To prevent needless worry and self-consciousness from festering, changes and differences need to be *normalized* and *desensitized* by easy acknowledgment and affirmative talk. When growth and development are perceived to be normal, body esteem is enhanced.

For a variety of reasons (including ignorance), perceived differences frequently lead to prejudicial and discriminatory responses. Studies show that teasing, taunting, and harassment about body size and shape are common in elementary and middle schools. Far from benign, these behaviors cause both an immediate and long term loss of body esteem and self esteem. Policies and protocol for zero tolerance of sexual and racial harassment should be expanded to include size and shape.

TEACH FOR THESE OUTCOMES

Students will know:

- Change is natural.
- Developmental changes occur for preteens and teens.
- There are ways to manage change more smoothly.
- This unit will apply to them personally.
- They can expect adults to provide them with answers to questions about body change.
- They can expect adults to enforce zero tolerance for teasing about size and shape.

Student attitudes will be:

- Adults will help me learn how my body will change as I grow up.
- It helps to know my classmates will be changing and growing in many of the same ways I will.
- I can look forward to many of the ways my body will be changing and growing.
- I hope *all* girls/boys can feel OK about how their bodies are or will be growing.
- Teasing someone who is growing faster or slower is hurtful behavior.
- Standing up for someone who is being teased shows wisdom and respect for differences. It is also the mature and honorable thing to do.

CONCEPTS NEEDED TO TEACH THIS LESSON

- Preteens will enter a new and important stage of growth and change called *puberty*.
- Most of when and how we grow is pre-determined, and therefore not in our control.
- Differences are not good or bad. A wide range of differences is natural and normal.
- Growth is not limited to height and weight but also affects the shape of bodies. This HBI Unit will focus on the many changes in outward appearance that occur with puberty.
- Body changes in puberty will be accompanied by changes in body image.
- Change is natural, but transitions require coping skills. Healthy coping skills include:
    - Getting information about what to expect.

- Hearing others talk openly about changes without embarrassment but with respect for modesty and privacy.
- Discovering others are going through changes as well. Developing a classroom climate that encourages positive peer support.

- Pre-pubescent children may have some anxiety about the body changes that lie ahead. This anxiety can be channeled into an investment in learning about what to expect.
- Pre-pubescent and pubescent children, especially girls, may have anxiety about gender-mixed discussions related to external body parts. Educators should be sensitive to this.
- Teasing about size and shape is not benign. Adults have a responsibility to enforce zero tolerance of this behavior.

CRITICAL CONCEPTS

To set the stage for this HBI Unit, students (and, as far as is possible, parents and guardians) should clearly understand the following:

- This unit will focus on changes in appearance with puberty. Lessons will not teach about reproduction.
- Pubescent changes cannot be halted or postponed. Most changes can only be observed and managed. Some changes may be influenced (positively or negatively) through choices about hygiene, nutrition, exercise, sleep habits, and other self-care options.
- The purpose of this HBI Unit is to help students feel good as their bodies change. They will learn what to expect and the choices to make for healthy body images.
- Peer support is an important tool in managing change.
- Teachers will maintain the highest standards for students' emotional safety in classroom and for playground discussions resulting from these lessons (see *Suggested Lesson Script # 10*).

VOCABULARY WORDS

- puberty
- pre-determined
- stress
- body image
- programmed
- normal
- natural

LESSON PREPARATION AND MATERIALS

Materials	Preparation
▪ Each student should have a file folder in which to put handouts and worksheets for this Unit, and one plain sheet of construction paper. ▪ Review and copy the handouts you will use: I-A, I-B, I-C, and I-D for classroom and home education. Also copy the *Home Education* slips. (Reminder: Perforated versions of handouts to remove for photocopying are in the Appendix.) ▪ Make overheads that you will use, choosing from I-A, I-B, I-C, and I-E. Before copying, use the key from the *Suggested Lesson Script* to fill in the blanks on I-B and I-C.	▪ Read the entire *Suggested Lesson Script.* ▪ Familiarize yourself with handouts and rhythm for reading the poems. ▪ Prepare to discuss the ground rules for emotional safety you will require. ▪ Prepare to instruct students to begin the creation of their own *Body Image Building Blocks* model, cutting the blocks from HANDOUT I-D and pasting it in the proper position onto the sheet of construction paper in their folder.

LESSON SUMMARY

- INTRODUCE: Change is *normal,* natural, and inevitable. Bodies and *body image* change in puberty.
- READ HANDOUT I-A — *Terry the Tadpole Learns Tools for Change.*
- DEFINE: *Pre-determined* growth means it occurs outside of our control. Changes over which we have no control can be stressful.
- HANDOUT I-B (optional)—*Tools for Coping with Change* (Use overhead if desired.)
- HANDOUT I-C (optional)—*This Body Image Unit Will Help Me in These Ways* (Use overhead if desired.)
- EXPLAIN: Concepts taught in *Tools for Coping with Change* will be used throughout the *HBI* Unit.
- SET LIMITS: Talk about changes or differences should never include teasing. Brainstorm ground rules for emotional safety in class and on the playground.
- REASSURE: Depending on your plan, reassure students that discussion of gender-sensitive issues (Lesson 3) will occur in gender-specific classes.
- INTRODUCE: *Body Image Building Blocks* and the use of HANDOUT I-D.
- ASSIGN HOME EDUCATION.

SUGGESTED LESSON SCRIPT

1. **ASK for examples of change.**

   Distinguish certain from uncertain change.

   Examples:

   - Certain: day/night, seasonal changes, life span of plants or animals
   - Uncertain: moving, losing a friend, finding $100.00, learning to read

   ASK: What changes have occurred for *you* since you were born? Were they certain or uncertain?

2. **DETERMINE: Change is natural. We cannot prevent it.**

3. **EXPLAIN:**

   In the next few years you will be growing in new ways that will gradually change the way you look. This is certain. You will not only grow taller but will grow in new ways that will change many things about your appearance. This is an important time in your life called *puberty.* Every single healthy person goes through it.

4. **DISCUSS: *Puberty* and *body image***

   Puberty is an "in-between" time. In puberty, bodies gradually change from that of a child into that of an adult. Because appearance changes over a period of years throughout puberty, your body image—or *the way you feel and think about your body*—will change, too. These lessons will help you to know what to expect *so your body image will remain positive.* They will also help you to learn *how to support each other* as you all go through changes together.

5. **INTRODUCE HANDOUT I-A (or use overhead): *Terry the Tadpole Learns Tools for Change***

   This poem is about Terry the Tadpole. Terry has feelings about going through "in-between" changes in her body. See what you can learn about what helped her feel good about those changes. (Read the poem to students.)

6. **DEFINE: *Pre-determined***

   Until her teacher told her the facts, Terry was worried about a change she saw occurring to her body.

- She did not know the growth of her leg was normal and expected.
- She did not know this change was pre-determined, or set up ahead of time
- She did not know this change was going to occur for *all t*adpoles.

Predetermined means something is programmed, or set up ahead of time, to happen a certain way. All living things are programmed to grow as they do. Terry had no control over this. But as Terry learned, *it can help to know what to expect, it can help to know that others are having the same experience, and it can help to talk about these shared experiences right out loud.*

Human bodies do not change as much as tadpoles do as they grow. But when and how human bodies grow and develop *is* pre-determined. One of the important natural stages of human growth is called *puberty*. Because each person's growth is pre-determined for him or her *we cannot control when and how our bodies grow either.* Like Terry, we can only *learn what to do to stay healthy* and watch what happens.

7. ACKNOWLEDGE: Change can be *wonderful* and *stressful* at the same time.

TELL: Growing from a child into an adult offers wonderful and exciting opportunities.

ASK: What are some of the wonderful and exciting things that come with growing from a child into a teen (and eventually adult)?

(Students will have many ideas. Be sure all of the following points are included. Examples are provided here in case students need help. Points are listed in order from most to least obvious.)

- Bodies usually become taller, heavier, and stronger. As a result, they can do many new things that a child's body cannot do.
  - For example, run or throw a ball much farther, stay up later without becoming tired, lift heavy objects, reach the top of a locker, sit in the front seat of a car with airbags, win at tug of war, drive a motor boat, etc.

- Brains contain more information. In addition, it becomes possible to better organize information and do things in increasingly complex ways.
  - For example, a child's brain might be able to enjoy a simple toy or game, but a more mature brain will be able to enjoy a more complicated game. While a child's brain can make a sandwich, a teen or adult brain can make a whole dinner, with appetizers and dessert!

- Brains can consider complex reasons to do or not to do something. Teens and adults therefore have more responsibility for decisions that affect their own and other's welfare.
  - For example, a child may do his or her homework, knowing the teacher will check it, but a teen or adult will do the work because it is important to learn, whether or not anyone checks it. A young child may tease another child if no adults are watching, but a maturing child will know it is important to be kind and supportive regardless. *(Note: Reflect back on this later in the lesson when discussing the norms your class will adopt to make sure everyone feels safe and accepted.)*

TELL: Growing from a child into an adult can be stressful, too.

TELL: Stress is a tension that occurs when there is a *lot* to learn or manage all at once. Even good changes can be stressful. This is especially true if changes occur over which we have no control.

ASK: What are some of the stressful things that come with growing from a child into a teen (and eventually into an adult)?

- Would anyone like to tell about a change that caused stress in his or her life?
- What helped with the stressful feelings?

8. **ADVISE: There are some things that almost always ease the stress of change:**
   - Get the facts. It can help to know what to expect.
   - Learn who to ask or where to go for more information as new questions come up.
   - Talk to others who are going through or who have had similar changes to get reassurance you are not alone.
   - Use what you have learned to make sure that others are reassured as well. Mutual support is helpful for everyone.

READ POEM: OVERHEAD 1-B–***Tools for Coping With Change***

Here is a poem to help you remember this advice. (Read the poem to students in a rhythmic way.)

ASK:

- What helped Terry when her *body image* was changing? (It helped to learn the facts, talk with others, find out she wasn't alone).
- How did Terry end up feeling about her body image?

9. **EXPLAIN:**

We are about to begin a new unit on body image. The purpose is to help you feel good about your body.

(Optional) TELL: Here are some of the ways this unit will help you: (Use HANDOUT I-C— Students fill in the underlined words.)

Key for I-C:

THIS BODY IMAGE UNIT WILL HELP ME IN THESE WAYS:

1. I will feel comfortable knowing my body is growing in a normal and healthy way.
2. I will understand my growth is *pre-determined.* That means it is set up ahead of time to be a certain way.
3. I will understand what makes one person's body look different from another's.
4. I will understand no one has control over when and how growth happens. It is important not to judge appearances during puberty—or any other time.
5. I will understand what I can and cannot control about my size and shape.
6. I will understand how to have a good body image (how I think and feel about my body).

10. **DISCUSS expectations for classroom discussions. For example:**

In this unit we will be talking about many different, normal, healthy body changes. We will also be talking about many different kinds of healthy body types. Since you all will be going through changes, you will *all* benefit from learning how to understand and be comfortable with this together.

No one will ever *have* to talk out loud during this HBI Unit, but we want you to know how to talk to each other in ways that are helpful, never hurtful.

BRAINSTORM NORMS for a safe and supportive environment.

Help students to compose a list that includes their ideas for the norms they would like to have in their classroom both during and after this unit. Post the list in a clearly visible place. Invite students to suggest additions to the list as each lesson is completed. Here is a list composed by one class:

"Be respectful, listen, never laugh unless the person means it to be funny, no guests (in the classroom during these lessons), no teasing after class or on the playground, ask questions if you don't know something—someone else may have the same question and be afraid to ask. If someone is being teased, tell the person who is doing it to stop. If they don't stop, tell the teacher."

ANTICIPATE GENDER-SPECIFIC CLASS DISCUSSION *(Depending on your plan for Lesson 3):*

TELL: Sometimes it may feel most comfortable for girls to talk only to other girls about body changes, and boys to talk to only boys. We will have times for this. Most of the time you will find it is OK, even helpful, to talk in a mixed group. We will do both in this Unit.

STATE ZERO TOLERANCE for teasing during or after these lessons and your plan to enforce consequences.

To be an effective tool, zero tolerance must be more than an intervention with negative consequences. Be prepared to talk with children, helping them to understand what is not OK about their behavior. Teasing is not only ignorant; it is an unkind and dishonorable thing to do.

11. INTRODUCE the *Body Image Building Blocks*:

Show students the *Body Image Building Blocks*—OVERHEAD I-E or an enlargement you have made for your classroom.

Distribute HANDOUT I-D. Students should cut the *Building Block* for this lesson from HANDOUT I-D and paste it onto a sheet of construction paper to begin constructing their own replica of the *Body Image Building Blocks*. After each lesson, students should add the Building Block for that lesson. Be sure that students place their blocks into 3 tiers, adding the corresponding labels: 1) "These are facts we must accept," 2) "These behaviors make us strong," and 3) "This advice is wise to follow."

Have students store their *Body Image Building Blocks* materials in a folder or envelope.

12. ASSIGN HOME EDUCATION:

Assign HANDOUTS I-A, I-B, and I-C to be read at home with caregivers. Consider offering extra credit for signed and returned Home Education slips.

I-A TERRY THE TADPOLE LEARNS TOOLS FOR CHANGE

Terry was a tadpole.
She lived in Silver Pool.
Every day she went to swim
With pals from her own school.

But one day Terry woke up,
Felt a pang of awful horror.
A leg was growing out of her
Where none had grown before!

Terry thought this must be bad,
She felt she was a freak.
She didn't know the facts, and so
Her fear just made her weak.

She tried to hide her leg,
But she was sure it had to show.
She felt like staying home.
She didn't want her friends to know.

The next day in the classroom
Teacher jumped into the pool
And said, "Today's the day you'll learn
You'll all be hopping soon."

"The facts are not uncertain.
For a while you may feel odd.
You're not quite tadpoles anymore,
But neither grown-up frogs."

Ms. Frog taught what would happen,
While not for everyone the same.
A few brave tadpoles raised their hands
And said they'd noticed change.

Some had legs that grew on bellies.
Some were growing fatter butts.
Some were getting bigger muscles.
Some felt awkward, like a klutz.

Some even wondered right out loud
What was wrong with them?
They hadn't noticed anything
From head to tail-end fin!

The teacher had the answers —
Terry knew she could feel great!
They had a lot in common.
It was *normal*—a tadpole's fate!

When Terry told her family
How she'd woken feeling strange,
How the teacher said it right OUT LOUD,
It wasn't strange, but CHANGE!

Her family told their stories
Of how they'd felt anxious, too.
How they had wondered, "What's the deal?"
When their body change was new.

They said at first they'd worried, too,
When friends grew more or less.
Taller, shorter, fatter, thin,
Each different than the rest.

Terry was glad to have the facts
And glad that she had talked.
The answers helped to calm her —
Now she knew that soon *she'd* hop.

Her body sure was changing,
Her friends would soon change, too.
It would take some time to get there,
But she knew now what to do.

She had to wait and watch and wonder
How her looks would be.
Meanwhile, just play and learn and grow
And keep herself HEALTHY.

I-B TOOLS FOR COPING WITH CHANGE

When your body starts to grow
from a child into a teen,
you will want to know the facts about
what will be happening.
You will want to get good answers
from the grown-ups you can trust;
those who have your health at heart
will give you answers you can trust!

It will help to hear from classmates
who are growing now with you.
You'll see you're not alone,
but just one of the group.
These body image lessons
will help you day by day
as you watch your body grow
in a healthy, "just right" way!

I-C

HEALTHY BODY IMAGE LESSONS WILL HELP ME IN THESE WAYS:

1) I will feel comfortable knowing my body is growing in a

n _ _ _ _ _ _ and **h** _ _ _ _ _ _ way .

2) I will understand my growth is pre-determined. This means

it is **s** _ _ - _ _ ahead of time to **b** _ a certain way.

3) I will understand what makes one person's body look **d** _ _ _ _ _ _ _ _ from another's.

4) I will understand it is important not to **j** _ _ _ _ appearances during puberty or any other time.

5) I will understand what I **c** _ _ and **c** _ _ _ _ _

c _ _ _ _ _ _ about my body's size and shape.

6) I will understand how to have a good **b** _ _ _ **i** _ _ _ _ (feel good about my body).

I-D BODY IMAGE BUILDING BLOCKS

UNIT INTRODUCTION: The way we look will change as we grow up

LESSON 1: People become unhappy trying to control something that is not in their power to control. As for looks, it's best to make the most of who we were born to be.

LESSON 2: The way we look is only one part of us. We need to pay attention to *all* of who we are.

LESSON 3: There are many different normal ways for looks to change in puberty. Sooner or later, most girls and boys will gain weight and fill out.

LESSON 4: Most of the way we look is determined before we are even born: taller, shorter, fatter, thin—all are normal, all built in!

LESSON 5: Each person's body works to grow and maintain a weight that is natural for him or her.

LESSON 6: Hardly anyone looks as perfect as the models in advertisements. I will be careful not to compare myself or others to them.

LESSON 7: Weight-loss diets are not a good idea. We can hold back hunger for a while but will eat more to make up for it later.

LESSON 8: Satisfy hunger completely with enough wholesome food at regular at regular meals and snacks.

LESSON 9: It's important not to sit too much in our free time. Being active is one of the best things we can do for our health and self-confidence.

LESSON 10: Choose role models you admire for things deep inside and who make you feel good about who you are.

ALL LESSONS: Support each other in having a healthy body image, in eating well, and in being active.

I-E

The Body Image Building Blocks

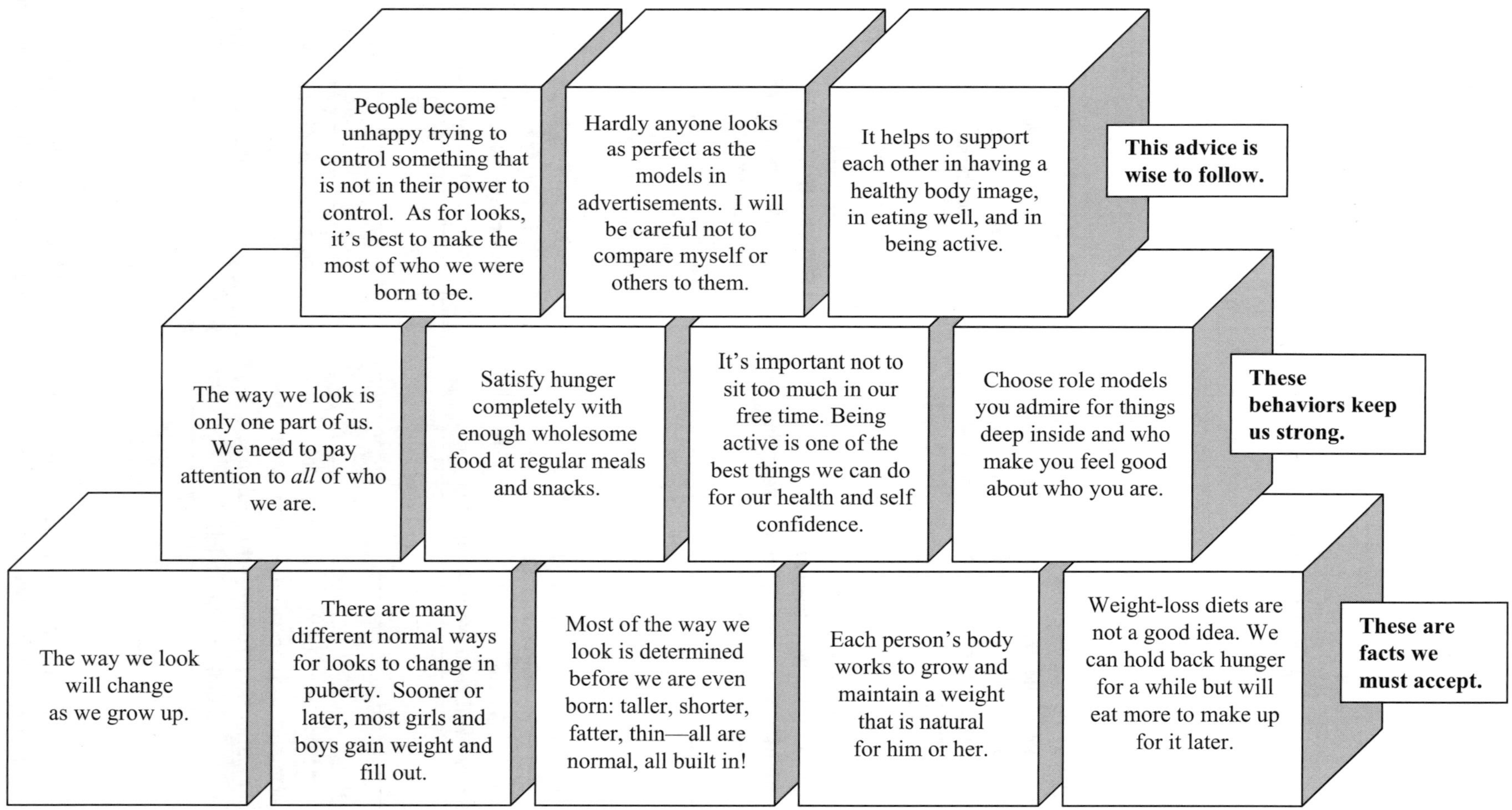

LESSON 1

GAINING PERSPECTIVE

The Development of Unrealistic and Negative Body Images in Western Culture

> **Body Image Building Block:**
> *People become unhappy trying to control something that is not in their power to control. As for looks, it's best to make the most of who we were born to be.*

LESSON OBJECTIVES

The story included with this lesson introduces students to virtually all of the concepts that will be covered in this *Healthy Body Image* unit. Future lessons will refer to this story to illustrate core concepts.

Through a metaphorical story of the Namuh ("human" spelled backward), students will learn how a group of well-intentioned but misguided beings can unwittingly develop and identify with ideals that in the end are destructive to the very culture itself. The Namuh demonstrate many of the ways that negative body image attitudes and unhealthy eating behaviors have developed in our culture. Happily, the story also reveals that it wasn't always like this and that a far better way is possible. Students will be caught up in the story and, in the discussion that follows, will recognize the following points:

- They have heard a metaphorical history of the unhealthy shift in beliefs, attitudes, and behaviors related to body image and eating that has occurred in the past four decades in their own culture.
- Clearly identifiable forces have contributed to this shift toward unhealthy body image and eating.
- Awareness may help them to resist these unhealthy pressures.

Students will understand the relevancy of this lesson to their own lives and will become motivated to invest in learning about healthy body image.

BACKGROUND

Body dissatisfaction is so common today, many people do not realize that the pervasive and intense body discontent now found among American women and adolescent girls did not exist before the 1960s. While men and women have always been interested in looks, and one particular body type or another has been in vogue throughout recorded history, the current extreme value placed on appearance and the intense pressure on women to be unrealistically thin in order to achieve desirability is unprecedented. Compared to the 1960s, when 30% of American women reported unhappiness with their sizes and shapes, 75% of American women currently struggle with this. Few figures are available prior to that time, presumably because there was little pressing need to gather them. In a very short time, it has become "normal" for girls to grow up afraid eating will make them fat—and therefore, undesirable. Boys, too, have joined the bandwagon. In 1972 only 18% of males expressed dissatisfaction with their upper torsos, but by 1996 this had risen to 38% and in 2005 to nearly 50%.

Ours is not the only culture in which destructive attitudes and behaviors have become the custom. Consider the similarities between today's body image attitudes and the following examples:

- Until 1911, bound feet were considered to be essential for females in China. The painful binding, maintained from age four until feet were fully grown, aimed to create three-inch "lotus feet," rendering a girl's feet practically useless and confining women to home. At first practiced by only the very rich, this custom spread over the years to even poor farming families. Unbound girls were considered unsuitable for marriage.
- Brass spiral rings of increasing length are still placed on the necks of the Pa Dong Hill tribe girls in Northern Thailand to prevent them from marrying outside the tribe. Rings force down the girls ribs as they grow, making their necks appear very long. The *long-neck women*, who wear the rings into old age, defend this custom, saying it is tradition.
- During the 19th century corsets were laced so tightly, wearers could scarcely breathe. The use of the corset was driven by the social expectation that women would have a fashionable figure, and girls as young as two to four years of age were trained in their wearing. While not all women were expected to be slim, laces were drawn tight enough to create an hourglass shape, supposedly an indication that the wearer took her appearance seriously.

Whether these practices are considered to be more or less extreme than those resulting from today's body image norms, it's useful to think about how such obviously destructive ideals can come to be embraced by an entire culture. When students learn that today's unrealistic body image and eating attitudes have only recently developed and understand the inevitable unhappiness these cause, their investment in a healthier alternative will increase. While much remains to be understood about this rapid historical transition, even a rudimentary perspective can be helpful. This story of the Namuh provides a backdrop for students to critically examine and consider the body image pressures that surround them today.

Many concepts that are the focus of future lessons are introduced in this lesson.

TEACH FOR THESE OUTCOMES

Students will know:

- Humans have physical, social, and emotional needs and limitations.
- Mass marketing can influence what people *believe* they need, want, or can do. People can be led to believe they need something or should be something that is not realistic for them. This causes unhappiness and may interfere with physical and emotional health.
- It is important to have perspective on today's body image, dieting, and eating norms. Specifically, students will consider the negative effects of:
  - Disproportionate emphasis on image over substance.
  - Unrealistic disregard of the biological limits to our control of body size and shape.
  - Ignorance or denial regarding the counterproductive effects of weight loss diets.
  - Prejudicial attitudes regarding fatness.
- Body image attitudes/prejudice matter, and can influence happiness and health.

Student attitudes will be:

- I can admire people who meet a certain standard of beauty or brawn without feeling I should try to imitate them.
- Looks affect first impressions, but what is essential may not be seen right away.
- I do not need to be slim, buff, "beautiful," or "handsome" to be attractive.
- I accept who I am.
- I would not want anyone to feel bad about how he or she looks.
- People are meant to be many different sizes and shapes.
- Restricting food and denial of hunger is neither healthy nor a good way to lose weight.
- Even if my friends go on diets, I will not feel that I should, too.

CONCEPTS NEEDED TO TEACH THIS LESSON

- Humans have basic needs, universal to all: physical, social, and mental/emotional. Of particular relevance to this unit are the physical need to satisfy hunger and the social/emotional need to be included and accepted and to belong.
- Denial of a basic need or prolonged, disproportionate focus on one need at the expense of another will result in negative consequences.
- Entire cultures can come to value ideals that conflict with basic needs. The likelihood of this is greatly enhanced when distorted ideals are communicated very quickly to large numbers of people through mass media.

- Mass media is funded primarily by sponsors whose purpose is to sell products. Naturally, images to promote these products in the most appealing light are chosen. In the past four decades the use of stereotypically beautiful human images to enhance the appeal of products has proven very successful.
- Mass production of carefully chosen, unusually symmetrical, perfectly proportioned, artfully crafted, and computer-altered images of people has altered our perception of what people need in order to be deemed socially desirable. As such, mass marketing has been a major force in the creation of a disproportionate focus on appearance as a criterion for desirability and has further created an unrealistic standard which the culture now defines as the "right look."
- Because mass media is so pervasive and persuasive in its appeal to human needs, it is essential for people to develop critical thinking and coping skills in order to resist identification with a proliferation of images that are unrealistic.

CRITICAL CONCEPTS

This story introduces virtually all of the building blocks in the *Model for Healthy Body Image.* As such, it is a primer for the curriculum. Students enjoy the story and quickly understand the metaphorical significance. In addition, it is referred to frequently in future lessons. If copied and sent home, it is a home education tool that is not only appealing, but extremely potent in its broad presentation of critical concepts.

If time allowed for only one lesson to be presented from this curriculum manual, Lesson 1 offers the best opportunity to teach all of the *Body Image Building Block* concepts.

LESSON PREPARATION AND MATERIALS

Materials	Preparation
▪ Copy HANDOUT 1-A for each student to draw/color during the story (optional). ▪ If possible, copy the entire story for each student to read with you in class and to take home to read and discuss with their families. To limit the cost of copying, consider binding copies into books to use from year to year.	▪ Familiarize yourself with the story. ▪ The story is most effective if read in one sitting of about 17 minutes. ▪ Integrate discussion questions to break up the time spent listening. ▪ Be aware the story is a *metaphor* based on an evolution that has occurred in American culture; it is not actual history. ▪ Use your best dramatic reading voice!

LESSON SUMMARY

- READ AND DISUSS: *How the Namuh Learned to be Content with Who They Were.*
- ADD: *Body Image Building Block.*
- ASSIGN HOME EDUCATION.

SUGGESTED LESSON SCRIPT

1. **READ *How the Namuh Learned to Be Content with Who They Were.***

   Students may draw and color HANDOUT I-A as you read and/or read along if you have copied the story for take-home family education.

2. **DISCUSS the story questions. Strive for:**

   - **Historical perspective**—The story is a metaphor for a transition that has occurred in *our* culture. Today's pervasive body image values did not always exist and do not need to be the norm in the future.
   - **Personalization**—People can unwittingly be hurt by identification with unrealistic mass-marketed images. Students should understand this risk exists for them personally, especially if they do not learn critical-thinking skills.
   - **Critical thinking**—Students should development awareness of the influence of mass marketing on individuals and groups (further developed in Lesson 6).
   - **Introduction to the role of internal hunger cues**—Students should consider the predictable counterproductive effects of restrictive dieting behaviors (further developed in Lesson 7)

3. **INFORM students that this story will be referred to in future lessons.**

4. **ADD the *Body Image Building Block*** for Lesson 1 from I-D to the students' models.

5. **ASSIGN HOME EDUCATION:**

   If resources allow, send a photocopy of the story home to be read with families along with a Home Education slip to be signed. The story is also available in *Real Kids Come in All Sizes: Ten Essential Lessons to Build Your Child's Body Esteem* (Random House/Broadway Books, 2004).

How the Namuh Learned To Be Content With Who They Were

By Kathy Kater

Once upon a time in a world not really so far away, there lived the Namuh, who happened to be quite a lot like us. The Namuh had their share of life's ups and downs, with good days and bad, happy times and sad. But they had learned to take the good with the bad and understood what they could and could not control. They were content.

Now, the Namuh lived in towns and in the country where they worked and played together. Their children went to school, played games as all children do, and looked forward to growing up to do all the things that grown-ups can do, like stay up late, make the rules, and raise their own families of little Namuh.

One day in the world of the Namuh a photographer was feeling a bit down. He wished to become a very successful photographer. He hoped to sell many portraits so he could make a lot of money and afford to live in a big house. He was a good man and good at his business, too. Even so, he felt his business was not growing as much as he would like. He needed a new idea to attract people to his photo studio.

Now, the Namuh took great pride in their family heritage, and family portraits from many generations before hung on their walls. The photographer thought and thought until he decided to show off some of his best family portraits in the front window of his store. He hoped people passing by would like them so much, they would want a portrait of their own family. He also decided to try something that had not been done before. He paid the newspaper—which until then had no pictures—to print some of his best photos. This way all the readers of the newspaper would see his good work and be inspired to have their portraits taken. He carried out his plan, and, sure enough, his business doubled in no time!

When customers came from far and wide, they told him it was *not* the portraits of the grown-up Namuh that had caught their eye in his advertisements. No, it was the portraits of cute, smiling children they oohed and ahhed about. Well, children are always adorable, no matter what, aren't they? And so the photographer continued to advertise his photos, but more and more he used photos of beautiful, young children—for that is what brought in the business.

Time went by, and the photographer was doing very well. Nevertheless, he wanted to do even better. He was only taking pictures of children, and he wanted to expand his business to include adults. So he wondered, "Why is it that Namuh like photos of children the best?" Well, it wasn't enough for him to know that pictures of baby *anythings* are always the cutest. Of course baby animals and children *have* to be the cutest things, don't they? That's their job! It makes us want to pick them up and hug them, play with them, make them smile, and take good care of them. Think about it for yourself. Baby kittens, big-eyed puppies, human babies—even new young seedling plants coming through the ground—they all make us say, "Ooooh, look! Big eyes in a little face, sweet little mouths, perfect turned-up noses, soft, smooth skin, or silky, fuzzy fur." Now, doesn't it just make you smile to imagine it?

"That's it!" he thought. "Young and cute are what people like to look at. When they see what they like, they feel happy. Then they want to own it for themselves. Young and fresh and delicate and smooth and perfect, without any lumps or bumps or wrinkles!"

When the photographer realized this, smart man that he was, he had a new idea. "What if I took photos of grown-up Namuh to advertise my business but selected only those who still have the youngest-looking faces, with smooth skin, delicate features, and turned-up noses? I'll search until I find rare Namuh females with very slim, child-like bodies—tall but not really rounded, the way most adult females are, so they'll look even younger and slimmer! In my studio, I can make them look perfect with special lights and cosmetics. Then other grown-up Namuh will want me to take their pictures, too, and my business will double!"

But then he thought, "Would people like grown-up Namuh men to appear cute like little boys? Hmmm." Namuh usually liked their men to be big and strong so they could do the heavy work on the farms. And so he decided to concentrate only on young, cute, and slim Namuh females. He was sure this would succeed.

The photographer paid the newspaper to print his advertisements and settled back to see if his idea would work. Sure enough, people flocked to his business. They especially oohed and ahhed about the beautiful photos of grown-up Namuh females in his advertisements. They wanted their own portraits to look that way.

The photographer was doing very, very well. He bought a big, big house and a different car for every day of the week. He was happy.

Now, one day a neighbor, who had a toothpaste factory, met him on the street. "How do you do it?" he asked—for he wished he could do as well with his toothpaste sales. Since the photographer was a good man, he decided to share his idea with the toothpaste maker. "Cute," he said. "You've got to make your toothpaste cute! That's what I did!"

The toothpaste maker had his doubts, but he didn't think the photographer would steer him the wrong way. So he went back to his factory and set to work. Soon he had the photographer take pictures of his toothpaste tube all dressed up, with little legs and arms sticking out and a big toothy, smiling face on the front! Oh, it was cute! He advertised his toothpaste in all the newspapers and magazines and on the TV, too. Sure enough, his sales increased. But not as much as he had hoped.

Time went by. One day the toothpaste maker was having lunch with some business friends: a car maker, a clothing salesperson, a lawn furniture designer, and an orange juice salesperson. Who should walk into the restaurant but the photographer! "Join our table," he said to the photographer, hoping to ask for more advice. "I've had success with my cute packaging but not as much good fortune as you. What do you think I should do?"

The photographer was happy to help if he could. So he thought and he thought. Finally he said, "Maybe it's not cute packaging or cute songs so much as cute, young children or beautiful young-looking women that attract people to buy. Maybe you need to have photos of cute children or young, perfectly beautiful, smiling women holding your toothpaste in your advertisement. Then people will feel, if they buy your toothpaste, their smiles will look forever young and fresh like the images of the models in the pictures!"

All the business people showed up at his studio the very next day. And so, the photographer took pictures of toothpaste, orange juice, cars, tennis rackets, and lawn furniture, all arranged with lovely, slim, young women who had that special childlike appeal—which he made even more appealing and perfect with his special effects. But it was what happened next that the photographer never, ever could have imagined.

By now the advertisements with unusual models were everywhere: on TV, in newspapers, in magazines, billboards, on the product labels themselves. The lovely ladies in all the ads all seemed to be saying the same thing, "Look at me! If you buy this product, you'll be as appealing and special as I am!"

Well, it wasn't long before all the Namuh females began to notice that all the models and actresses looked one certain way. They were a lot like young fluffy kittens or playful, happy puppies,or rosy-cheeked, soft-skinned children—people just couldn't get enough of looking at them. Movie and TV show makers had caught on, too, so now almost all the actresses were chosen for that same young and perfect look. Whenever people looked at pictures of them, they oohed and ahhed and felt happy.

At first the female Namuh enjoyed the images of the exceptional and beautiful Namuh models as much as anyone. Oh, some of them thought it would be fun to look like the models in the ads and on the TV, but they knew most Namuh don't really look like that.

But as years went by and the ads with the rare Namuh models were *everywhere*, the feelings of the young Namuh females began to change. Seeing those pictures of beautiful women smiling at them almost from the day they were born . . . Well, the Namuh females began to think that maybe that was the way *they* were supposed to look!

After a while, it came to be that the young Namuh girls no longer remembered that there was a time when there were many different ways to look and all Namuh were happy to be who they were. Now most Namuh girls grew up to believe they should compare their looks to the models and look forever young, slim, and perfect.

Of course, almost none of them could look as perfect as the models. So naturally they could not help feeling badly about themselves in comparison. But when the Namuh females compared themselves to how completely slim and trim the models were, they saw an opportunity. You cannot change the color of your skin, the shape of your face, or your height—but if you eat less, you can lose weight. Isn't that right?

It wasn't long before more and more of the Namuh females were on strict diets to be thinner. In fact, everyone was so hopeful that diets would give them a slim body like the beautiful models, just about every female was dieting. Since almost no one was naturally as thin as the Namuh models, even the slim Namuh dieted—just in case. Hardly anyone felt she could relax and eat normally. Dieting became the normal thing to do! No one felt happy anymore because they were all trying so hard to be thinner.

Now that the Namuh females felt anxious about their looks, they began to buy a lot of cosmetics and other products to make up their faces, color their hair, and try to hide all the ways they now felt imperfect. When they bought clothing, instead of looking for clothing they felt would be fun to wear, they tried to fit into the clothing they saw looking great on the models. Well, I wish I could say this was as bad as it got because things got even worse.

All those dieting Namuh women began to feel what any dieting person feels: *hungry!* Well, this should be no surprise, but these Namuh had lost all common sense. Hungry? They began to feel something was *wrong with them* when they were hungry! Can you imagine such a thing? When they finally become so hungry from all the dieting that they couldn't stand it, you can guess what happened. What happens to any creature that is so hungry? When they would finally let themselves eat, planning, of course, to eat just a little, they couldn't stop—not for a long time and not until well after they were quite stuffed.

Now, you would think they would understand this is the natural thing to do, wouldn't you? Of course, anyone has to eat and eat and eat after getting so hungry—don't you agree?

But they did not understand this. Instead, they felt horrible about having eaten so much. They decided it meant they should try to diet more and be even stricter about it because by now most blamed themselves. They believed their hunger was the problem. They felt like gluttons around food and thought their overeating proved it. They did not stop to think anyone would be extra hungry if she didn't eat enough. So, back to dieting they went.

Well, guess what? They did so much dieting and so much overeating to make up for it, many of them overate themselves right into larger and larger sizes! The thinner they tried to be, the fatter they got. The ones who didn't get fat—well, they were still afraid food would make them get fat. Everyone was miserable. Can you imagine what they did? What would you do?

One day the Namuh women—who had been so busy feeling bad and comparing themselves to the models and to each other that they had almost forgotten how to talk to each other—started talking. Not about their diets or how fat they felt but *really* talking about how unhappy they were. They asked, "Is this how it is suppose to be when you grow up?" They missed how it had been when they were children. Some could recall when they simply ate plenty of good food and then went out to play. They remembered they had felt so satisfied after eating, they could go until the next meal without being hungry! They noticed the photos hanging in the houses of their parents and grandparents and aunts and uncles. They realized that these grown-ups were all different sizes and shapes and had many, many different looks and styles.

They said, have you noticed that every kind of animal in the world is so *cute* when it's young? Whenever anyone looks at kittens or puppies—even little boys—they ooh and ahh. But when little animals or little boys grow up, their looks change. Those cute little ones don't just get taller; they fill out, too! While some are still good-looking, people don't ooh and ahh at them anymore. Most simply look average—not beautiful or ugly. People love them, just the same.

They asked, "Why are *we* all trying to keep on looking like puppies and kittens and young monkeys? It's time for us to look like who we were meant to be. People are born to be all different sizes and shapes—big, small, round, and soft, with shapes like pears, apples, or carrots, or willow trees; muscled or dainty, short and tall, with imperfect faces to top it all!"

The Namuh females decided it was not worth it to spend their lives feeling bad because they could not be something they were not meant to be. Now, just as they had never felt bad that they were not rich or famous—because they had not expected it of themselves—they came to understand that, to be happy, they should not expect to look other than the way they were born to look.

Finally they realized what they had tried to do could not work. Finally, they could stop feeling like failures! Instead, they felt free to become the best they could be in all ways, enjoying the bodies they were born to have.

They dressed and decorated themselves their own special ways, understanding that Namuhs could look attractive in lots of different ways. They bought things they needed or liked, rather than to copy the models. They ate lots of different foods until they were full, and then they went on to play, work, and school. In the end, the advertisers weren't quite so rich. But they had not meant to cause such harm. They were glad that everyone was happier and healthier, content to be who they were.

***Namuh* Story Discussion Questions**
Discuss these and your own questions.

1. What do you think about how the Namuh females came to feel bad about themselves? Why do you think this happened?

2. Do you think what happened to the Namuh could happen in our culture?

3. Can you imagine a situation in which you might feel the way the Namuh females felt?

4. What did you think when the Namuh females felt there was something "wrong with them" when they became "so hungry" from dieting?

5. Have you ever known anyone who has complained that they were hungry all the time, or who became crabby when he or she was on a diet?

6. The Namuh females realized that almost none of them was born to look like the models and that trying had only made them unhappy. What do you think about this?

7. Have you ever become unhappy trying to do or be something that you later realized was not right for you (at least, not without more effort than it was worth)? What was that like? What did you decide to do? How did that feel?

8. In this story, almost all of the Namuh females talked together and decided to stop trying to be something that they were not meant to be. What if only a *few* of the Namuh females had decided this, but everyone else continued? Would there have been a different outcome?

9. Could the advertisers have done anything differently to increase their sales? What?

10. Why do you think the author called these people "the Namuh?" (It is *Human* spelled backward.)

1-A

The Namuh were beings who hung many portraits on their walls. Draw a portrait of two or more people of different sizes and shapes who are important to you.

Portrait

LESSON 2

IDENTITY AND COMPETENCY

More Than the Way We Look

Body Image Building Block:

The way we look is only one part of us. We need to pay attention to all of who we are.

LESSON OBJECTIVES

As students consider the many diverse aspects of their identities, this lesson will reinforces a balanced sense of the whole self. Looks are only one part. Students will:

- Consider the relative merit of the Namuh's singular focus on appearance as a measure of worth.
- Conclude that undue focus on one aspect of identity results in an unbalanced and constricted way of living.
- Create an art project expressing diverse aspects of their own identities.

BACKGROUND

Keeping the relative value of appearance in perspective is a primary contributor to healthy body image. This protective factor is frequently lost as today's children experience media and peer pressures that encourage excessive preoccupation with looks. For example, when asked what else was important to her (besides looks), a beautiful-by-any-standard eighth-grade girl answered:

> *Well, in grade school I liked volleyball. But now. . . I know you won't really believe this, but looks are everything in my school. If I don't lose 10 pounds this summer, I might as well not even go to high school.*

Preoccupation with and insecurity about appearance is bad enough, but today's children learn from an early age that they should *act as if* they are not troubled by this. This cover-up makes it difficult to realize how many young students are struggling. A wrenching split between the "real me" and a public persona that presents what it is believed the world wants to see has become all too common. This disconnect from the true self is a significant risk factor for a host of problems, including eating disorders, alcohol and other drug abuse, early sexual activity, depression, and anxiety. Even if such serious disturbances are avoided, children who are preoccupied with presenting the "right" external appearance lose valuable years during which the most important developmental tasks should be discovery and expression of "who I am" rather than "how I look."

When children are able to maintain a balanced sense of identity based on *many* attributes, overall self-confidence is enhanced and strengthened. A strong sense of self as *more than the sum of his or her body parts* will empower resiliency in the face of unhealthy pressures.

TEACH FOR THESE OUTCOMES

Students will know:

- There are many aspects to their identity.
- Disproportionate focus on one aspect of identity results in unbalance.
- Combined parts are stronger than one alone.
- Knowledge of many aspects of self creates a more stable personality.

Student attitudes will be:

- I have a lot to offer.
- I can do a lot of things.
- There are some things about me that I can change or improve.
- There are some things I was born with, and they will always be part of me.
- My worth does not depend on my looks. How I look is only one small part of who I am. I have other valuable attributes.
- Beauty is only skin deep.
- I am someone who is worth getting to know.

CONCEPTS NEEDED TO TEACH THIS LESSON

- Each person has many attributes. Among these are knowledge, feelings, and values as well as abilities, talents, personal preferences, personality characteristics, physical traits, strengths, and weaknesses.
- Some attributes are inherited and are not open to control. Others are influenced by learning and experiences.
- Recognizing many aspects of identity enhances a stronger, more stable sense of self.
- Undue focus on one attribute can put a person at risk for unhealthy attitudes and behaviors.
- It is normal to want to be known and valued for many aspects of identity.

CRITICAL CONCEPTS

Recent studies suggest that an identity drawn from diverse sources contributes to resiliency in the face of stress. Activities that require students to identify different aspects of their identity are empowering for children as they grow.

VOCABULARY WORDS (underlined in the lesson script)

- formula
- identity
- attributes
- balance

LESSON PREPARATION AND MATERIALS

Materials:	**Preparation:**
▪ Copy HANDOUTS 2-A and 2-B. ▪ Acquire an old deck of playing cards (a few singles will be torn in the demonstration) or a stack of pre-cut cardboard rectangles—enough so that it is impossible to tear through the stack. ▪ Materials for HANDOUT 2-B—*Balanced Identity Mobile*: Follow the suggested design, or devise your own. It is important that the end result demonstrates balance. For the design described here, each student will need: 1. A paper plate 2. 21 paper clips 3. 10 pieces of string cut into 10- to 12-inch lengths (colored is nice.) 4. Glue and construction paper to provide backing for the 2-B—*Identity Cards*.	▪ Read the *Suggested Lesson Script.* Complete a demonstration model of 2-B, using aspects of your own identity (see diagram). You will use the mobile you have constructed to demonstrate the importance of balance. ▪ This lesson can be completed in one longer or three shorter sections, as follows: Part 1—Present the core concepts; students complete HANDOUT 2-A. Part 2a—Students fill out 2-B, glue the page on construction paper, and cut out the rectangles into cards. Part 2b—Students construct their *Balanced Identity Mobile.* Part 3—Share the mobiles. Do not skip this part of the activity.

LESSON SUMMARY

- REVIEW the Namuh story, which illustrates a *formula for feeling bad.*
- DEFINE IDENTITY: Identity is made up of all the many aspects of who we are.
- DEMONSTRATE the strength of many versus few.
- COMPLETE HANDOUT 2-A—*Your Identity: Many Parts Make You Strong.*
- DEMONSTRATE the benefits of a balance of attributes, using the teacher's pre-made *Balanced Identity Mobile.*
- COMPLETE HANDOUT 2-B—*Attributes of my Identity,* and construct the *Balance Identity Mobile* (or alternative representation.)
- STUDENTS SHARE their *Balanced Identity Mobiles.*
- ADD: *Body Image Building Block.*
- ASSIGN HOME EDUCATION.

Construction of the Balanced Identity Mobile

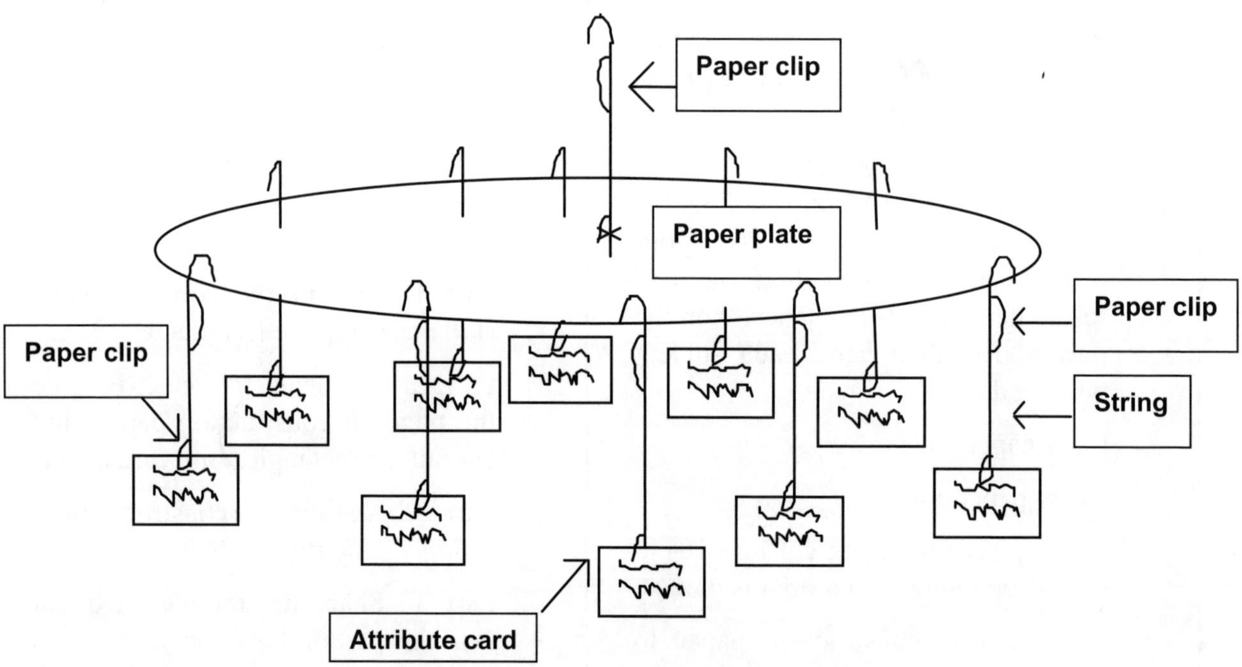

Instead of the mobile, students may combine the 2-B Identity Cards into a collage. If this is done, develop a means of discussing the concept of balance.

SUGGESTED LESSON SCRIPT

PART 1—CORE CONCEPTS AND SELF-SURVEY

1. **IMAGINE:**
   - Something you enjoy but for which you only have an average talent.
   - Someone who is an *expert* at that same activity.
   - You had to decide how to feel about yourself by comparing your ability to the expert's ability.
   - This would be a *formula for feeling bad.*

2. **REVIEW the main point of the Namuh story.**

   The Namuh females became unhappy when they compared themselves to a "look" that they liked but that was not realistic for most of them.

   ASK: Could anyone feel good with this formula?

   TELL: Today we will talk about a *formula for feeling good* about who you are.

3. **DEFINE IDENTITY:**
   - Who you are is made up of many parts. What are some of those parts? (Intelligence, personality, physical ability, creativity, etc.)
   - What we know about the different parts of who we are makes up our sense of identity.
   - Our sense of identity can be strong or not so strong. Which would feel best?

4. **DEMONSTRATE: The strength of many versus few.**

   Using the old deck of playing cards or stack of cardboard rectangles, tell students that the individual cards represent all the many parts of a person. Ask a volunteer to demonstrate how easy it is to tear any one or even a few of the cards in half. Then put all the cards in a stack. Allow students to try to tear the stack of cards. (Be sure you have enough so it is impossible.)

   EMPHASIZE: Like the cards, when it comes to who you are, the *more parts you know about and pay attention to*, the stronger you will be.

- The Namuh forgot that all of the parts of their identity were important and became overly concerned with one part (looks).
- Of course they became unhappy. *Anyone would.*

5. DO: HANDOUT 2-A—*Your Identity: Many Parts Make You Strong*

It is important for each of you to stay as strong as possible (like this whole deck of cards) to be healthy and happy. This survey will remind you that there are many valuable parts to your identity.

PART 2—BALANCED IDENTITY MOBILE ACTIVITY

1. INTRODUCE ACTIVITY: HANDOUT 2-B—*Balanced Identity Mobile*

To help you maintain a balanced sense of yourself, each of you will be making a *Balanced Identity Mobile*. Using your survey 2-A, choose two or more attributes from each category that are important to you. Write your choice on the corresponding 2-B—*Attributes of my Identity* card for that category.

Some of you will have more attributes in some categories than others. That's because you are different. Everyone has different preferences, interests, strengths, and weaknesses. It's very important not to compare yourself to anyone else. (Push students to list more than one attribute in each category.)

2. GUIDE students in constructing their mobiles.

3. DEMONSTRATE a balance of attributes (parts of identity):

While students work, teachers may demonstrate their own pre-made Balanced Identity Mobile. *Lift several cards on one side to show what happens if we focus attention on only one or a few parts of ourselves: the mobile becomes unbalanced and tips. Offer examples of the ways in which too much of even a good thing can cause a lack of balance in life. This is an important opportunity to broaden your students' perspectives. For example, students may quickly suggest that too much TV, playtime, or staying up late could be problems. But it is also true that too much studying, generosity (at one's own expense), or perfectionism may result in serious problems as well. Use only examples from your own or a stranger's life and ask students if they can suggest ways to correct the imbalance.*

PART 3—DISCUSSION

1. **SHARING:**

   Most of us want to be known for the many different sides of who we are. Who would like to be first to tell us about his or her mobile? (Every child should share his or her mobile.)

2. **CONCLUDE (Have your *Identity Mobile* at hand):**

   Some parts of your identity will stay the same throughout your life. You may have been born with certain characteristics that will remain with you. Some aspects of your identity were learned as part of your family, cultural, or religious life. Some of these aspects may change as you grow into an adult.

   Knowing yourself and balancing the many parts of who you are will keep you from tipping over throughout your life. (Again lift attributes from one side of your *Identity Mobile* to demonstrate the tilt—then replace them to show the return to balance.)

   Balance will help you to be strong and to resist formulas for feeling bad.

3. **HANG the mobiles in your classroom and refer to them as this unit progresses.**

4. **ADD** the *Body Image Building Block* for Lesson 2 from I-D to student's models.

5. **ASSIGN HOME EDUCATION:** Encourage students to share 2-A—*Your Identity: Many Parts Make You Strong* at home, stressing the importance of all the many parts of who they are. They may tell their caregivers about the mobiles they have made and that they will bring them home to share at the end of the *Healthy Body Image* Unit. Ask for a signed and returned Home Education slip.

2-A YOUR IDENTITY: MANY PARTS MAKE YOU STRONG

Check or circle all of the items below that are part of who you are.
This may include:

- All of the things you enjoy doing, whether or not you do them well.
- All of the things you do well, even if you do not do them often.
- All of the things you have never tried but dream of doing in the future.

I AM PHYSICALLY ACTIVE

I can:

____ Run
____ Throw
____ Catch
____ Have energy to be active for a long time
____ Dance
____ Jump
____ Climb
____ Lift heavy things

I enjoy:

____ Skiing
____ Swimming
____ Gymnastics
____ Basketball
____ Football
____ Horseback riding
____ Track
____ Walking
____ Playing outside
____ Skating
____ Bicycling
____ Wrestling
____ Tennis
____ Soccer
____ Volleyball
____ Hockey
____ Dancing

List other physical activities or specific sports that are part of who you are:

____

____

____

I HAVE INTELLIGENCE. I CAN DO:

____Math
____Foreign language
____Reading
____Creative Problem Solving
____Spelling
____Science
____Writing
____ History
____Other____________________________

____

I TAKE PRIDE IN MY APPEARANCE

____ I take care of my health, eat well, stay fit, rest
____ I comb or brush my hair
____ I keep clean my hands and face
____ I like to wear my favorite colors
____ I like clothes that say something about me
____ I wear hats, jewelry, or other "decorations"
____ I like to appear friendly

Color of my hair__________________________

Eyes_______________ Skin____________

My hair is: Short Medium Long
Curly Straight

Overall size (for my age): Big Small Average

Another thing about my looks is:__________

____

I AM CREATIVE OR ARTISTIC

_____ I like to draw, paint, or color
_____ I write poetry or stories
_____ I dance
_____ I am in theater
_____ I sew
_____ I build things or do crafts (What kind?)
_____ I am musical (In what way?)

List other creative or artistic abilities:

____

____

____

2-A Page 2

I AM OPEN TO LEARNING	I AM A CITIZEN (part of my community)
____I try new things	____I am respectful ____I pitch in to help
____I learn from mistakes	____I am responsible ____I work up to my ability
____I like to solve problems	____I participate (do my part)
____If something is hard, I keep at it	____I take care of the environment
____I finish projects or assignments	____I think about others as well as myself.

I HAVE RELATIONSHIPS

____ I am friendly
____ I am caring
____ I am reliable
____ I am loving
____ I am kind
____ I Communicate well
____ I include people who are not my best friends
____ I have fun ideas

____ I have interests to share
____ I am a team player—do what I'm asked for the sake of the team
____ I can be a leader, take charge
____ I can laugh at myself and at my mistakes
____ I care about how people feel
____ I can resolve conflicts

____ I am fun to be with
____ I enjoy humor
____ I like to learn new things
____ I am polite
____ I can be serious
____ I am a good listener
____ I share

I MANAGE MY PHYSICAL AND EMOTIONAL HEALTH

____I shower or bathe regularly
____I eat healthy food
____I am physically active
____I play safe
____I play smart
____I think about healthy choices
____I know what I need and ask for it

____I take time to relax
____I have realistic expectations of myself
____I can accept it when things don't work out
____I organize and manage my time
____I organize and manage my belongings
____I am able to make decisions
____I can say no and disagree if I need to

I have many feelings:
_____happy
_____sad
_____afraid
_____hurt
_____angry
_____excited
_____anxious
_____grateful

I HAVE MANY INTERESTS (Add as many as you like!)

____I collect things (list things that you collect):
____
____

____I have a pet (what kind(s)?________________

List other hobbies and interests:
____
____
____

I enjoy: _____ Cards or other indoor games
____Miniature golf
____Scuba diving
____Computers
____Building things
____Magic
____Cooking
____Have a pen pal
____Reading
____
____
____

2-A Page 3

I HAVE VALUES AND/OR BELIEFS ABOUT LIFE Do you have a religious faith? What is it called? ____ Do you have strong cultural or ethnic ties? What are they? ____ List a few of the values you think are most important in life: ____________________ ____
MY PREFERENCES OR FAVORITES: (You may list one or more than one)
Color
Food
Drink
Quiet activity
Busy activity
Person
Teacher
Animal
Way to dress
Memory
Hobby
Sport
Fruit
Vegetable
Subject in school
Song
Game
TV show
Movie
Book
Hero

2-B

ATTRIBUTES OF MY IDENTITY

Choose two or more attributes from each category of your identity survey (2-A) that are most important to you. Write your choices in the appropriate rectangles below. You may write attributes on both sides of each card if you wish. Glue this page to a sheet of construction paper to make it stronger. Cut the rectangles into cards. Use the supplies provided by your teacher to make an Identity Mobile. Use your Identity Mobile to remember there are many parts to who you are—even more than are included here.

I am PHYSICALLY ACTIVE.	**I am CREATIVE OR ARTISTIC.**
I take PRIDE IN MY APPEARANCE.	**I have INTELLIGENCE. I do:**
I LEARN NEW THINGS.	**I am a CITIZEN (part of my community). I am:**
I have OTHER INTERESTS.	**I have RELATIONSHIPS.**
I manage my HEALTH and well being.	**I have VALUES AND/OR RELIGIOUS BELIEFS.**

LESSON 3

HOW YOUR APPEARANCE WILL CHANGE IN PUBERTY

Body Image Building Block:
There are many different, normal ways for looks to change in puberty. Sooner or later, most boys and girls will gain weight and fill out.

Please consider the following three points as you approach this lesson:

1. If your class has already had a unit on body changes in puberty, it is likely that several Critical Concepts regarding body size that are included in this lesson were not addressed. These should be covered before moving on to the next lesson.

2. It is strongly recommended this lesson be presented in gender-specific classes or that time be allowed for gender-specific discussion groups after the lesson. This will promote the following objectives:
   - Regardless of grade, children are likely to participate more freely in discussion.
   - Girls and boys will feel an increased sense of positive connection with their own gender: "We are in this together!"
   - Respect for individual modesty—at its peak for girls in grades four through six—will be honored.
   - Students should be informed of these objectives for the gender-split class and that the lesson content for boys and girls is the same.

3. If you are planning a unit on Family Life (sex education), it should *not* be paired with this lesson.

LESSON OBJECTIVES

Students will understand the changes in appearance to expect with puberty

While appearance is only one aspect of identity, changes in puberty naturally heighten children's interest in how their bodies look. This lesson, along with Lessons 4 and 5, promotes healthy, realistic expectations, attitudes, and responses when appearance becomes a central focus. Students will learn:

- The *outward changes* in appearance to expect during puberty for both boys and girls.
- They can feel free to talk about these changes with each other and trusted adults. Reassurance and sound information about body development is available.
- Their questions are normal and shared by many.
- Self-consciousness and worry can be reduced by learning what is normal and expected.

Students will understand the proper use of words to describe body sizes

The words *fatter* and *thinner* accurately describe *all* bodies but are rarely used without judgment. This lesson strips these words of their "bad/good" value. Students will learn:

- *All* people are innately or *naturally* pre-disposed to be fatter, thinner, or in-between.
- Use of words "fatter" or "thinner" may accurately be used only to *describe* a body type, never as a judgment of "good" or "bad."

NOTE: Future lessons will teach students that they can trust that their body size and weight are right for them when they eat well and have an active lifestyle, not when they achieve a prescribed size or appearance. Since students may make comments or raise questions during Lessons 3, 4, and 5 about weight management, teachers should be well-versed on how this is addressed in Lessons 7, 8, and 9 prior to proceeding.

BACKGROUND

Pubescent changes

Many adults are uninformed about the expected outward physical changes that are a normal part of puberty for both boys and girls. This, coupled with our society's fat-phobia, means that children, especially girls, receive virtually no enthusiastic support for the entirely normal and expected rounding out and weight gain that is part of their pubescent development. Lacking both facts and encouragement to feel good about the changes underway, girls at this tender age routinely respond by comparing their budding bodies to the unrealistic culturally sanctioned thin-idea. Since that ideal reflects a body type that almost none of them will or should expect to maintain, most normal-weight girls learn to feel bad about their healthy, growing bodies. In turn, many respond to messages that encourage various weight-loss techniques and begin to engage in unhealthy weight-loss behaviors.

Developing boys are also left uneducated to compare bodies to lean and buff cultural ideals. Magazines, action figures, and movie stars suggest males can easily achieve these sculpted bodies through simplistic formulas: *"Only four weeks to be the trim, muscular guy you've always known you could be!"* When findings show that the chest of a life-size G.I. Joe would have increased from 44.4 to 54.8 inches and his biceps from 12.2 to 26.8 inches between 1973 and 1998, we cannot be surprised if boys acquire unrealistic expectations.

It is hoped that as children are guided to compare their bodies to what is normal, healthy, and diverse, rather than to externally prescribed "ideals," they will be better prepared to begin puberty with realistic, non-judgmental expectations and healthy body images.

Overt use of culturally loaded words

It is understood teaching children and adults to use culturally loaded words describing fatness in an accurate, nonjudgmental way is a very delicate process. Initially almost everyone will continue to hear the descriptive words "fat" or "fatter body type" as condemning (he or she must eat too much), while "thin" is viewed as "good" (virtuous, in control). Teachers are urged to reconcile their own personal prejudices ahead of time and to become sensitive to and very clear about the correct, matter-of-fact, value-free use of these words. You might want to practice saying words out loud until you can say them comfortably and non-judgmentally. For example:

> *"Some people are naturally thinner. Some people are naturally fatter. I am fatter than my sister Mary but a little thinner than my sister Laura. At the same time, my sister Tracy is quite a lot fatter that any of us. But we all eat well and are very active and fit, so I'm confident we are the right size and shape. How much fatness do you think is right for you?"*

TEACH FOR THESE OUTCOMES

Students will:

- Learn the natural changes in appearance that occur with the onset of puberty.
- Recognize that individual differences in development are normal.
- Learn that developmental body changes are not open to control or interruption through healthy means.
- Recognize that innate body-type pre-disposition is not open to judgment.

Student attitudes will be:

- I feel comfortable with the way my body is growing.
- It helps to talk with people whom I can trust about how my body shape will change as I grow up.
- People cannot control when and how their body is set to change and grow.
- Some of the ways that boys and girls develop are different and some are the same.
- All people are naturally pre-disposed (set up to be) fatter, thinner, or in-between.
- To say someone is fatter or thinner is a way to describe, not judge, them.
- It is normal for girls to gain body fat during puberty.

- Since my body will keep on changing over several years, I can't worry too much about how I look along the way.

CONCEPTS NEEDED TO TEACH THIS LESSON

Puberty brings expected changes in common for both boys and girls

- Once the growth spurt begins, growth is more rapid than ever before in life. The previous average of two inches per year in height now may be four inches or more in one year.
- Growth and development are usually not proportionate; some parts grow faster or slower. Feet often grow to full size first, for example, followed by legs and arms and later the spine and other bones. Ears and chins grow before other facial features. If children are not told, they may worry that these odd proportions may be permanent.
- For a while bodies may look, feel, and be awkward because of disproportionate growth.
- It is normal to gain weight and body fat during puberty.
- Fatter and thinner are *descriptive words*, not judgments. They have come to be used as judgments in our culture. This is based on pervasive ignorance about many of the determinants of weight, as well as generalizations about eating behaviors and lifestyle choices.
- Some boys and girls will develop much later or earlier than others. Timing will not affect the end result. A few individuals will remain small even as adults.
- Skin changes occur gradually as oil and sweat glands become more active. This may result in oily hair and acne in addition to increased perspiration and stronger body odor.
- Body hair will grow in new places: in the pubic area, underarms, and on arms and legs.

Puberty results in changes specific to GIRLS:

- Most pre-pubescent girls are very interested in how their bodies will be developing.
- The average age for the onset of development is 10 to12; the common range is from 8 to15.
- It is normal during puberty for girls to gain body fat rapidly. It is normal for a girl to gain 20% of her body weight in fat, or up to 20 pounds or more in one year. This is part of the healthy, rounding out of a girl's body as it grows into the body of a young woman, and should *never* be confused with "getting fat."
- Girls may get fatter before getting taller, or the other way around.

- At first, the additional fat may be dispersed evenly throughout a girl's body. It will then appear to redistribute as height is gained, and roundness becomes more localized in buttocks, thighs, and bust.
- Later, and more slowly, pelvic bones widen and become denser, broadening the hips
- Developing girls may gain 40 to 60 pounds in only two to four years. This is normal but may be interpreted with alarm when the prevailing cultural message is that weight gain is bad.

Puberty results in changes specific to BOYS:

- Pre-pubescent boys vary in their levels of interest in their bodies' growth and development. However, interest seems to be on the rise along with the rise in "ideal" male images in the media.
- The average age for the onset of outward development is 12 or 13.
- Once growth begins, boys quickly catch up to girls, with most growing taller and eventually more muscular than most girls.
- Boys may get fatter before getting taller, or the other way around.
- Growth in height precedes muscular growth by a few years. Boys get taller before they fill out.
- There are normal breast changes for boys. Besides the darkening and widening of the nipple and a somewhat tender, flat lump under the nipple, more than half will have a bit of swelling of their breasts. This is temporary and will go away in one to two years. Boys need the facts about this or they may worry needlessly that they are developing breasts.
- Boys often do not fill out completely until 18 to 22 years.
- Boys' voices may change around 12 to 13 but can change as late as 15 years.
- Boys will gradually begin to grow facial hair and, for some, chest hair.

CRITICAL CONCEPTS

Until now, it has been rare for children to be educated and reassured about the out-of-proportion body growth that is so natural to the pubescent stage of development. It is even less common that young students are educated about the *normal gain in weight* that is expected with puberty, especially in the form of fat for girls. Since boys and girls *routinely* get somewhat fatter before they get taller, it is critical that they be informed of this to counter messages that otherwise suggest to them that this is bad. Research clearly shows that misinterpretation of normal pre-pubescent and pubescent change is a major contributor to the onset of body image disturbances. It is also critical to introduce the words *fat* and *thin* as descriptive words as opposed to judgments. This basic diversity education should be integrated into all relevant curricula.

LESSON PREPARATION AND MATERIALS

Materials:	**Preparation:**
▪ Copy HANDOUT 3-A for each student. While the handout is several pages, it is a worthwhile tool for both students and their families. ▪ A three-hole folder for each student to "bind" 3-A.	▪ Read the *Suggested Lesson Script*, including the *Book Text.* ▪ If possible, present this lesson to gender-specific groups. A male teacher is preferred for boys and a female for girls. ▪ Discussion will occur most freely if this lesson is presented by a teacher who is comfortable with the material and with whom students have a relationship. ▪ This lesson is particularly dense and may take two class periods. It commonly generates a lot of discussion and includes a *Write a Book* project. ▪ Some teachers more time is available for discussion when they fill in the answers to 3-A in their own hand-writing, and photocopy this "master copy" to distribute to students. The class then reads and discusses the book (and takes it home to read with parents) without students having to fill in the blanks. ▪ Teachers have found it helpful to make overheads of the *Write a Book,* with blanks filled in, providing a visual model for students to follow in completing their own books. ▪ If time allows, students may want to design original covers for their books.

LESSON SUMMARY

- EXPLAIN: We will learn the outward changes in *appearance* to expect with puberty. (This will not be "sex education.")
- INTRODUCE/DO HANDOUT 3-A—The *Write a Book* activity. Students write books as you provide and discuss information from the *Book Text Key.*
- ENCOURAGE questions and discussion as puberty material is presented.
- ADD: *Body Image Building Block.*
- ASSIGN HOME EDUCATION.

SUGGESTED LESSON SCRIPT:

1. **EXPLAIN:** We have been talking about maintaining a balanced sense of who you are. Even so, we will now begin several lessons that will focus on only one part of you—appearance. The purpose, however, is to help you keep this in balance.

   Your bodies will soon begin to change and grow. This is an important time! When things change, they call for more attention than when they stay the same. We learned from Terry Tadpole that *not understanding change made her worry. Information helped her relax.* To help *you* keep your feelings about puberty in balance, we want you to know what to expect.

2. **DISTRIBUTE and INTRODUCE the *Write a Book* Activity 3-A—*How Appearance Changes in Puberty*.** In this lesson we will talk about how looks change during puberty. You will become the expert and write a book on this subject.

3. **ASK:** Your book will be written for kids—but anyone who wants the facts about puberty will be able to learn from it. Do you think the grown-ups where you live already know everything about puberty?

   TELL: While many grown-ups know about puberty (they *did* go through it!), many grown-ups today did not get all the facts about how and why bodies *look* the way they do as they grow. After you read your book with your parents or caregivers, you will be *sure* you both have the right information.

   DIRECTIONS FOR TEACHERS:

   Read the Book Text Key for How Appearance Changes In Puberty (see page 46) *out loud slowly and carefully. As you read, words that are* ***underlined*** *will be filled in by students in their Write a Book. Allow time for questions and discussion.*

   Emphasize *the following themes as you discuss the material:*

   1. The age range for puberty varies among individuals. Variations are normal.
   2. Differences are not "good" or "bad." They are simply different.

4. **ADD the *Body Image Building Block*** for Lesson 3 from I-D to the students' models.

5. **ASSIGN HOME EDUCATION:** Encourage students to share their books at home. Ask for a signed and returned Home Education slip.

BOOK TEXT KEY: How Appearance Changes in Puberty

Dear Puberty Expert,

There is a lot to learn about how kids' bodies grow during puberty. I have some ideas, but I don't know if they are correct or true for everybody. Some kids in my class are already growing in new ways. I heard you had a class on this, and you might have the answers to my questions.

1. *Does everybody go through puberty sometime?* **Yes** No
2. *Will growth be more than just getting taller?* **Yes** No
   As you develop you will also be **filling out.**
3. *Is everybody supposed to change at the same time?*
   Everyone changes at **different** times, according to their own inner "body **clock,**" or pre-determined **schedule.**
4. *Do boys and girls change at the same time?* Yes **No**

Compared to each other:				*Average age*	*As early as*	*As late as*
GIRLS change:	**sooner**	same	later	**10 to 12**	**8**	**15**
BOYS change:	sooner	same	**later**	**12 to 13**	**9**	**15**

5. *So it's normal for many girls to be taller than many boys at our age?* **Yes** No
6. *I heard someone say my friend is having a "growth spurt." What is that?*

   Growth spurts are when you grow **faster** than ever before. During puberty, instead of growing about **2 inches** per year, you may grow **4 inches** or more per year. You may hear your family say, "You are growing out of your clothes too fast." But you can't help it!
7. *Is it better to start puberty sooner or better to start later?* (circle)

   Better sooner Better later **Not better either way**
8. *Why doesn't everybody start puberty at the same time?*

   How and when we grow **is not** something anyone has control over. The timing for this is **pre-determined** before birth. Whether you start your growth spurt earlier or later (*circle*) **will not** affect how big or small you will be in the end.
9. *What if I'm really early or late in starting puberty? I don't want to be different.*

   Differences in body changes **are not** something that can be judged as **good** or **bad**. No one has control over when or how these changes occur. It is like the color of your eyes, or how fast your hair grows. It is not something anyone should ever have to feel bad about. Even if it would be easier to change at the same time or in the same ways as your friends, differences are a **normal** and **necessary** part of life.

10. *What if someone teases me?*

It may mean they do not understand the facts about **puberty**. Or once in a while a person may intend to be mean. You could try **ignoring** or even **educating** them. Or you could try telling a **friend** and getting his or her **support**. If that doesn't help, you should ask a trusted **adult** to stop the teasing.

11. *Please tell me all the details about puberty change.? Will I grow everywhere all at once?*

Some parts of your body will grow **faster**, while other parts will grow **slower**. It is different for everyone, but here is the usual order:

- First **feet**. Feet can be full-size long before you are!
- Then **arms** and **legs**.
- Then **back bone** and other bones.

12. *What exactly will make me "fill out"? What should I expect?*

It is **normal** to **gain weight** from adding **body fat** and **bone mass** during puberty. In later teen years, you will also gain **muscle.**

13. *Isn't fat bad?*

Sometimes fatness is talked about as if it were just plain "bad." There are at least three reasons why this idea is not accurate. Many people need to learn the ABCs of body fat:

A. The body **cannot live** without fat. It is critical for health. Fat lubricates our joints and protects our vital organs. Body fat is also needed to help the body absorb vitamins needed for health. *In addition, 60% of the solid part of the brain is made of fat.* Last but not least, fat is the body's storage container for energy. We will learn more about this later.

B. **All** people are naturally pre-disposed (set up before they are even born) to be **fatter**, **thinner,** or in-between. When something in our nature is pre-disposed, there is a *very strong* tendency for it to be a certain way. This is not in our control. If a fatter person is **eating well**, is **active**, and is **fit,** then his or her fatness is probably just right. No matter what people say or think, a naturally thin pre-disposition is *not* better than a fit and healthy fatter one; just different. The important thing is to be fit at any size.

C. It is not only ignorant to judge a person's pre-dispositions as bad; it is not fair. When we state that someone is fatter or thinner this should *only* be a way to **describe** that person, never a way to **judge** him or her as "good" or "bad"—as if size could be "right" or "wrong." This would be the same as judging someone because of their eye or skin color, or because they are very good at music but not at sports.

D. Because so many people have learned incorrect information about body size and weight, we will be talking more about this in later lessons.

14. *Girls develop earlier than boys. Are there other differences for girls ?* **Yes** No

LET'S TALK ABOUT CHANGES FOR GIRLS

1. While everyone is different, it is normal for girls to gain body fat in puberty. Girls may gain **20 pounds** or more in one year. This does not mean they are getting fat.

2. *Why do girls gain more body fat than boys?*

   This is the beginning of the normal, healthy rounding-out of a girl's body as she grows into a young woman. Nature **intends** most adult women to carry more body fat than most boys and men. This is part of a woman's special design for bearing children and *should not* be confused with becoming unhealthily fat.

   It is perfectly **normal** for a woman to have a more **rounded** figure than a man. Puberty is when this rounding-out begins.

3. *What does a girl's body do with the added fat?*

   At first a girl may develop a layer of fat **all over**, like an extra layer under the skin. Then it will begin to be more obvious in certain parts: **breasts, hips, and thighs.**

4. *Do girls get taller before they add fat, or rounder first?*

   Either way. Everyone is different. Some may get rounder first and only later gain height. Others may get quite tall and thin first, later adding curves or roundness.

   A **few** girls will remain very thin and not very rounded all their lives, whether they are taller or shorter. But, despite what people think, a very thin body (*circle)* ***is not*** the most common or natural body shape for a woman.

5. *Are there any other changes for girls that boys don't share?*

   Girls' pelvic bones (just above their hips) very gradually begin to **widen.** This is essential for a woman to be capable of having a **baby** when she is an adult. For example, this occurred to allow your **mother** to have you. Wider pelvic bones are the **second** reason why women normally have bigger hips than men.

   Overall, girls develop different shapes than boys. Following are some ways girls may grow early in puberty. **(Draw the following graphic on the board for students to copy.)**

IN PUBERTY, GIRLS MAY GROW:

Taller first	Rounder first	Not much taller or rounder	Taller and rounder	The most common adult female shape: narrower at the shoulders, wider at the hips

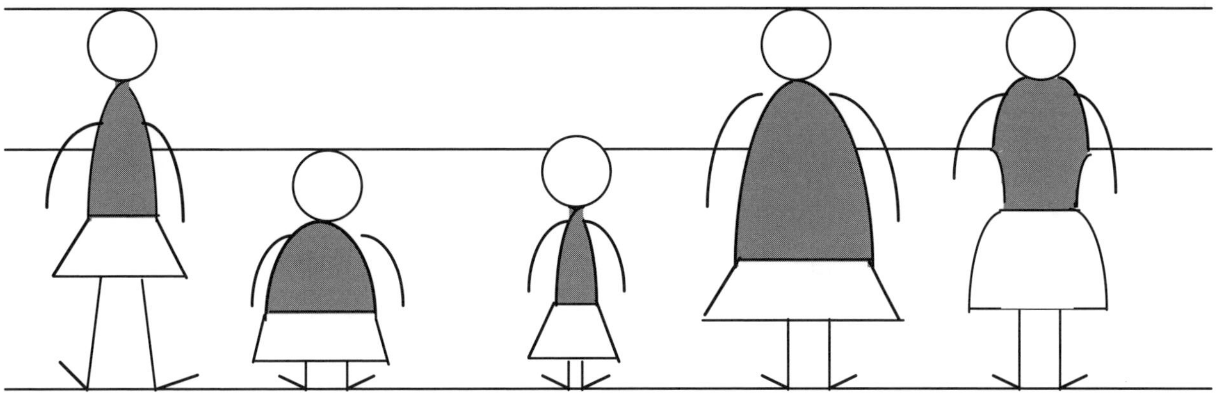

LET'S TALK ABOUT CHANGES FOR BOYS

1. *Aren't men usually bigger than women? How can boys begin their development later than girls?*

   Once outward growth begins, boys quickly catch up. Most, but not all, boys eventually become **taller** and more **muscular** than most girls.

2. *Is it normal for boys to gain body fat during puberty, too?*

   Often **Sometimes** Rarely

   Some boys become fatter before they get taller. However, as boys grow taller, many stretch out their fatness into a taller, slimmer body. While there are natural differences, most adult males carry (circle) ***less*** body fat overall than most females.

3. *What other changes occur for boys?*

   Later in puberty, **shoulders** can become wider and eventually more muscular. However, boys usually do not **fill out** their bodies until later teen years. Then, they will begin to look less like boys and more like adult males. **(Draw for students to copy.)**

IN PUBERTY, BOYS MAY GROW:

Fatter first	Taller and fatter	Not much taller or fatter	Taller, always slim	The most common adult male shape: broader at the shoulders than at the hips

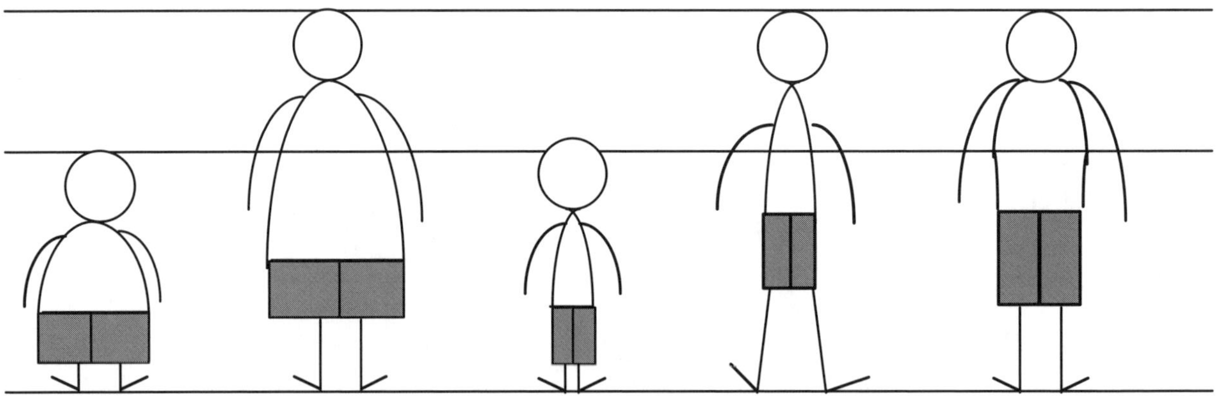

4. *Anything else?*

   More than half of all boys will have some **<u>breast swelling</u>** in puberty. This is normal and does *not* mean they are developing breasts. The swelling will go away in one to two years. Boys do not need to worry about this.

5. *What happens to a boy's voice during puberty?*

   When a boy's voice box has grown larger, usually by age 14 or 15, his voice becomes **<u>deeper</u>**. This may happen somewhat suddenly or in a gradual, less noticeable way. Some boys experience a **<u>cracking</u>** of their voices as they go through this change. Their voices may become high-pitched or squeaky unexpectedly.

6. *Isn't that embarrassing? What if a boy gets teased?*

   There is no reason to be embarrassed because voice changes are simply part of growing up. But teasing is always wrong unless the person being teased is genuinely having fun.

7. *Aren't there some other outward changes for both boys and girls in puberty?*

   <u>Yes</u> No

LET'S TALK ABOUT CHANGES THAT BOYS AND GIRLS HAVE IN COMMON

1. *What are some changes boys and girls have in common?*

   Boys and girls grow hair in new places: First **<u>pubic</u>** and underarm hair, then on **<u>arms</u>** and **<u>legs</u>**, and, for boys only, eventually **<u>face</u>** and **<u>chest</u>** hair. Also, two glands become more active: **<u>oil</u>** and **<u>sweat</u>**.

2. *What about the glands?*

   When oil glands are more active, you may notice your hair gets oily faster. Also, many kids have some pimples or skin acne when they are further along in puberty.

   When sweat glands are more active, we perspire more. Also, perspiration may have a more **grown-up** odor. When oil and sweat glands become more active, kids usually need to bathe or shower and wash their hair more often. You may want to ask a parent or guardian for deodorant.

3. *It sounds like this puberty business goes on for a while. I guess it doesn't happen overnight.*

   That's (circle) **true** **false.**

4. *It also sounds like different parts of the body grow earlier or later—even more or less than other parts. If some bones grow faster than others, I add body fat before I get taller, or if I get taller before I fill out, won't I look kind of funny or out of proportion?*

   Yes No **Maybe**

   It may take several years before you see how you will end up looking.

It is important to understand that the way you grow in puberty may not be even.

For example, your arms, and legs may grow long, while your backbone is still short. Your feet may be as big as an adult's feet, even two or three years before the rest of you grows taller. Your ears and chin may grow before the rest of your face.

For a while the way you look may be very different from how you will end up. One day you may look in a mirror and enjoy seeing the changes. Another day, you may not be so happy about them.

It may help to know many kids feel this way at one time or another. Most kids feel a little awkward or clumsy when some parts of their bodies are growing faster than other parts. Remember, you are not a finished product yet! That is why teasing about body changes is especially unfair and hurtful. Remember Terry the Tadpole and picture him as half tadpole and half frog. Puberty is not a time to judge or worry about looks. It is a time to be amazed at the many wonderful changes your body is going through as you are growing up.

THINK ABOUT IT THIS WAY:

It probably took from **5** to **8** years for you to gain your first fifty pounds, and longer yet to get to be four feet tall.

When you start your growth spurt, you may very well gain another **50** pounds in only two or three years, and a foot or two of height in just a few years. That's a BIG change.

My advice is:

A. **relax**

B. **stay healthy**, and

C. give your body time to show you how it's going to grow.

If you will:

A. **eat well**

B. **stay active**, **strong,** and **fit**, as well as

C. **watch**, then you will see your body develop naturally into the size and shape it was born to be.

Remember the *Tools for Change* we learned in our first body image lesson.

When your body starts to grow
from a child into a teen
You will want to know the facts about
what will be happening.
You will want to get good answers
from the grown-ups that you trust;
those who have your health at heart
will give you answers you can trust!

It will help to hear from classmates
who are growing now with you.
Then you'll see you're not alone,
but just one of the group.
These body image lessons
will help you day by day
As you watch your body grow
in a healthy, "just right" way!

3-A

HOW APPEARANCE CHANGES IN PUBERTY

By

____

Age ______

HOW APPEARANCE CHANGES IN PUBERTY

Dear Puberty Expert,
There is a lot to learn about how kids' bodies grow during puberty. I have some ideas, but I don't know if they are correct or true for everybody. Some kids in my class are already growing in new ways. I heard you had a class on this, and you might have the answers to my questions.

1. ***Does everybody go through puberty sometime?*** **Yes No**
2. ***Will growth be more than just getting taller?*** **Yes No**

   As you develop you will also be ______________________ ______________.

3. ***Is everybody supposed to change at the same time?***

   Everyone changes at ______________________ times, according to their own inner "body ______________________," or pre-determined ______________________.

4. ***Do boys and girls change at the same time?*** **Yes No**

Compared to each other:				Average age	As early as	As late as
(Circle. Fill in the ages) GIRLS change:	sooner	same	later	_______	_______	_______
BOYS change:	sooner	same	later	_______	_______	_______

5. ***So it's normal for many girls to be taller than most boys at our age?*** **Yes No**
6. ***I heard someone say my friend was having a "growth spurt." What is that?***

   Growth spurts are when you grow ______________________ than ever before. During puberty, instead of growing about ____________ ______________________ per year, you may grow ____________ ______________________. You may hear your family say, "You are growing out of your clothes too fast." But, you can't help it!

7. ***Is it better to start puberty sooner or better to start later?*** **(circle)**

Better sooner **Better later** **Not better either way**

8. ***Why doesn't everybody start puberty at the same time?***

How and when we grow (circle) **is** **is not** something anyone has control over. The timing for this is ________________ - ____________________________ before birth. Whether you start your growth spurt earlier or later (circle) **will** **will not** affect how big or small you will be in the end.

9. ***What if I'm really early or late in starting puberty?*** *I don't want to be different.*

Differences in body changes: (circle) **are** **are not** something that can be judged as________________________ or __________________. No one has control over when or how changes occur. It is like the color of your eyes, or how fast your hair grows. It is not something anyone should ever have to feel bad about. Even if it would be easier to change at the same time or in the same ways as your friends, differences are a ______________________________and a ______________________________ part of life.

10. ***What if someone teases me?***

It may mean they do not understand the facts about ____________________________ or once in a while a person may intend to be mean.

You could try ____________________________________ or even ____ them. Or you could try telling a ________________________and getting his or her _________________________.

If that doesn't help, you should ask a trusted _____________________________ to stop the teasing.

11. ***Please tell me all the details about puberty changes. Will I grow everywhere all at once?***

Some parts of your body will grow ______________________________, while other parts will grow _________________________________. It is different for everyone, but here is the usual order: First ________________________________. Feet can be full-size long before you are! Then_________________________________ and

______________________________. Then______________________________ ________________________ and other bones.

12. ***What exactly will make me "fill out?" What should I expect?***

It is ______________________________ to _____________________ ______________________________ from adding ____________________ _________________________ and _________________________________ ____________________________ during puberty. In later teen years, you will also gain some _________________________________.

13. ***Isn't fat bad?***

Sometimes fatness is talked about as if it were just plain "bad." There are at least three reasons why this idea is not accurate. Many people need to learn the A B Cs of body fat:

A) The body _______________________ ____________________ without fat. It is critical for health. Fat lubricates our joints, and protects our vital organs. Body fat is also needed to help the body absorb vitamins needed for health. In addition, 60% of the solid part of the brain is made of fat. Last but not least, fat is the body's storage container for energy. We will learn more about this later.

B) __________ people are naturally pre-disposed (set-up before they are even born) to be _______________________, _________________________, or in-between. When something in nature is pre-disposed, there is a *very strong* tendency for it to be a certain way. If a fatter person is _________________ _____________, __________________, and _____________, then his or her fatness is probably just right. No matter what people say or think, a naturally thin pre-disposition is not better than a fit and healthy fatter one; just different. The important thing is to be fit at any size.

C) When something is not in a person's control, then it is ignorant to judge it as "bad." It is also not fair. When we state that someone is "fatter" or "thinner," this should only be a way to ____________________________ that person, never a way to __________________________ them as "good" or "bad"—as if size could be "right" or "wrong." This would be the same as judging someone because of their eye or skin color, or because they were good at music, but not at sports. Because so many people have learned incorrect information about body size and weight, we will be talking more about this in later lessons.

14. ***Besides developing earlier than boys, are there other differences for girls?***

Yes **No**

LET'S TALK ABOUT CHANGES FOR GIRLS:

1. ***While everyone is different, it is normal for girls to gain body fat rapidly in puberty.***

   Girls may gain ________________ ______________________ or more in one year. This does not mean they are getting fat.

2. ***Why do girls gain more body fat than boys?***

   This is the beginning of the normal, healthy rounding out of a girl's body as she grows into a young woman. Nature ______________________ adult women to carry more body fat than most boys and men. This is part of a woman's special design for bearing children, and should not be confused with becoming unhealthily fat. It is perfectly ________________________ for a woman to have a more ________________________ figure than a man. Puberty is when this rounding-out begins.

3. ***What does a girl's body do with the added fat?***

   At first a girl may develop a layer of fat ___________ __________________, like an extra layer under the skin. Then it will begin to be more obvious in certain parts: ____________________________, ________________________, and ______________________.

4. ***Do girls get taller before they add fat, or rounder first?***

   Either way. Everyone is different. Some may get rounder first, and only later gain height. Others may get quite tall and thin first, later adding curves or roundness. A ____________________ girls will remain very thin and not very rounded all their lives, whether they are taller or shorter. But, despite what people think, a very thin body (circle)

   is **is not** the most common or natural body shape for a woman.

5. ***Are there any other changes for girls that boys don't share?***

Girls' pelvic bones (just above her hips) very gradually begin to ______________________________. This is essential for a woman to be capable of having a ______________________________________ when she is an adult. For example, this occurred to allow your ________________________________ to have you. Wider pelvic bones are the ____ reason why women normally have bigger hips than men. Overall, girls do develop different shapes than boys. Following are some ways girls may grow early in puberty. *(Draw the figures according to scale.)*

IN PUBERTY, GIRLS MAY GROW				
Taller first	Rounder first	Not much taller or rounder	Taller and rounder	The most common adult female shape: narrower at the shoulders, wider at the hip.

LET'S TALK ABOUT CHANGES FOR BOYS

1. ***Aren't men usually bigger than women? How can boys begin their development later than girls?***

Once outward growth begins, boys quickly catch-up. Most, but not all boys eventually become ______________________________ and more _________________________________ than most girls.

2. ***Is it normal for boys to gain body fat during puberty too?*** (circle)

Often **Sometimes** **Rarely**

Some boys become fatter before they get taller. However, as boys grow taller, many stretch out their fatness into a taller, slimmer body. While there are natural differences, most adult males carry (circle) **more** **less** body fat overall than most females.

3. ***What other changes occur for boys?***

Later in puberty, ______________________________ can become wider, and eventually more muscular. However, boys usually do not ____________________ ____________________ their bodies until later teen years. Then, they will begin to look less like boys and more like adult males. (Draw the figures according to scale.)

IN PUBERTY, BOYS MAY GROW				
Taller first	Rounder first	Not much taller or fatter	Taller and always slim	The most common adult male shape: broader at the shoulders than at the hips.

4. ***Anything else?***

More than half of all boys will have some____________________ ______________________________ in puberty. This is normal and does not mean he is developing breasts. The swelling will go away in 1 to 2 years. Boys do not need to worry about this.

5. ***What happens to a boy's voice during puberty?***

   When a boy's voice box has grown larger, usually by age 14 or 15, his voice becomes ____________________. This may happen somewhat suddenly, or in a gradual and less noticeable way. Some boys may experience a ____________________ of their voices as they're going through this change. Their voices may become high-pitched or squeaky unexpectedly.

6. ***Isn't that embarrassing? What if a boy gets teased?***

   There is no reason to be embarrassed, because voice changes are simply part of growing up. But teasing is always wrong unless the person being teased is genuinely having fun.

7. ***Aren't there some other outward changes for both boys and girls in puberty?*** (circle)

   Yes **No**

LET'S TALK ABOUT CHANGES BOYS AND GIRLS HAVE IN COMMON

1. ***What are some changes boys and girls have in common?***

   Boys and girls grow hair in new places. First ____________________ and underarm hair, then on ____________________ and ____________________, and for boys only, eventually ____________________ and ____________________ hair. Also, two glands become more active: ____________________ and ____________________.

2. ***What about the glands?***

   When oil glands are more active, you may notice your hair gets ____________________ faster. Also, many kids have some pimples or skin acne when they are further along in puberty. (More about this in later grades.) When sweat glands are more active we perspire more. Also, perspiration may have a more ____________________ ____________________ odor. When oil and sweat glands become more active, kids usually need to bathe or shower and wash hair more often. You may want to ask a parent or guardian for deodorant.

3. ***It sounds like this puberty business goes on for a while. I guess it doesn't happen overnight.***

   That's: (circle) **true** **not true.**

4. ***It also sounds like different parts of the body grow earlier or later than others. If some bones grow faster than others, if I add body fat before I get taller, or if I'm getting taller before I fill out—won't I look kind of out of proportion?*** (circle)

   Yes **No** **Maybe**

   It may take several ____________________ before you see how you will end up looking.

It is important to understand that the way you grow in puberty may not be even.

For example, your arms and legs may grow long, while your backbone is still short. Your feet may be as big as an adult's feet, even 2 or 3 years before the rest of you grows taller. Your ears and chin may grow before the rest of your face.

For a while the way you look may be very different than how you will end up. One day you may look in a mirror and enjoy seeing the changes. Another day, you may not be so crazy about them.

It may help to know many kids feel this way at one time or another. Most kids feel a little awkward or clumsy when some parts of their body are growing faster than other parts. Remember, you are not a finished product yet! That is why teasing about body changes is especially unfair and hurtful.

Remember Terry the Tadpole and picture him as half tadpole and half frog. This is not a time to judge or worry about looks. It is a time to be amazed at the many wonderful changes your body is going through as you are growing up.

THINK ABOUT IT THIS WAY:

It probably took from ____________ to ____________ years for you to gain your first fifty pounds, and longer yet to get to be four feet tall. When you start your growth spurt you may very well gain another __________ pounds in only two or three years, and more than another foot or two of height in that same amount of time. That's a *BIG* change in a short amount of time.

My advice is:

A) ________________________ B) ____________________ _________________________,

and C) give your body __________________________ to show you how it's going to end up.

If you A) ________________________ _________________________, B) stay) __________________________________ , ___________________________________ , and ________________________ as well as C)____________________________, you will see your body develop naturally, into the size and shape it was born to be!

Remember the *Tools for Change* from our first body image lesson:

When your body starts to grow
from a child into a teen
You will want to know the facts about
what will be happening.
You will want to get good answers
from the grown-ups that you trust;
those who have your health at heart
will give you answers you can trust!

It will help to hear from classmates
who are growing now with you.
Then you'll see you're not alone,
but just one of the group.
These body image lessons
will help you day by day
As you watch your body grow
in a healthy, "just right" way!

DRAW A PICTURE OF YOURSELF AS A BABY, At 5 YEARS OLD, AND NOW.

Think about all the things your body can do now that it could not do when you were younger!

Me as a baby	Me at 5 years old
Me NOW!	

LESSON 4

GENETICS

How Body Size and Shape are Determined

> **Body Image Building Block:**
>
> *Most of the way we look is determined before we are even born: taller, shorter, fatter, thin-- all are normal, all built in!*

LESSON OBJECTIVES

This lesson provides a foundation for understanding the limits to external control over body size and shape through healthy means. In an environment that directly encourages the belief that fashion is the best dictator of the "right" body size and shape, the objectives of this lesson are critical.

Students will learn:

- Genetic pre-disposition is the greatest single determinant of body shape and size.
- The degree to which weight and shape can be influenced by external choices is limited by innate factors.

BACKGROUND

Despite clear evidence to the contrary, the belief that human weight and shape are first and foremost influenced by food consumption and physical activity has become deeply imbedded in the American culture. Silence in challenging this fallacy has resulted in transferring to children inaccurate and dangerous assumptions about the extent to which people can healthily manipulate weight and shape at will. These assumptions promote weight prejudices based on ignorance. They also encourage risky eating behaviors that can contribute to malnourishment, disordered eating patterns, unhealthy weight gain, and obesity.

Disregard for the facts of genetic heritage contributes to widespread distain for many normal and healthy body types and to other eating disorder risk factors, especially in girls. Currently, a majority of children grow up feeling they are to blame if they do not have the "right" (lean) body type. In turn, cultural pressures endorse self-defeating and dangerous restrictive eating behaviors based on the belief that these can be an effective solution. Dieting for weight loss results in numerous problems, not the least of which is disruption of the natural weight regulatory system and unhealthy weight gain (see Lesson 7).

It is hoped that, as children become clear about genetic pre-disposition for body shape, they will take to heart the healthy *limits* to their control. In turn, they will be free to focus on the effective choices that enhance confidence and competency in discovering a weight that is healthy and natural for them (see Lessons 8 and 9).

As children face the pressures in today's society to idealize certain body types, a knowledge of genetic diversity and the genetic basis for their own particular body types will strengthen their resiliency and resistance. It will be clear to them that the healthy response to cultural pressures to embody one particular shape will be, "Get real!"

TEACH FOR THESE OUTCOMES

Students will know:

- Genetic programming is in place before humans are born.
- Genetic influence is the greatest determinant of body shape and size.
- There is enormous natural diversity in body size and shape.
- There is a limit to the degree to which weight and shape can be externally controlled by healthy means.
- There are many common misconceptions about control over body size and shape that result in prejudicial attitudes.
- Clues to our own genetic heritage can be seen in our appearance, and that of their biological relatives..

Student attitudes will be:

- A lot of the way I look was determined before I was born.
- While we may prefer a different body shape, we have to accept who we're born to be.
- I accept myself for who I am.
- While eating and fitness habits may influence our weight, the influence will be limited by our genetic predisposition.
- If I eat well and stay fit and strong through physical activity, I can be confident of a healthy weight at any size.

CONCEPTS NEEDED TO TEACH THIS LESSON

- Genes are like biological computers, programmed to tell our bodies how to grow.
- Genes are inherited from biological parents and can be dominant or recessive.
- From 50% to 80% of the influence for body size and shape is genetic. This includes:

  - Bone structure: the length, width, and thickness of bones, which determine the shape of the body's frame, skull and facial structure.
  - The base proportion of fat to lean tissue in the body.
  - The location of the fat stores.
  - The base metabolic rate (see Lesson 5).
- Healthy options for influencing physical appearance are limited to a healthy lifestyle, good grooming and hygiene, and personal style (see Lessons 7, 8, and 9).
- Many in our culture believe we have more control over body size and shape than is realistic. This reflects either a lack of information or denial of the facts.
- Many fatter people have optimal eating and lifestyle habits, and many thinner people do not. Therefore, whether a person is "over" or "under" their natural weight range cannot be determined by simply observing that they are fatter or thinner. (This concept is demonstrated experientially in Lesson 5.) A careful analysis of eating behaviors and lifestyle is necessary to make a diagnosis of "overweight" or "underweight."
- Body type pre-disposition may not be apparent until the late teen years.
- The physical attributes observed in biological parents and grandparents can provide clues to the attributes a child may develop. The attributes of children who do not know their biological parents (adoptees) provide evidence of some genetic attributes of those parents (hair type and color, skin and eye color, talents, etc.)

CRITICAL CONCEPTS

Children today are rarely exposed to the factual, biological information contained in this lesson, or, if they are, they are generally not directly encouraged to apply the information to themselves. Therefore, if time constraints require condensing the HBI Unit, this lesson should not be omitted. It is possible conceptually to combine Lesson 6 with this lesson, although teachers have reported that it is the experiential nature of both Lesson 5 and Lesson 6 that is memorable to children.

VOCABULARY

- programmed
- pre-determined
- genes
- genetic inheritance

LESSON PREPARATION AND MATERIALS

Materials:	**Preparation:**
▪ Make overheads of 4-A and your own *Pictorial Family Tree* to use as examples. ▪ Copy 4-B for Home Education. ▪ Copy 4-C and 4-D for each student.	▪ Read the *Suggested Lesson Script.* ▪ Prepare your own *Pictorial Family Tree* as a model for students. ▪ Prepare to manage the activity for children not with biological parents.

LESSON SUMMARY:

- PROVIDE: A working knowledge of genetic programming.
- TELL: Genes are inherited from parents and are programmed to determine body growth.
- TELL: Many think the main things that influence body size and shape are eating behaviors and activity levels. However, the greatest influence is genetic.
- DISCUSS HANDOUT 4-A: Genes determine bone structure and variables influencing fatness and thinness.
- DO HANDOUT 4-B—*Pictorial Family Tree.* Children will consider their genetic heritage.
- ADD: *Body Image Building Block.*
- ASSIGN HOME EDUCATION.

SUGGESTED LESSON SCRIPT

1. **ASK:** Who knows how to program a VCR?

   A VCR can be *programmed* to turn itself on while you are away, tape a program that you don't want to miss, turn itself off, and have the tape ready when you want to watch it later.

2. **CONCLUDE:** If you know about programming a VCR, you know what it means to be programmed: something is set up ahead of time in a way that *pre-determines* what it will do later.

3. **DETERMINE: Bodies are programmed.**

   ASK: Has anyone been told that you look like someone in your family?
   How do you think you came to look like that person?

EXPLAIN:

- In your body you have genes that are like the computer in the VCR.
- Thousands of genes (too tiny to see) are inherited (come from) our biological parents before birth.
- Groups of genes work together to tell our body when to grow, how to grow, and when to stop growing.

4. **CONCLUDE:** More than anything else, our looks are determined by genes. This includes our facial features, hair and eye coloring, and the size and shape of our bodies. In order to understand what controls how we look, we have to understand our *genetic inheritance.*

5. **INFORM:** The study of genetics can be very complicated. However, the basic facts are simple. You inherit the genes that program your body from either or both parents.

   For example: (Consider sketching descriptive pictures on the board as you talk)

   - You might inherit long legs from your Mom or your Dad.
   - You might get your hair color from your Mom but it's curliness from your Dad.
   - You could inherit your facial features and chubby fingers from your Mom and your musical talent and your big feet from your Dad.
   - Genes can "skip" a generation. You might inherit a talent or look from a gene that your parents "carry" from a grandparent or even a great-grandparent—even though they themselves do not have that characteristic!
   - Your aunts, uncles, and cousins inherited their genes from your grandparents, too. They may have some of the same genes and traits you do.

   ASK: Who has been told they look like a brother or sister, grandparent, uncle, or cousin? (Encourage children to offer examples from their genetic heritage.)

6. **DISCUSS THE INFLUENCE ON BODY SIZE:** Many people believe the *main* thing that influences how big or small, fat or thin a person is, is what they eat and how much they exercise. These do have an influence, *but not as much as you might think. More* influence comes from your genes.

7. **PROVIDE THESE DETAILS:** (OVERHEAD 4-A)

   Regardless of eating or activity, genes will determine how long, short, thick, narrow, or wide your bones will be.

   - Bones are the frame for the rest of your body.

- Bones determine height but also (for example):
    - How wide your shoulders and hips are.
      (Reminder: As a rule, girls' hip bones grow wider than boys' in puberty.)
    - How long your back is compared to how long your legs are.
    - How long your fingers are, etc.
- You could have long legs, short arms, wide feet, and narrow hips—it all depends on the genes you inherited.
- Bones also shape your face—your nose, cheeks, and the shape of your head.

Regardless of eating or activity, genes will determine whether you will generally be more or less fat. This might be:

- Overall thinner or fatter.
- Thinner or fatter in some parts of your body than other parts. (Examples: fatter thighs/ smaller breasts, fatter waist/thinner hips, plumper cheeks/thinner calves)
- Almost any combination is possible.

8. ASK: How many normal body sizes and shapes do you think there could be?

ANSWER: There are thousands of genes to inherit, millions of combinations.

There are more normal body sizes, shapes, and looks than you can imagine.

9. OBSERVE:

- Look around. See for yourself. Some are tall, some short, some thinner, some fatter, some have long legs and a short body, some have short legs and a long body, etc.
- The range of what is normal and healthy is as varied as you can imagine.

10. RECOGNIZE: You are probably curious how your body is programmed to grow.

It's too soon to tell. But we can imagine some of the possibilities. If you know your biological family, you can get some clues from looking at parents and grandparents. If you do not know your biological family you can look at yourself for clues to some genes your parents *must* have had.

11. ACTIVITY: 4-D—*Pictorial Family Tree* (Use 4-C to get kids started.) This activity is best if done as homework with the help of parents.

A. Guide the children in drawing their pictorial family tree, going back to their grandparent's generation or even before. They can use 4-C as a guide, and the overhead you have made of your own *Pictorial Family Tree.* Students should draw and color as many physical characteristics for relatives as possible, such as curly or straight hair, hair color, eye color, relative body size and shape, etc., as well as special talents.

B. ***If children do not know their genetic heritage:*** Think twice before skipping the activity. Instead, help students focus, not on their absent birth parents, but on the concept that their bodies did come from somewhere. They can *assume* many things about their genetic heritage. Help these children look at and think about themselves. Then have them imagine and draw a *Pictorial Family Tree* that includes characteristics their blood relatives *must* have had—because *they* have those characteristics! For example, a student with black hair should draw a set of birth parents, one of whom must have had the genes for black hair (musical ability, blue eyes, athletic ability, etc.).

NOTE: Many teachers are concerned this will be a sensitive subject for some students, and your own judgment is best with your students. However, many, if not most, adopted or foster children will feel affirmed in your recognition that they are *not* different in this way. They *do* have a genetic heritage, just as anyone as anyone else.

C. Since they have not yet developed their grown-up bodies, students can only think about the possibilities for their body-shape inheritance. Discourage children from drawing any conclusions, such as, "Since my parents are tall/short or slim/fat, I will be too."

12. ADD the *Body Image Building Block* for Lesson 4 from I-D to the student's models.

13. ASSIGN HOME EDUCATION: Send HANDOUTS 4-B, 4-C, and 4-D along with the Home Education slip for parents to sign.

4-A OVERHEAD

Regardless of eating behavior or activity, *genes* will determine the following:

1. How *l—o—n—g*, **short**, narrow, or **wide** your bones will be.

   This will affect your height but also how long your arms and backbone are, how wide your shoulders and hips are, how big your feet will grow, the shape of your nose, the rest of your skull, and MORE.

2. **Whether you will be more, medium, or** less fat.

   This could be overall thinner or fatter, or thinner in some parts and fatter in other parts.

4-B HOME EDUCATION

WHAT DETERMINES THE SIZE AND SHAPE OF BODIES?

- Many things may influence weight and shape. But most of the way we look is determined before we are born: taller, shorter, fatter, thin—all are normal, all built in!
- The internal "programming" for our body's size and shape is genetic. This means a natural weight range and overall body shape is *built into* our bodies before we are born.

REGARDLESS OF EATING BEHAVIOR OR ACTIVITY, *GENES* WILL DETERMINE THE FOLLOWING:

1. **How *l—o—n—g*, short, narrow, or wide your bones will be.**

   This will affect your height but also how long your arms and backbone are, how wide your shoulders and hips are, how big your feet will grow, the shape of your nose, the rest of your skull, and MORE.

2. **Whether you will be more, medium, or less fat.**

   This could be overall thinner or fatter,
   or thinner in some parts and fatter in other parts.

PEOPLE BECOME UNHAPPY TRYING TO CONTROL SOMETHING THAT IS NOT WITHIN THEIR POWER TO CONTROL. AS FOR LOOKS, TAKE CARE OF YOUR HEALTH, AND MAKE THE MOST OF WHO YOU WERE BORN TO BE.

4-C

DO YOU KNOW WHO MAY HAVE PASSED THESE CHARACTERISTICS TO YOU?

CHARACTERISTIC	WHAT IS YOURS?	WHO IN YOUR FAMILY HAS THIS CHARACTERISTIC?
HAIR COLOR		
HAIR TYPE (straight, curly, etc.)		
EYE COLOR		
SHAPE OF NOSE		
SHAPE OF MOUTH		
SKIN COLOR		
Other Abilities or Talents: ATHLETIC		
MATHEMATIC		
ARTISTIC		
MUSICAL		
OTHER *(name other abilities you think may be inherited.)*		

4-D

YOUR GENETIC FAMILY TREE

I. Use the following plan to draw your own *Genetic Family Tree* on a *larger paper.*

A. FOR CHILDREN WHO KNOW THEIR BIOLOGICAL FAMILY:

Draw a *rough* picture of your blood relatives. Include brothers and sisters, parents and grandparents. If possible, also add aunts and uncles and great-grandparents. Get help from adults at home who may be able to describe relatives you do not know well. Show as many of the following as possible:

- hair color
- hair type (straight or curly)
- eye color
- skin color
- height (taller, medium, shorter)
- body type or overall shape (thinner, medium, or fatter)

It is not important that your drawings be artistic. What is important is that your pictures help you think about all the genes you have inherited that will determine how you will look.

B. FOR CHILDREN WHO DO NOT KNOW THEIR BIOLOGICAL RELATIVES:

If you or the adults you live with do not know your blood relatives, or know only a few, this activity is still a great one for you. Your genetic heritage is important. All you have to do is look at yourself. Then imagine and draw a Family Tree that includes characteristics your blood relatives MUST have had—because *you* have those characteristics! Let an adult or your teacher help you.

II. If you have special abilities or talents, you may have inherited these as well. Write them next to any people who also have those talents.

SAMPLE: (make yours large enough so you can sketch and color the characteristics.)

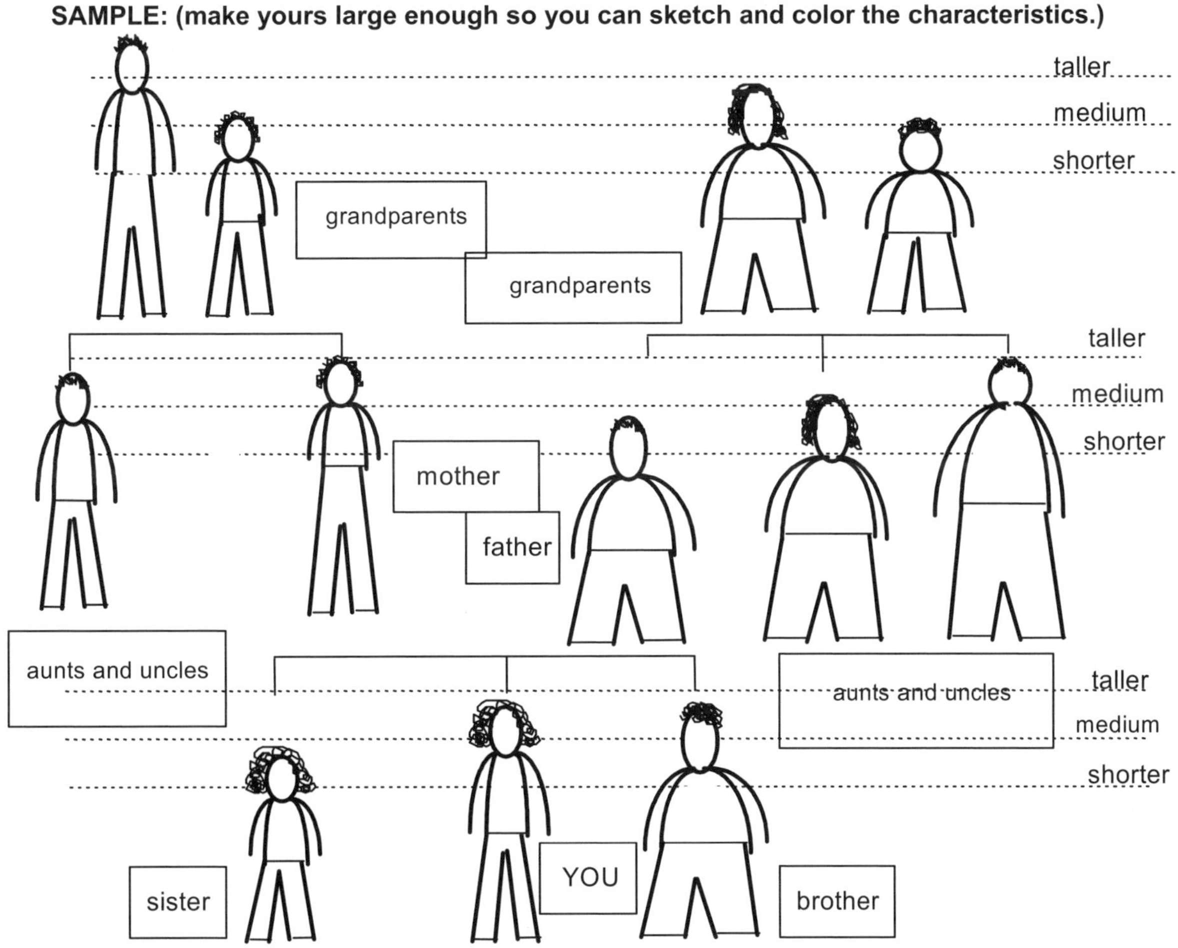

LESSON 5

INTERNAL WEIGHT REGULATION

The Metabolism Factor

Body Image Building Block:

Each person's body works to grow and maintain a weight that is natural for him or her.

LESSON OBJECTIVES

This lesson challenges weightism by demonstrating that genetic differences in the internal weight regulatory system naturally result in a diverse range of fat-to-lean bodies across a normal population. Children will learn:

- The body's internal weight regulatory system *limits* the degree to which fat stores can be permanently influenced by healthy means.
- Metabolism (the speed at which the body uses food energy, or calories) is *one example* of the body's internal weight regulatory system components.
- Metabolism (and other internal weight regulators) determines the fatness or thinness of a body as much as or more than consumption of calories or activity levels.
- It cannot be assumed that fatter people eat more or exercise less than thinner people.

BACKGROUND

Given the aversion to fatness that is fashionable today, combined with the fact that mature females are naturally more rounded than the accepted "ideal," it should be no surprise that young girls, even those of normal or low-weight, fear they are (or will become) "too fat." *Little do they know that the nature of fatness is extremely complex.* Students take their cue from the majority of adults who have come to believe that people are fatter entirely because they eat more and exercise less than people who are thinner. In light of this belief, it is understandable that many students feel they must begin to discount normal hunger cues our of their fear that normal eating will make them unacceptable.

While the complexity of fatness requires much more research, one thing is clear: even when food intake and activity are the same, body types remain diverse, with persons ranging naturally from quite fat to quite thin. This fact directly contradicts the myth that fatter people inevitably eat more or "too much." It is essential to correct this dangerous and prejudicial assumption and teach children instead that bodies *defend* diverse natural weights through an internal weight regulatory system that is not within our control. Many internal factors operate as part of this system to influence weight. However, a demonstration of one of these—the effects of metabolism—easily illustrates the fact that there are *limits* to each person's ability to comply with simplistic directives to "control weight."

It is hoped that as students accomplish the goals of this lesson, they will be more accepting of size diversity and trusting of their bodies' built-in ability to regulate weight with the help of positive lifestyle choices. In turn, students may be more motivated to eat well and be active for good nutrition, hunger satisfaction, energy, self-confidence, and enjoyment rather than to manipulate size.

The simplistic belief that fatter people "eat too much" contributes to mistrust of normal, healthy hunger as it becomes inaccurately assumed that hunger needs to be controlled rather than satiated. In Lesson 7 students will learn how myths that promote restrictive eating for weight loss contribute to disordered eating.

TEACH FOR THESE OUTCOMES

Students will know:

- Each person's body works to grow to and maintain a weight that is natural for him or her.
- One way the body maintains weight is through a mechanism called *metabolism.*
- Different people have different rates of metabolism (from fast to slow).
- Different rates of metabolism will affect how much food the body uses for immediate energy and how much is stored as reserve energy, or fat.
- If everyone ate exactly the same food and was active in exactly the same ways, people would still have diverse shapes and sizes, ranging from quite fat to quite thin, depending upon their naturally predisposed, base rate of metabolism.
- It is not safe to assume a thinner person eats less and exercises more or a fatter person eats more and exercises less.
- It is not safe to assume that a thinner person is healthier and a fatter person is less so.

Student attitudes will be:

- Understanding metabolism makes it easy to understand that people naturally range from fatter to thinner.
- My normal, healthy body size could be fatter or thinner.
- You can't make assumptions about people's eating habits or activity level based on their appearance alone.
- Judgments based on a person's size are not right.

- Hunger feels the same to people who are fat or thin.
- I accept myself for who I am.

CONCEPTS NEEDED TO TEACH THIS LESSON

- Many complex factors contribute to fatness or thinness. It is clear that the body has an internal weight regulatory system that goes far beyond former formulas for weight regulation The disposition for fatness or thinness varies tremendously from one person to the next, even when food intake and activity levels are identical. Likewise, when identical twins are raised separately, weights remain remarkably similar, even when cultural influence and lifestyle patterns are very different.
- Just as genetics determine bone structure and where fat is stored, the internal weight regulatory system is genetically predisposed. One of the best known components of this system is *metabolism*—the rate at which calories are used in the body.
- Activity level, the proportion of muscle tissue in the body, caloric intake, and some medications may increase or decrease the rate of metabolism, but the degree of influence through healthy means is limited. Base rates of metabolism are diverse, ranging from fast to slow, and seem to be fairly consistent for individuals over their life spans. In general, children with slower rates of metabolism grow up to become adults with slower rates of metabolism
- While metabolism is not the only factor regulating weight, learning about the effects of metabolism offers an example whereby we can understand why one person's body may be consistently fatter, regardless of eating and activity, while another's is consistently thinner.
- Food is like fuel for a car. Bodies need food energy to keep the "motor" going. Food that is not used by the body (metabolized) right away is stored in the body in the form of fat. This kind of fat provides a "reserve tank" of fuel for the body. It also serves as a lubricant for bones, pads the joints, keeps the skin smooth and soft, and is needed for the body to absorb vitamins that are not water-soluble.
- Hunger is a complex drive that, among other things, is linked to the immediate glucose needs of the brain as well as to the type of nutrients needed by body cells at a given time. There is no basis for the common belief that fatter people should be less hungry than thinner people.
- Given *identical healthy eating and activity patterns,* under otherwise normal conditions, a person with a slower metabolism will convert food into energy more slowly, store more "reserve" fuel, and be fatter than someone with a faster metabolism. In other words, with healthy choices, a fatter body is the natural outcome for a person with a slower rate of metabolism who is genetically predisposed to carry a higher proportion of fat-to-lean tissue. Under equal circumstances, a person with a faster metabolism will naturally be thinner.
- "Overweight" is defined as "more weight than is normal or necessary" (Webster). Given the great range of normal diversity in the internal weight regulatory system, use of the

words "overweight" or "underweight" would accurately need to reflect "more or less weight than is normal for each individual." What is *normal* for each individual can only be determined by a careful evaluation of a person's lifestyle and eating patterns. Therefore, the *casual* use of these words based on appearance is inappropriate.

- The use of the words "overweight" or "underweight" based on appearance alone arises from the false assumption that fatness cannot be normal and therefore must reflect unhealthy eating and/or activity patterns.

SPECIAL POINTS

Weight and size *are not behaviors* and therefore cannot be "controlled" or prescribed according to an external standard. However, certain behaviors influence both weight and health. Lessons 7, 8, and 9 address three behavioral factors that contribute to a healthy weight:

1. Avoidance of dieting.
2. Satisfaction of hunger through wholesome eating.
3. Limited sedentary habits and increased physical activity.

The belief that size can and should be manipulated at will by eating and activity choices has led to widespread nutritional deficiencies, disordered eating, excessive consumption, and eating disorders in our population. These behaviors are clearly linked to a rise in health problems. Therefore, it is a core objective to teach children to value and make healthy choices regardless of size.

Certain medical conditions or medications may induce unstable eating behaviors that may contribute to overweight or underweight. However, in otherwise healthy individuals, *most overeating or undereating that results in overweight or underweight occurs in response to a failure to eat well.* For example:

1. Reactive overeating to compensate for the restricted eating of a weight-loss diet (see Lesson 7).
2. Discounting the primary purpose of eating for nutrition and energy in favor of eating for entertainment (see Lesson 8).
3. Eating or not eating as a perceived need to maintain autonomy by resisting authority figures or cultural pressures. The purpose is to differentiate, to defy, to achieve a sense of control, and/or to assert independence. For example, if the perceived message is, "You have to eat less/more, lose/gain weight, eat/be different than you are, etc." The reactive response might be, "Then I'll eat it all" or "Then I won't eat anything."
4. Similar to #3, but rather than being an assertive stance of individuation, overeating or undereating occurs in response to some other real or perceived threat or loss. As with #3, food loses its primary purpose as an enjoyable, nutritional substance, and instead becomes an *object to control* (to eat or not to eat) results in a temporarily sense of being "in control" in the face of difficult emotions, such as anger, grief, anxiety, loneliness, or ambivalence. Both psychological and physiological changes that occur with overeating, undereating, or ritualistic eating are known to contribute to this soothing effect.

CRITICAL CONCEPTS

Core concepts from this lesson could be integrated into Lesson 5. However, in field tests, teachers who simply explained the concepts to students reported students *did not believe them.* In contrast, surveys with students who played *The Metabolism Game: Eat Your Lunch* showed they *got it.* In addition, this game is memorable. In response to a survey question, "What did you like best about the Body Image Unit?," a fifth-grade girl responded:

> *"I liked best the metabolism game. Everyone is different and has a different speed of metabolism and it showed a reason why some are fatter and some are thinner."*

VOCABULARY

- metabolism
- overweight
- underweight

LESSON PREPARATION AND MATERIALS:

Materials:	**Preparation:**
▪ Copy HANDOUT 5-A for Home Education. ▪ For *The Metabolism Game: Eat Your Lunch!* copy HANDOUT 5-B for each student and sufficient copies of 5-C for the normal distribution you have pre-planned for your class. (See #4—Preparation) ▪ Have two envelopes and tape for each individual.	▪ Read the *Suggested Lesson Script* and learn how to play *The Metabolism Game*: Eat Your Lunch! While there appear to be many instructions, these directions are no more complicated than for any card or board game. Instruct students to cut (color optional) 5-B and put their "lunch" in an envelope prior to the lesson. ▪ Plan a normal distribution of slow to fast metabolic rates for your class using the Directions for Assigning Metabolism Rates. Attention to detail is important for the desired outcome.

LESSON SUMMARY

- DETERMINE: The body needs "reserve" energy (stored fat). Consider historical and biological perspective on this.
- REVEAL CULTURAL MYTH: Many believe that fatter people inevitably eat more (too much) and exercise less (too little) in comparison to thinner people.
- REVEAL THE FACT: Eating and exercise can influence weight. But weight is adjusted by internal regulators that are not in our control. One example of this is metabolism

- DEMONSTRATE THE FACT: Play *The Metabolism Game: Eat Your Lunch!*— a 25-minute game that shows the effects of varied rates of metabolism on the storage of body fat, challenges common prejudices about fatness, and introduces the concept of the hunger drive.
- DISCUSS AND RELATE TO LIFE: People naturally range from fatter to thinner. This is largely influenced by internal regulators, of which metabolism is a major component. Diversity reflects nature more than the success or failure of people.
- ADD: *Body Image Building Block.*
- ASSIGN HOME EDUCATION.

If students ask:

While devices are under development, there is still no easy, cost effective way for most ordinary people to measure their unique metabolism. Accurate measures are possible only under laboratory conditions. While formulas exist (such as 9 calories per pound of body weight), these formulas are based on an average, and only perpetuate simplistic myths about the relationship between eating and weight by discounting the vast range of individual differences. Furthermore, even if an individual's metabolic rate were to be measured and found to be low or high, this information would be of questionable use, since their large or small hunger drive will continue to be a driving force. Efforts are better spent teaching young students to make mindful choices that promote health, regardless of metabolic rate or size.

SUGGESTED LESSON SCRIPT

1. **ASK:**
   - What happens if you drive your car but don't put gas in it? (It will stall or die.)
   - Why? (A car gets energy to run from fuel, or gas.)
   - What would happen if we went through our days but didn't put food in our stomachs? (First we'd get weak. Eventually, we'd die.)
   - Why? (A body gets energy to live from food.)
   - If your car ran out of gas, would it get weak first or die right away? (Die.)
   - Why do you think we don't die right away if we don't eat?

2. **TELL:** A person's life has more value than a car. Nature built bodies in a way to store "reserve" or "back-up" energy in the body. This way, when there is no food, we will feel weak. But we will not die for many days.

ASK: Who can tell me how the body stores its "reserve" energy? (The body stores energy as fat.)

3. **HISTORICAL/CULTURAL PERSPECTIVE**

When there is enough to eat, we may forget how important it is that the body can store energy in the form of fat.

Food was not always as plentiful or available as it is for most of us today. There are many places in the world where there is still not enough food. When enough food is not available, the body's "reserve" energy (fat) can mean the difference between life or death. If the body could not store fat, all the cave men and women would have died, and we would not be here today. *We should be thankful for fat!*

4. **INTRODUCE:** Today we are going to learn one of the things that influences how much fat a body stores. This lesson will help you understand why some people are naturally fatter or thinner that others.

5. **REVEAL THE MYTH:** Many believe the *only* reason people are fatter or thinner is that fatter people eat more and exercise less than thinner people.

Eating and activity can *influence* weight. But this is not the whole picture. We know also that genes program bodies to store more or less fat. The *biggest* reasons for weight differences are built into the body. Each person's body fights very hard to maintain a pre-set weight range that is right for him or her. Today we will learn an example of how the body does this by learning about *metabolism*.

6. **BACKGROUND:** The body uses energy from food to live. The *speed* at which a body uses food is called the *rate of metabolism.* Here's how it works:

TELL: Metabolism is like a fire, or furnace in the body.

- What happens if you put dry sticks on a very big fire? (They burn quickly.)
- What happens if you put the same number of dry sticks on a small fire? (They will also burn but more slowly.) (*Note: Feeding a fire of any size also makes it burn hotter.)*

DEDUCT: The size or heat of the fire determines how fast the sticks will burn. In a similar way, metabolism "burns" the food that is put into the body.

- What would you expect to happen to food eaten by a person with a very hot "metabolism fire"? (Food energy is burned quickly.)
- What would happen to food eaten by a person with a cooler or smaller "metabolism fire"? (Food energy is used but more slowly.)

CONCLUDE: Each person's rate of metabolism determines how fast food is used in the body.

7. **ASK:** When food is used more slowly because of a slower metabolism, what happens to the food while it is *waiting* to be burned? (It is stored as fat.)

ASK: Some people have fast rates of metabolism. Some have slow. What do you think determines each person's rate of metabolism?

TELL: Several things can make our metabolism speed up or slow down *to some degree.* For example, when we are active and eat enough to satisfy our hunger, our metabolism speeds up, and when we are inactive and do not eat enough, our metabolism slows down.

Even so, for the most part, metabolism is programmed by *genetics*. Our beginning (basal) rate of metabolism is inherited. Different people with different genetic programs will have different metabolisms. Each individual burns food at his or her own rate—fast, medium, or slow.

8. **SITUATION:** What would happen if three different children, all with the same activity level—one with a fast metabolism, one with a medium, and one with a slow metabolism—ate exactly the same food? (They would have less, medium, or more fat to store.) *Let's see what this would look like.*

9. **PLAY the Metabolism Game:** ***Eat Your Lunch***

(NOTE: This game has proven to be an extremely effective experiential teaching tool. It is strongly recommended because student beliefs are frequently changed by its powerful visual lesson. Some teachers who at first decided *not* to play the game found students didn't believe the concepts *until* the game was played.)

If you do not play the game, skip to #10 to finish the lesson.
If you play the game, skip to #12 below.

10. SHOW: A normal bell curve: *Most people have a medium rate of metabolism*

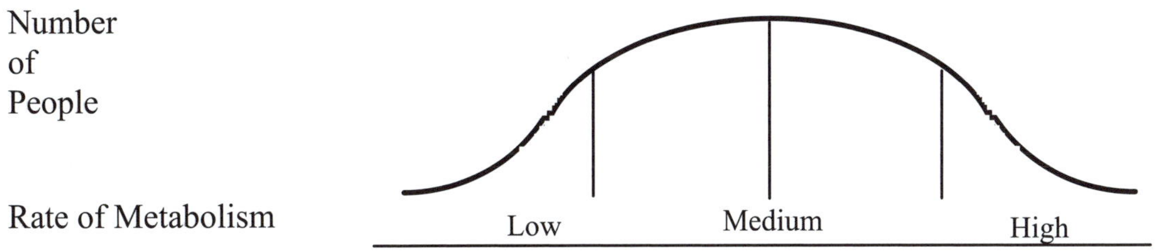

11. DISCUSS:

- *Most* people have a rate of metabolism that is medium—*a little* higher or a little lower than average.
- A *few* have a *very* high or *very* low rate of metabolism.
- Everyone gets hungry.
- If people ate exactly the same food (and had the same activity level), each would use that food at their own rate of metabolism. They would be fatter or thinner, as a result.

12. CONCLUSION:

Myth:	Many assume people are fatter or thinner *entirely* because of how much they eat or how active they are.
Truth:	Eating and activity can influence weight but not as much as people think.
Truth:	Another reason why one person's body has more or less fat is that each one's body works to grow and maintain a weight that is natural for him or her
Truth:	Making choices to eat well and stay strong and fit are more important than how fat or thin the end result is.

13. ADD the *Body Image Building Block* for Lesson 5 from I-D to student's models.

14. ASSIGN HOME EDUCATION: Send Handout 5-A, and the Home Education slip to be signed and returned.

THE METABOLISM GAME: EAT YOUR LUNCH!

This is an experiential game demonstrating:

1. THE EFFECTS OF VARIED RATES OF METABOLISM ON BODY SIZE. Note that metabolism is but *one* of the factors influencing weight and therefore serves as an example only.
2. AN INTRODUCTION TO HUNGER
3. AN INTRODUCTION TO FAT PREJUDICE

Game summary: Students will participate in a game in which they will be assigned one of five metabolism rates, from slow to fast. They will all be provided with and "eat" the same mock lunch. As student's "burn" their mock lunch over a condensed time period, the effects of their different metabolic rates will be visually demonstrated. The children will watch as some children burn their lunch quickly, while others are still storing food on their bodies even after a much longer period of time. Discussion will follow, concluding that fat prejudice reflects ignorance of innate diversity. During the discussion the teacher will provide introductory information about how hunger is triggered.

GAME TIME: Approximately 25 minutes, including set up, *not* including discussion.

PREPARATIONS AND MATERIAL: At least five people are needed. Each student will need "lunch" **5-B**, two plain envelopes, and tape. To save time, students can prepare materials (See below, #1) ahead of time.

Directions for assignment of Metabolism Rates: Each student will be assigned a metabolism rate **5-C** (see "sensitivity directions" below). Distribute the Metabolism Rate Directions according to a standard distribution of a normal bell curve. For example: If you have 10 students, assign metabolism rates as follows:

Rates:

1: **x** 1 student, *very slow rate*
2: **xx** ____ 2 students, *moderately slow rates*
3: **xxxx** _______ 4 students, *average rates*
4: **xx** ____ 2 students, *moderately fast rates*
5: **x** 1 student, *very fast rate*

IMPORTANT: Sensitivity directions: The goal of this lesson is to reduce fat prejudice. It is assumed that, prior to the lesson, fat prejudice may exist among students. Therefore, teachers should not assign a slow rate of metabolism (Rates 1 and 2) to children who appear to have inherited a slower metabolism rate (fatter children), and who may have already been victims of prejudice.

GAME SCRIPT

1. DIRECT: *We are going to play a game to see what happens when people eat the same food but have different rates of metabolism. To play, each of you will "eat" the same pretend "lunch"* (6-B).

- *Cut-out your lunch, then cut it into pieces along the dotted lines. Each piece will count as one "bite." There should be 16 "bites."*
- *Write the word "Stomach" on one envelope and tape it with the flap-side out and open on your clothing, over your stomach. You may now "eat your lunch" by putting the food pieces into your stomach.*
- *Write the words "Metabolism Energy Converter" on the second envelope, and tape it on your clothes flap-side out and open where you can easily reach it—perhaps just below your stomach.*

TELL: *Metabolism of food does not occur in an organ, like the stomach. Actually, it is directed by your brain and occurs in every cell of your body. We are picturing your metabolism as an actual place or "furnace" in the body only for the purpose of understanding how it works.*

2. HAND OUT metabolism rate directions: *Here is your metabolism rate. You must keep your rate a secret! Your lunch will metabolize or be used at your assigned rate. In the end we will all see what happens.*

3. INFORM: *In real life, food takes several hours to be digested in the stomach and then to be metabolized. Also, different foods are digested and metabolized faster or slower than others. For the purpose of this game, we will pretend all of our food will digest at the same speed and that, for every few seconds of real time, 15 minutes of digesting and metabolizing time will pass.*

4. DIRECT: *Every time you hear my signal, you should follow your Metabolism Rate Directions to move bites of your lunch from your stomach into your "Metabolism Furnace."*

(You may want to use a bell to signal the passing of time for the digestive and metabolizing process. Allow enough time between signals for students to complete the transfer of food pieces. There will be 16 signals total. Announce the time as follows:)

Signal 1: *About 15 minutes have passed. Move food from your stomach into your Metabolism Furnace according to your assigned directions.*

Signal 2: *About 30 minutes have passed. Move your food.....*

Signal 3: *About 45 minutes..., etc.* (Continue through Signal 8, which represents 2 hours.)

At Signal 8, students with metabolism rate #5 (fast metabolism) will have emptied all food from their stomachs into their Metabolism Furnace. Tell these students to write "2 hours" on their Metabolism envelope. They may now sit back and watch what happens to students with slower metabolism.)

Signal 9: *About 2 hours and 15 minutes..., etc.* (Continue through Signal 10.)

At Signal 10, or "2 1/2 hours," students with metabolism rates #1 to #4 will still have food in their stomachs. **Instruct them as follows:**

Your stomach would have fully digested all your lunch by now. Since it is digested, but your body has not yet needed it for energy, you will have to store it somewhere. Take the food remaining in your stomachs and store it (tape it) somewhere on your body or clothing where we will be able to see what happens to it.

5. ASK (as the children are storing the digested food): *Since the food you are storing has been digested in your stomach, do you think it still looks like bites of food?* (No.) *What do you think it looks like when it is ready to store in your body?* (Fat.)

6. REMIND: *A natural amount of body fat is important. You all have it and need it. Fat is not a "bad thing" when it is the normal result of good choices about eating and activity. Body fat is reserve energy. It keeps you going so you don't "run out of gas" before your next meal.*

7. RESUME: *Now that your stomach is empty, you will take food from your Reserved Energy Storage to put in your Metabolism Furnace as we continue.*

If you run out of "reserve energy," write the time that is announced at that signal on your Metabolism Furnace envelope.

8. COMPLETE THE PROCESS:

Signal 11: *About 2 hours, 45 minutes have passed. Move food from your Reserved Energy Storage into your Metabolism Furnace according to your assigned directions.*

(Continue through Signal 16, or "4 hours.")

9. ASK: *It has now been 4 hours since you last ate. Who would be hungry?*

CONCLUDE: Most children would be hungry by now. But let's see what has happened to the food eaten by individuals with different metabolism rates.

- After the final signal, children with rates #1 and #2 will still have food taped (stored) on their bodies. They should leave it in place.
- Have individuals or groups report their status, i.e., when they ran out of food or how much food they have remaining. Groups should stand together and in order, 1-5, while the effect of their metabolism is discussed. In this way, they will provide a visual bell curve.

SUMMARY OF RESULTS

GROUP 1 - Slowest metabolism: 1/2 of lunch is still stored as fat

GROUP 2 - Moderately slow metabolism: 1/4 of lunch is still stored as fat

GROUP 3 - Average metabolism: Lunch fully metabolized in 4 hours

GROUP 4 - Moderately fast metabolism: Lunch fully metabolized in 3 1/4 hours

GROUP 5 - Fast metabolism: Lunch fully metabolized in 2 hours

10. DISCUSSION QUESTIONS

Group 5:

This group has had an empty stomach for 2 hours, and they metabolized all of the energy provided by their food. How do you think they would be feeling now? (Very hungry.)

What emotions do you think they would be feeling? How do you feel when you are very hungry? (Crabby, impatient, distracted, with difficulty concentrating.)

Group 4:

This group burned all their lunch, too, but only 45 minutes ago. How do you think they are feeling? (Probe for all the same ways. They would be just as hungry. They haven't eaten in 4 hours and their stomachs have been empty for the same amount of time.)

Group 4 and 5:

Do you think these two groups have faster or slower metabolisms? (Faster.) *Which is fastest?* (Group 5.)

Since these groups of children burned up all their food quickly, even long before it was time to eat again, what influence do you think that will have on their body size and shape—will they be fatter or thinner? (Thinner.)

Group 1 and 2:

These children still have food stored on their bodies. What do you think that means? (They have a slower metabolism. Their lunch was not fully metabolized in 4 hours, and some is still stored.)

Are you sure it doesn't mean they ate more food than Group 4 or 5? (It does not—although, this is a common myth when people have more food energy stored.)

With the reserve energy you can see on their bodies, do you think these children would be hungry? (Provoke discussion with the following question:)

How could they be hungry with all this food still hanging around? (Reserved energy—fatness—does not affect hunger. The brain reads hunger primarily from the digestive system.)

TELL: *Of course they are hungry! Their stomachs have been empty for as long as anyone's.*

Since they are as hungry as Groups 4 and 5, they will need to eat soon, too. If they are genetically pre-disposed to metabolize their food more slowly, what type of natural, healthy body size and shape are they predetermined to have? (Fatter.)

Group 3 standing:

What about these children? Do you think they are hungry? (Yes. Their stomachs have been empty, too.)

Do you notice there are more children in this middle group than in any other? Why do you think that is? (Solicit responses about what is "average." More people have average rates of metabolism.)

How do you think their metabolism is likely to influence their body size and shape? (Not fat, not thin, but in-between.)

SUMMARY: People with average rates of metabolism will tend to use *most* of the food they eat *most* of the time, and their normal, healthy bodies will be average—-not very fat, not very thin—but in the middle.

• An average teenage or adult woman stores some fat on her body that gives her curves. This is how *most* adult females look. An average teenage boy or man will store less fat than most females, but every healthy body stores some.

• It is natural for some people to have a little higher- or a little lower-than-average metabolism. A few people will naturally have a *very* high or *very* low metabolism. Many things influence why people are quite fat or very thin. But the internal weight regulatory system provides a major influence.

It is a myth that all people would be the same size and shape if everyone just "ate right and exercised." All bodies should be well fed and exercised for the sake of health. But bodies will always come in many different sizes!

5-A WHAT IS THE MAIN INFLUENCE FOR FATNESS OR THINNESS?

Understanding the Internal Weight Regulatory System

If you forget to put gas in your car, it will stall—unless you have a "reserve" tank of gas.

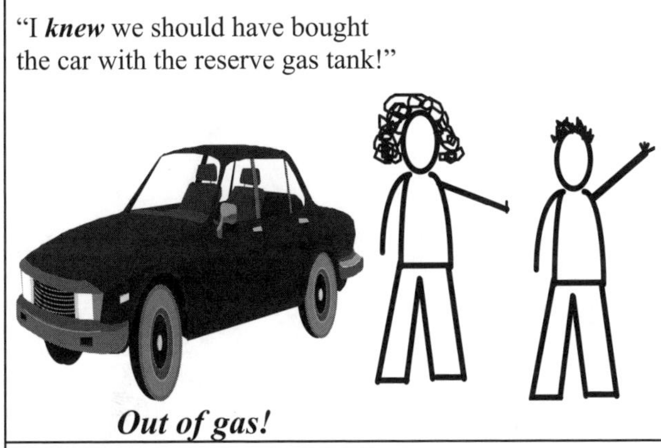
"I ***knew*** we should have bought the car with the reserve gas tank!"
Out of gas!

Fortunately, nature built in a way for bodies not to "stall" when there is not enough to eat. Fat is fuel that is stored "in reserve." Why do some people store more of it than others?

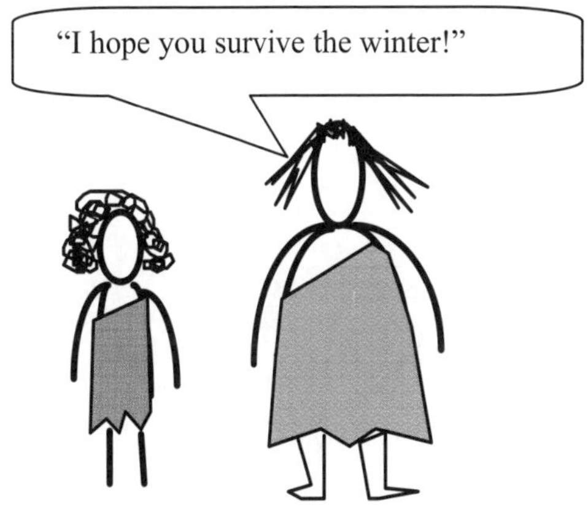
"I hope you survive the winter!"

People often assume that people are fatter or thinner entirely because of how they eat or how active they are. But this is a myth.

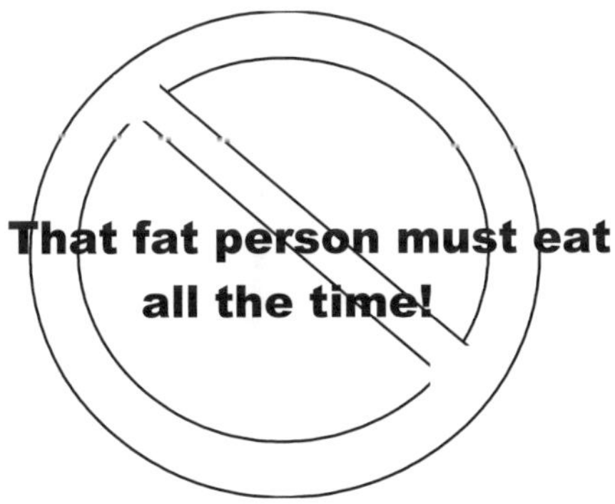
That fat person must eat all the time!

Bodies work from the inside to grow and to maintain a weight that is natural for each one. For this to work, we must listen to the messages our bodies send.

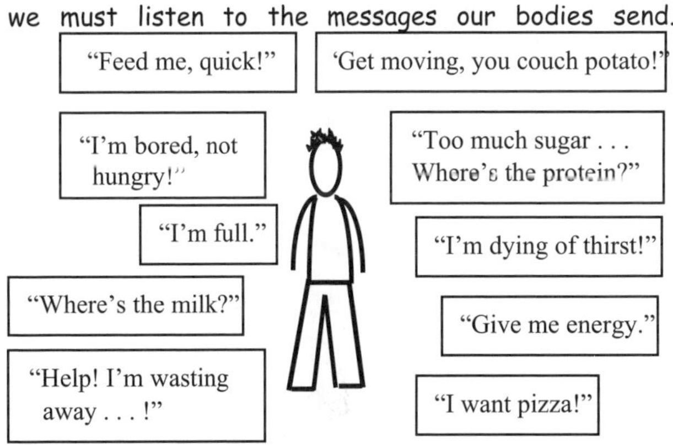

If everyone ate exactly the same food and was active in exactly the same ways all the time, they would still be many different shapes and sizes.

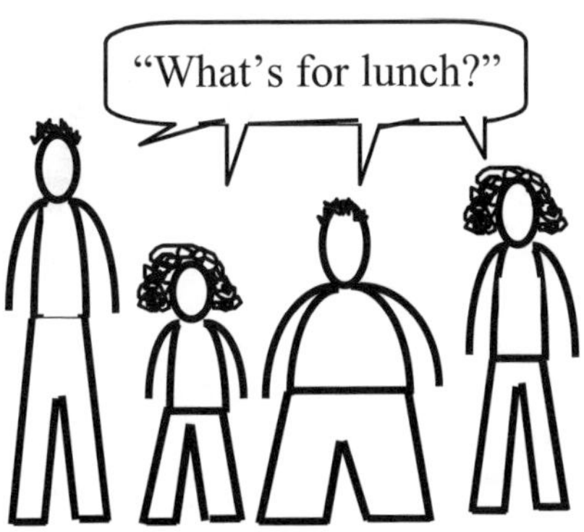
"What's for lunch?"

Same-age friends

Eat well and be active for nutrition, energy, satisfaction of hunger, and enjoyment.

Trust your body to find a healthy weight for you.

5-B

LUNCH

1) Cut out the foods below for your lunch.
2) Cut up the foods into “bites” along the dotted lines. You should have 16 portions, or “bites,” of lunch when you are finished.

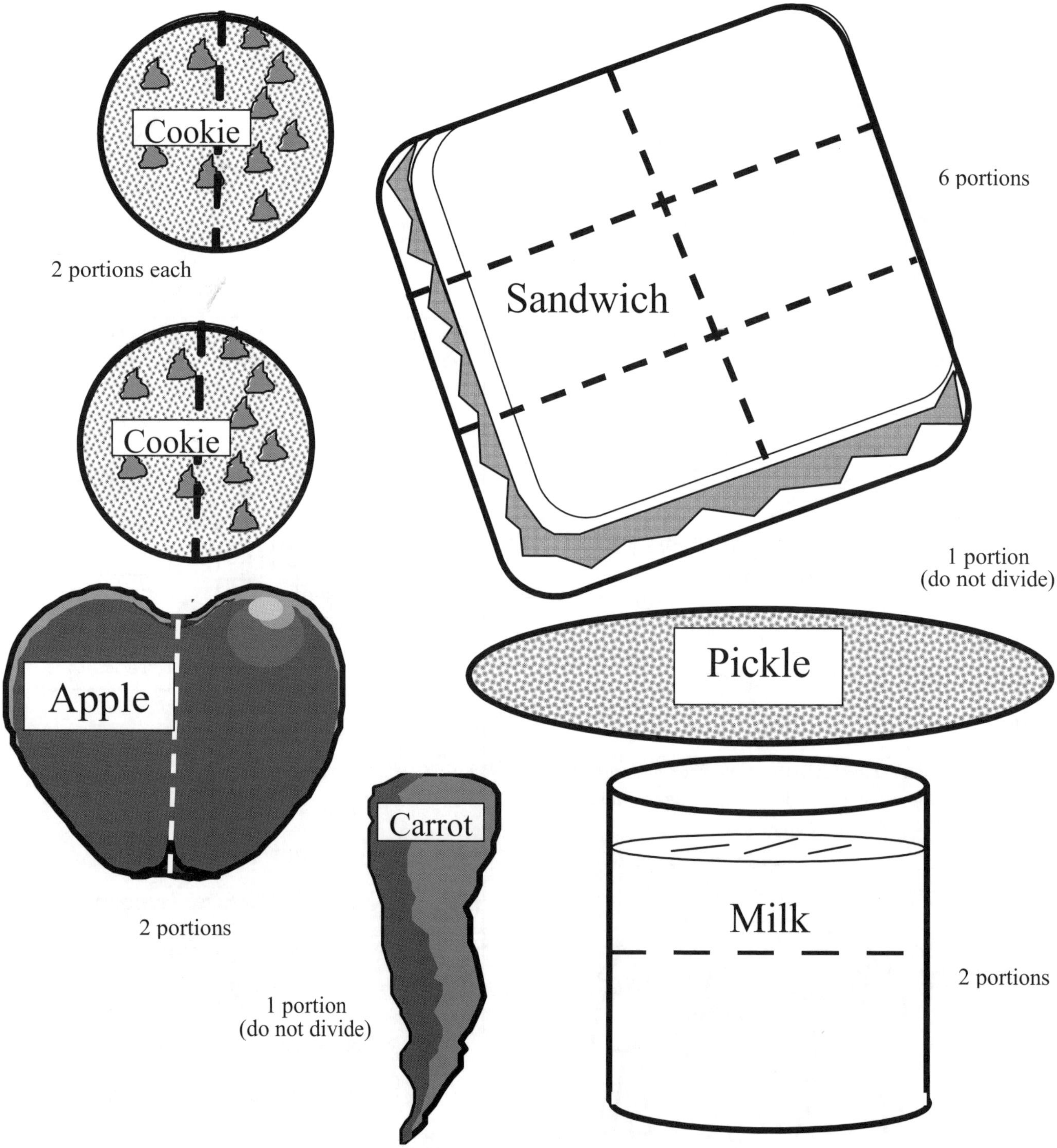

5-C

METABOLISM RATE HANDOUT

(Copy and cut the number needed according to a normal distribution, as directed.)

METABOLISM RATE DIRECTIONS 1

Your body will metabolize your food at this rate:
ONE BITE EVERY OTHER "15 MINUTES"

You will put one bite of your lunch into your body's Metabolism Energy Converter *every other* time your teacher signals.

METABOLISM RATE DIRECTIONS 2

Your body will metabolize your food at this rate:
ONE BITE EVERY "15 MINUTES" — except YOU WILL SKIP EVERY 4TH "FUELING"

You will put one bite of your lunch into your body's Metabolism Energy Converter every time your teacher signals—*except* you will skip every 4th signal.

METABOLISM RATE DIRECTIONS 3

Your body will metabolize your food at this rate:
ONE BITE EVERY "15 MINUTES"

You will put one bite of your lunch into your body's Metabolism Energy Converter every time your teacher signals.

METABOLISM RATE DIRECTIONS 4

Your body will metabolize your food at this rate:
ONE BITE EVERY "15 MINUTES" — except for EVERY 4TH "FUELING," when you will "burn up" 2 bites.

Every time your teacher signals, you will put one bite of your lunch into your body's Metabolism Energy Converter—*except* you will put 2 bites into the converter every 4th signal.

METABOLISM RATE DIRECTIONS 5

Your body will metabolize your food at a rate of
TWO BITES EVERY "15 MINUTES"

Every time your teacher signals, you will put two bites of your lunch into your body's Metabolism Energy Converter.

LESSON 6

"SOLD" ON LOOKS

The Influence of Mass Media

Body Image Building Block:

Hardly anyone looks as perfect as the models in advertisements. I will be careful not to compare myself or others to them.

LESSON OBJECTIVES

Students will consider the relative value of looks. They will think about why it is—when they have been taught that beauty is only skin deep and that we should not judge a book by it's cover—that people spend so much time and energy worrying about appearance. As they discover that people are more influenced by what they *see* than what they are told, they will begin to understand the powerful role *visual* media has had in this question.

Mass media serve many purposes (entertainment, education, political influence, etc.). But we often forget that, above all, mass media is almost always used to sell or promote something to very large audiences. For example, the SuperBowl is meant to entertain, but the opportunity to view it exists only because of the wish of advertisers to bring together an enormous pool of potential consumers.

In this lesson, children will learn that mass media images purposefully tell stories in order to collectively influence what people value, how they will feel about themselves based on these stories, and what their approach to life will be—including their beliefs about appearance and its role. In particular, students will learn how media:

- strategically creates images (that may not be what they seem)
- in order to provoke emotions, alter beliefs, and thereby shift attitudes and perspectives
- resulting in a perceived need
- that can best be met by a product.

Mass media includes all messages distributed to the general public for the purpose of selling something. The means include television, movies, radio, music, billboards, store window displays and photos, internet advertising, and web sites selling products or attitudes to viewers. Students will learn to interpret the most common photo advertisement themes. For example, "See how (compared to the model in this picture) you are lacking in something? In order to 'have what it takes' (like the model), you need improvement. Then you, too, can be (happy, successful, beautiful, rich . . . , etc.). To improve, you need . . . (our product)."

Students will become discerning about ads and resistant to being "sold" messages that are contrary to health and self esteem. In particular, students will develop resistance to ads that directly or indirectly promote a particular way to look. The lesson capitalizes on the innate desire in children to maintain what is right and true and on their righteous resistance to being manipulated. It is intended that students will feel a degree of indignation as they consider that mass communication is often used to exploit the normal human wish be accepted and to belong. Students will develop a stake in becoming "media-wise."

BACKGROUND

Studies have shown that American girls and women compare themselves to the unrealistic images of women that are pervasive in mass media, and feel deficient as a result. Men and boys are also affected, and we can expect this to increase, given many marketing objectives. When marketing is understood, it is no longer perplexing that a group of people, who individually value the deeper substance of our humanity, collectively feel and act as if "image is everything." While we know that "beauty is only skin deep," and "you cannot judge a book by its cover," it is also true that "one picture is worth a thousand words."

Historical perspective can help us to understand this inconsistency between what we know to be true about diversity and integrity, on the one hand, and our insecurity about our looks, on the other. While looks have always been of interest, prior to the explosion of mass media in the 1950s, people primarily looked to other ordinary people as the standard for comparison. While unusually "beautiful" people always stood out and their images were displayed in advertisements and in moving pictures, people were exposed to these relatively unaltered photo images at a rate of a few per day or week.

The average person today sees hundreds of carefully chosen, artfully crafted, computer-altered, unusually symmetrical faces, and perfectly proportioned bodies per day—40 to 50 million by the time they are 60. Babies begin to view thousands of these faces and bodies as toddlers. All these crafted images carry an implicit and often explicit dual message: *Beautiful people have beautiful lives* and *Happiness can be purchased by having the "right" look.* Ads and magazines selling fashion or beauty products (commonly purchased by teen girls) send direct messages pushing the importance of this "correct" standard of beauty: *Create the Right Face for the New Year!; Don't Get Caught With Those Saddle Bag Thighs!; Lose Ugly Fat Now!*; etc.

As a result, standards have changed dramatically in a very short time. The well-groomed, "nice-looking" person, who, not long ago, served as a more realistic standard, is scorned by teens as "ugly" in comparison to today's "ideals." A study of current body measurements of female models found the majority have a body weight 23% below normal for women in their age groups. Symbolizing "beauty" for all, they in fact represent a body type natural for fewer than 3% of the female population. Still, the message they carry is, "If you do not look like this, you are not trying hard enough . . . (this product will help!)."

It takes effort to locate a popular women's magazine that is not promoting the latest weight-loss diet or "quick-fix" to (for example) "burn fat and flatten your tummy while you sleep!" Barbie™, who would be grotesque if she came to life, is still idolized by young girls who are *not* clear that she is a fantasy. Many middle school girls deny that their body image is affected by media messages but describe the "ideal girl" as 5 foot 7 inches tall, weighing 110 pounds with blue eyes and long, blond hair. There is no reason to wonder why so many females feel fat, unattractive, and insecure!

The male wish to be seen as attractive has been exploited less, but surveys suggest this is changing. Surrounded by a growing number of images of "ideally" handsome men with the "chiseled" body look, studies show men are feeling increasingly deficient in comparison.

American economics may have benefited from the marketing of the thin-ideal and the resulting anxiety about appearance, but much has been lost by the American public. We may be richer, but we are not thinner, and we clearly feel worse. Most adults seem resigned to the negative body scrutiny they learned as young teens—as if this is an irreversible and therefore permanent part of their identities. But when asked about the next generation, adults who have lived with body angst are clear that they do not want their children to carry this same burden. For this objective to manifest, students today must learn at an early age to critically examine some of the ways image biases are formed.

Even families who carefully monitor their children's media exposure may remain uninformed about the messages that will reach and profoundly affect the development of their children. Parents and guardians can screen what comes into their homes, but messages pushing the "right look and how to get it" slide by on the sides of buses, beam down from billboards, pop up on computer screens, stare out from bigger-than-life fashion photos at the mall, and display themselves on the covers of magazines at doctor's offices and the corner store. Given the inevitability of exposure, it is important even for well-protected children to learn to become media literate and for their parents to do so, as well. In addition to the Home Education handouts, you may wish to recommend books to parents on this topic (see Appendix) or offer an education event to discuss one of the recommended videos.

TEACH FOR THESE OUTCOMES

Students will know:

- Humans have universal needs and desires and, therefore, vulnerabilities.

- The purpose of advertising is to sell something. Advertisements are strategically designed to create a perceived need, vulnerability, or deficiency that can be best satisfied by the product that is offered.
- How to recognize and interpret media messages that promote the "right" appearance as a critical value.
- How to critique media messages that promote unrealistic and unhealthy expectations about looks.
- Looks matter, but deeper qualities are of higher, longer-lasting value.
- Media messages promoting the "right look" and "how to get it" are not benign. It is important to recognize and resist their persuasive influence.

Student attitudes will be:

- Hardly anyone looks as perfect as the models in advertisements. I will be careful not to compare myself to them.
- If I see advertisements that make me feel I'm not good enough, I'll remember this is part of the plan to convince me I need to buy that product.
- It helps me to remember that even movie stars and fashion models feel insecure about their looks when they compare themselves to their professionally enhanced images.
- I will think carefully before I let media messages affect how I feel or what I think.
- I can enjoy pictures of beautiful people and still feel confident about myself.
- I care about my appearance, but what matters most is who I am on the inside.

CONCEPTS NEEDED TO TEACH THIS LESSON

- Appearance is a part of who we are, and it is normal to want to feel attractive. Studies suggest there are species-specific, innate preferences regarding looks that influence initial attractions. In humans, even infants are consistently drawn to look more frequently and longer at images of faces with more symmetrical features and balanced proportions.
- Despite this, we know appearance is only skin deep. As a species, we have learned that "What is essential is invisible to the eye," (Antoine De Saint Exupéry, from The Little Prince). We value and enjoy beauty but know to teach our children that it is appreciation of deeper qualities of character that provide the greatest satisfaction in long-term relationships.
- At the same time, one picture is worth a thousand words. Studies show females who were intensively exposed for 20 minutes to multiple photos of typical fashion models became caught up in an "appearance is everything" mentality that resulted in an immediate drop in self esteem. Americans now see hundreds of these images of extraordinary, "ideal beauty" per day. The result is an over-attention to and over-valuing of appearance.

- Since the late 1950s, our daily life has been flooded with millions of pictures that accurately represent the physical appearance of less than 3% of girls and women and a very limited number of men. Make-up, lighting, and computer-imaging further enhance these images, routinely resulting in a fantasy image of a virtual person so "perfect" he or she could not exist in reality. This creates an impossible standard that most people are not aware of.
- The strategic use of such unrealistic images is particularly common for images of women. For example, Guess™ executive for advertising, Paul Marciano, has said:

  "I'm proud that my ads use real men—real cowboys, ranchers, truck drivers, and an actual matador. My field is day-to-day street life. I don't want to create fake pictures."

  Women, however, are another matter. In that regard, Marciano said:

  "We always use models. It's difficult to find real women who fit what we're trying to say. Real women—they aren't as cooperative as real men."
- Advertisers do not benefit if people believe they already have "enough" or are "good enough." They rely on advertisements that create a perceived deficiency in the viewer. This strategy may be very direct or very indirect, i.e. focusing little on the virtues of the product but presenting images or words evoking normal human needs (to belong, succeed, be happy, be attractive, etc.) Marketing outcomes have shown that this strategy is very successful in convincing customers that they (or their lives), by comparison to the image in the advertisement, "need improving" or "needs more of something." It then appears that the seller is simply providing a service by educating the viewer about what is "needed."
- The use of extraordinarily good-looking models in advertising is a central part of the above strategy. By setting a beauty standard that is virtually unattainable, the customer's perception of deficiency or need to be improved is easily evoked. When advertisements then promise, "You, too, can have . . . ," vulnerable audiences are eager to buy. In this way, even when the product being sold is unrelated to beauty, advertising themes draw the correlation between the product and "looking good."
- One out of eleven advertisements is specifically for a product or program to improve appearance. These imply directly or indirectly that products or actions (for example, dieting, cosmetics, clothing, liposuction, etc.) can change (improve) looks significantly or that they will provide the "right look." The implication is that anyone may have total control over his or her ay-to-day appearance by merely buying and/or using a product. This message is unrealistic and promotes a sense of failure that often drives the search for more products.
- Attempts to imitate "perfect" images result in feelings of failure and diminished self esteem, but increased sales.
- Mass media has become a primary purveyor of American culture. Studies show that the way youth feel about themselves is strongly influenced by mass cultural conditioning delivered via mass media.

- Students can learn to use historical perspective, knowledge of genetics, knowledge of marketing strategies, and critical thinking to accurately interpret media messages, develop resiliency, and resist a sense of failure and negative self-image.

CRITICAL CONCEPTS

Curricula for teaching media literacy are increasingly available, and your existing curricula may cover some of the same concepts presented above. The critical difference would be in heightening students' awareness of advertising strategies that are specifically designed to promote unrealistic expectations about body size, shape, weight, dieting, eating, exercise, and health, as well as feelings of insecurity and deficiency about looks. Since early adolescence brings a dramatic increase in exposure to media with this intent, a foundation for healthy body image demands that children become informed viewers. If your students have studied media literacy in general, consider starting with #5 in the Suggested Lesson Script.

VOCABULARY

- mass media
- computer imaging

LESSON PREPARATION AND MATERIALS:

<table>
<tr><th>Materials:</th><th>Preparation:</th></tr>
<tr><td>
<ul>
<li>Acquire full-page ads showing stereotypically "ideal" models—at least six ads for every three to five students, plus additional demonstration ads. Choose photos of both men and women who are selling a variety of products, but include several that specifically promote looks in order to sell a product. These ads are available in any magazine, but one or two fashion magazines will provide all you need. Call your public library for free outdated copies .</li>
<li>Copy 6-A for use as an overhead.</li>
<li>Copy 6-B & 6-C for Home Education.</li>
</ul>
</td><td>
<ul>
<li>Review the Suggested Lesson Script.</li>
<li>Familiarize yourself with 6-A—Understanding Advertising: Stories Told By Pictures.</li>
<li>Become fluent in interpreting ads, particularly messages promoting the importance of looks. The examples provided on the Home Education HANDOUT 6-B will help you.</li>
<li>While the material in this lesson may be presented in one period, consider spending two or even three class periods to allow time for students to become well acquainted with the concepts.</li>
</ul>
</td></tr>
</table>

LESSON SUMMARY:

- DISCUSS: Looks matter, but many things are more important.
- POSE A CONTRADICTION: Even though people know beauty is only skin deep, they may feel and act as if looks are extremely important.
- UNDERSTAND how mass media has become a force in this contradiction.
- DISCOVER how advertising influences attitudes about looks: Use 6-A—*How Stories are Told by Pictures in Advertising.*
- ACTIVITY: Translate and interpret stories in actual advertisements.
- RELATE to attitudes about looks in our culture.
- RELATE to the need for critical thinking about media influences in student's lives.
- ADD: *Body Image Building Block.*
- ASSIGN HOME EDUCATION.

SUGGESTED LESSON SCRIPT:

1. **DISCUSS: Do we need "good looks"?** Looks are only one part of us. Even so, people of all ages like to look good—handsome or pretty.

Girls and boys become more interested in looks as they grow up. Appearance makes an impression. We often smile when we meet new people to be friendly but also in hopes that people will be interested in getting to know us. It can be fun to dress a certain way or comb our hair a certain way to express our own personal *style.* A way of looking, or a style, can catch someone's eye and make them think, "That person attracts my attention." There is nothing wrong with wanting to express our own personal look or style.

ASK:

- Do we *need* "good looks" to be appealing?
- Are "good looks" the same as *personal style*?
- How important are appearances? Are they as important as smartness, kindness, or laughter? Are looks as important as family, sharing, taking care of the earth, health, or enough money? *Why not?*

ACKNOWLEDGE: Most know looks are only skin deep. They matter—but are not the most important thing—and not something we have very much control over.

ASK: (Push the point.) *Do looks matter a lot to people?* (It seems this is so!)

2. **PRESENT THE CONTRADICTION:** In the past 20 years, people in America have spent trillions of dollars on looks. If looks are not *that* important, why do we worry so much about them? Studies tell us people worry about looks much more now than they did 35 years ago.

Why has this changed?

- **One way people change is from what they are told.** Who has heard these sayings about appearances? What do these sayings mean?

  "You cannot judge a book by its cover."
  "Beauty is only skin deep."
  "Looks are deceiving."

- **Another way people change is a result of what they *see*.** Who can tell me what this saying means?

  "One picture is worth a thousand words."

3. **TELL:** It turns out that pictures have had a lot to do with changing how we feel about looks.

Read or otherwise convey the following background information to students:

The Power of Pictures

There has been a big change in our culture in the past 40 years because of pictures. Prior to the 1950s, people mostly had other ordinary people to look at in their every day life. If they saw pictures of people whose *extraordinary looks* made an impression, it was only once in a while.

In the 1950s, mass visual media became an almost overnight sensation, suddenly presenting millions of images of people through entertainment and advertising that appeared virtually *everywhere*. Television, movies, magazines, newspapers, and billboards became an everyday part of our lives, presenting each of us with hundreds of pictures every day—hundreds of thousands of pictures every year. Suddenly everyone was seeing more images of people in a year than anyone had ever seen before in a whole lifetime.

Since people learn more from what they see than from what they hear or read, it is not surprising that these pictures made a big impression. We now know that exposure to so many pictures of people has had a big affect on how people now think and feel about *looks.*

As you grow up, you will see more and more images of people both for your entertainment, but also in the form of advertisements whose purpose is to sell you something. Since these will make an impression on you, you will want be smart about how mass media influences your feelings about looks.

How Advertising Works:

Manufacturers pay millions of dollars to sponsor programs to attract an audience of people who will then see, hear, or read their advertisements and learn about the products they sell. But it is worth it to them if they can attract even more millions of people to buy their goods or services. *(Note: Your students may not be aware that, except for PBS, not one of their favorite TV or radio programs, magazines, or newspapers would exist without the sponsorship of advertisers. Consider a discussion of the word "sponsor.")*

Advertisers often use words to tell about their products. But advertisers know words are easy to ignore. For this reason, they try to include a picture because pictures tell *stories.* Why would a story help to sell a product?

Stories awaken *feelings* in people. Feelings make people relate personally to what they are seeing or reading. Certain kinds of feelings can make people feel they want, or even *need,* the advertiser's product. Advertisers spend a lot of money to make sure every detail in the ad contributes to a story that will make you feel you need the product they are offering.

4. EXAMPLES OF STORIES TOLD BY "ADS" USING HUMAN MODELS

VIEW: Overhead 6-A—*How Stories Are Told by Pictures in Advertising*

APPLY: *Using the prompts in 6-A, demonstrate the "stories" told by actual ads that you have chosen. First demonstrate how to interpret ads with models that are not directly selling beauty. Point out subtle details (the appearance of the model, facial expressions, postures, props, etc.) that reinforce how the story promotes a need for the product. Then show ads specifically selling beauty products.*

Present the "story" that advertisements with human models have in common: These ads are selling *different* products. But they all have a *common story.* Can you tell what it is?

The *Common* Story of Advertisements With Professional Models:

You need something. In fact, if you compare yourself and your life to what you see in this picture, you will know there is a lot you could improve upon. See how these models are completely happy, healthy, and appear in control? See how attractive they are? Without a doubt, they are having better lives than you. You can tell this because of how good they look. If you compare yourself and your life to what you see in these models, you will quickly know that you are missing something. The models and their products go together. If you buy the products, you and your life will be more like theirs.

5. ACTIVITY: Interpreting Stories Told by "Ads" Using Human Models:

Provide groups of three to five students with at least six or more ads for various products promoted by stereotypically beautiful or handsome models. In the time allowed, each group should interpret several "stories" told by their ad images.

Include "stories" that specifically sell beauty or looks: *Point out that ads for cosmetics, fashion, diets, or diet food/equipment particularly exploit human vulnerability with the following story line:*

> *"**You need to improve your looks in order to…**belong, be included or chosen, be seen as attractive and desirable, count or be heard, be visible, be loved, find a mate, be your "best," be happy, be seen as a good person, make money, succeed at anything, compete, etc."*

After groups have successfully interpreted the ad "stories," ask each group to interpret an ad to the large group. Be sure they note messages that affect feelings about looks.

6. DISCUSSION QUESTIONS:

Display several ads with beautiful/handsome models in full view of the whole class.

- Are these ads appealing to you? Do you like to look at them?
- What impression do the pictures give you about how people "should look?" (See HANDOUT 6-C— *Read and Discuss Advertising Strategy at Home* for a description of the current "right way" to look for men and women.)

These pictures are appealing to most people. We have now become used to them as a standard for beauty. Advertisers hope you will compare yourself to this standard and feel a need to improve yourself by buying their product.

Before you do, consider:

- Will the products make you look like the models? Why or why not?
- Will the products make you happy?
- How do you feel about yourself when you compare yourself to the models in the pictures?

7. **TELL AND ASK:** Almost everyone agrees that looks are not that important. Yet, like the Namuh, sometimes people worry about looks. We now understand mass media has had a big part in this.

   As you get older, you will probably become interested in looking your best. You will want to feel attractive and enjoy fun clothes and hairstyles.

   When this happens, be smart and pay attention to how your feelings will be influenced by stories told in advertising.

8. **(Optional) DISCUSS these quotes from posters created by fifth graders:**
   - *If I looked in a mirror, what would I see? I wish everyone would see the inside of me.*
   - *We look different. We feel the same.*

9. **ADD the *Body Image Building Block*** for Lesson 6 from I-D to the students’ models.

10. **ASSIGN HOME EDUCATION:** HANDOUTS 6-B and 6-C and the Home Education slip for parents to sign and return.

OPTIONAL ADDITIONAL BACKGROUND

Artistic Enhancement of Media Images

No one looks as good as the images in advertisements, not even the models themselves! Most people do not know that media images are "enhanced." This means, special make-up and lighting is used to make the models look better than anyone could look in real life. (To illustrate, if possible, show a before and after "Glamour Shot"–type photo.)

Computer imaging alters pictures. Computers can reshape a nose or carve roundness off hips, make a waist thinner or shoulders broader. In the end, not even the models look as "good" as their pictures.

A new media trick is to take the "best" parts of two or more models and put them together in one picture to make one "ideal" model. (Suggest how this could be true in some of the ads you have displayed—the legs may be one model's, the body another's.) Movies do this, too—showing one actress' body and another's face. (Note: There may be students in the school who can demonstrate the way this is done using a "Photo Shop"–type program on the computer.)

We now know that many models and movie stars feel bad about themselves when they compare the way they look in real life to their enhanced photos. Remember, media pictures are "created" to get you to buy the product. Be careful you do not compare yourself to these unrealistic photos.

The video Behind Closed Doors *vividly demonstrates computer altering of fashion photography. While the video is not entirely appropriate for young students, a clip from the middle of the video demonstrates how a very slim model is "perfected" by slicing a few inches from her leg and smoothing the wrinkles on her hands and waist. This video may be obtained at a nominal cost from the Remuda Ranch Treatment Center by calling 1-800-445-1900.*

6-A

HOW STORIES ARE TOLD BY PICTURES IN ADVERTISING

Our Product is for YOU:

moms, dads, teens, animal lovers, old people, tough guys, cool girls, teachers, dancers, athletes, gardeners, swimmers, cooks, etc.

You are a person who is or could be:

happy, safe, loved, popular, adventurous, cool, healthy, gorgeous, successful, etc., or lonely, stressed out, in pain, worried, etc.

You believe in:

family life, getting ahead, being good, taking care of yourself, winning, looking good, working hard, having fun, a religious faith, etc.

You want:

Beauty: **great hair, white teeth, beautiful eyes, to lose weight, thin thighs, big muscles, smooth hands, clear skin, long fingernails, young skin, the "right" look, etc.**

Popularity: **attractiveness, pizzazz, what it takes, etc.**

Power: **control, to be "in charge," money, wisdom, fame, prestige, the "right" image, etc.**

Interest: **a cause, fun, laughs, color, excitement, speed, quiet, energy, the meaning of life, etc.**

Balance: **time, health, comfort, peace of mind, etc.**

***You need:* OUR PRODUCT!**

6-B

READ AND DISCUSS AT HOME

How stories are told by pictures in advertising

OUR PRODUCT IS FOR YOU: moms, dads, teens, animal lovers, old people, tough guys, cool girls, teachers, dancers, athletes, gardeners, swimmers, cooks, etc.

YOU ARE A PERSON WHO IS OR COULD BE: happy, safe, loved, popular, adventurous, cool, healthy, gorgeous, successful, etc., or lonely, stressed out, in pain, worried, etc.

YOU BELIEVE IN: family life, getting ahead, being good, taking care of yourself, winning, looking good, working hard, having fun, a religious faith, etc.

YOU WANT:

Beauty: great hair, white teeth, beautiful eyes, to lose weight, thin thighs, big muscles, smooth hands, clear skin, long fingernails, young skin, the "right" look, etc.

Popularity: attractiveness, sparkle, pizzazz, what it takes, etc.

Power: control, to be "in charge," money, wisdom, fame, prestige, the "right" image, etc.

Interest: a cause, fun, laughs, color, excitement, speed, quiet, energy, the meaning of life, etc.

Balance: time, health, comfort, peace of mind, etc.

YOU NEED: OUR PRODUCT!

EXAMPLES: Product, Words, and Picture	Unspoken Story
Car: *"The only mini-van to earn five stars in the crash test."* Beautiful, smiling, slim mother dressed in the latest style, standing by a van with five smiling, good-looking kids.	You value your family and want to be a top-notch mom. You also want to be a fun, trendy, attractive lady. You can have the good looks that lead to happiness and a happy, attractive family if you buy our product!
Hair conditioner: *"No more tug of war!"* (*Before*: Ungroomed, mad mom with comb and tearful girl with messy hair and clothing. *After*: Well-groomed, attractive, hugging, happy pair.)	Relationships are important to you. You feel bad and guilty when you fight with your daughter. To help you daughter achieve the good looks that will make her love and admire you, just buy our product!
Antacids: *"How do you spell RELIEF?"* (Miserable, pudgy, balding man in a sweat-suit at football game. Next to him are two slim, handsome, well-dressed happy men with two very pretty women.)	You could be a fun, eye-catching guy. Why let indigestion make you unattractive? To enjoy life, be the good looking guy you were meant to be, and *attract a pretty date*, you *need* our product!
Toy: Two very attractive, bright-eyed, laughing girls with shiny hair and stylish clothes are playing together with a *brand-name toy*. They are surrounded by other happy, attractive children who are eagerly watching.	No need to be left out or worry that you might not have friends and be popular. Without a doubt you will be one of the attractive, happy, popular kids when you buy our product!
Weight-loss plan: *"Diet magic! Lose 30 pounds in 30 days with No Hunger!"* Two photos: One is a black/white, grainy photo of a fat, sad-looking, woman with uncombed hair and unstylish clothing. The other is a color photo of the same woman, now slim, wearing a swimsuit and walking with a handsome man.	Hasn't your fatness kept you alone and unhappy long enough? No need for you to be shunned Lose weight quickly and get the relationships you've been waiting for. To be slim and find happiness by next summer, just buy our product!

6-C READ AND DISCUSS ADVERTISING STRATEGY AT HOME

Advertisements featuring models with "ideal" looks contain this common story:
"You need something. In fact, if you compare yourself and your life to what you see in this picture, you will know there is a *lot* you could improve upon. See how these models are completely happy, healthy, and appear in control? See how attractive they are? Without a doubt, they are having better lives than you. *You can tell this because of how good they look.* If you compare yourself and your life to what you see in these models, you will quickly know that you are missing something. The models and their products *go together*. If you buy the products, you and your life will be *more like theirs."*

Advertisers want you to believe you need improvement and that their products will correct what you are lacking. Be careful before you "buy" this idea!

Advertisements suggest there is a "right way" for men to look. Is it realistic?
Male models look strikingly handsome. Their bodies have broad shoulders balanced over narrow hips. Often they have intense eyes that look cool, detached, and far away, or they seem to look right through you. The "take-charge" eyes above strong chins and straight noses suggest these men are tough, on top of things, and clearly have no insecurities or worries. Some even look a little mean. Do most men look like this?

Advertisements suggest there is a "right way" for women to look. Is it realistic?
Most female models look extraordinarily beautiful, sophisticated, sleek, and very, very slim. They have only smooth lines and no fat. Their clothes hang perfectly, without a lump or bulge. Their skin is completely clear, without a wrinkle or blemish; their mouths are perfectly drawn and colored; and their eyes are bright and even, with long, divided lashes. Every hair shines. Do most women look like this?

Think about it.
Do you think you should try to copy the look of beautiful models in photo ads? Should you look for a girlfriend or boyfriend who looks like a model? Why or why not?

Fewer than three in 100 women naturally have the "ideal" body type of models shown in most advertisements. More than 97% of women do not. This strategy is very successful in convincing the majority of women that, by comparison, they are "too fat" or otherwise inadequate. After creating this insecurity, advertisers claim that buying their product will help. What do you think?

Neither male nor female models look as "good" as their pictures. Media images are "enhanced." Special lighting, make-up, and computer imaging make models look better than anyone could look in real life. It is normal to want to feel special. Advertisers hope to "wake up" your natural wish for this when you look at images of "beautiful" people. Think twice before you are "sold" on the idea that a certain look will make you special.

LESSON 7
HUNGER AND EATING
What Is and Is Not in Our Control

> **Body Image Building Block:**
> *Weight loss diets are not a good idea. We can hold back our hunger for a while but will eat more to make up for it later.*

LESSON OBJECTIVES

This lesson teaches students why tuning out hunger for weight loss or weight control is rarely effective in the long run, and routinely contributes to eating problems, including weight gain. Students will learn the following:

- Five things are essential to life for mammals: air, water, food, sleep, and warmth.
- If any of the basic needs for life are not fully satisfied, there are reliable and predictable consequences.
- While primary drives can be restrained in the short run, drives for satisfaction of basic needs are virtually impossible to discount by emotionally healthy individuals over the long run without significant negative consequences.
- These consequences drive (compel) people to seek *enough* of what is needed. Drives exist to insure preservation of life, and what is enough is different for different people.
- The consequences of restrained or restricted hunger satisfaction compel people to respond to food in ways that are counterproductive to long-term weight loss, and routinely contribute to weight gain.
- In light of poor outcomes coupled with unhealthy or dangerous side effects, it is imperative to think critically about and avoid "dieting" for weight loss.

BACKGROUND

Hand in hand with the drive to be thin, "dieting" has become a statistically normal style of eating in America. This has occurred in spite of a well-substantiated body of research documenting the counterproductiveness of food restriction as a weight-loss method. While cutting calories or food groups routinely "works" for dropping pounds in the short run, long-term results consistently show dieting is not only ineffective; it has many negative, and even dangerous, lasting side effects.

The original, landmark studies documenting the predictable, negative consequences of a reduced-calorie diet were published in 1950 by Ancel Keys. Eating according to a plan that was nutritionally adequate but provided about 1570 calories, on average, Dr. Keys' subjects (male volunteers with no prior history of dieting for weight loss) showed extraordinarily similar responses: all quickly developed a relentless obsession and preoccupation with food, a loss of interest in and ability to concentrate on anything else, and a growing irritability and self-centeredness. As expected, all subjects lost weight on this 24-week experimental diet. However, when food restrictions were lifted, hunger showed itself to be ravenously overpowering. Subjects described an insatiable appetite, driving them to eat compulsively or binge well beyond the point of "fullness." Not only was all weight that had been lost quickly regained but, in several cases, additional pounds as well. Of particular note, the obsession with food as well as a fear of not getting enough, compulsive eating, and hoarding of food persisted long after food restriction had ceased.

A host of studies, clinical records, and anecdotal reports in the past 20 years have confirmed that the same results reliably occur in response to the common on-again-off-again "normal dieting" that is so prevalent in our culture. Outcomes show that over 90% of weight lost with any calorie restriction plan (which includes plans restricting food groups, such as the "low carb" diets) is regained, and very often with additional pounds. Dieters are several times more likely than non-dieters to experience significant weight gain (more than 22 pounds over the starting weight) over a 15-year follow-up period. Exceptions do occur and are pointed to as if these were the probable outcome. But the vast majority of dieters diet over and over again, trying to beat the unlikely odds. If dieting were more successful, this would not be the case.

Individuals who do manage to overpower or repress hunger over the longer term rarely do so without suffering the significant side effects: obsession and preoccupation with food and weight, anxiety and depression, rigidity, a constricted way of life, and, not infrequently, loss of physical health. Some individuals who suffer a mental illness, such as anorexia nervosa, may deny problems resulting from their restrictive eating, but those who recover from restrictive eating disorders almost always admit the terrible price they paid for their denial. In addition, it is extremely common even for those with anorexia to eventually experience a break-through of their hunger, followed by a transition to bulimia, chronic compulsive overeating, or a binge-eating syndrome.

In the same four decades since the drive to be thin and dieting for weight loss have come into vogue, America has become the fattest nation on earth. While this increase in body weights is a complex problem, it cannot be ignored that the primary "solution" for weight loss is ineffective in producing *lasting* weight loss for reasons that are elementary enough for a child to understand. In addition, dieting triggers a host of unhealthy or disordered eating problems. In recent years, the popular press has occasionally informed the public about "yo-yo" dieting. However, most people remain generally uniformed about the failure of weight-loss diet plans, as well as remaining ignorant about the expected counterproductive side effects of restricted eating. As a result, most dieters and many healthcare providers continue to point to the short-term "success" of calorie restriction, and blame individual weakness for long-term weight-loss failure. In light of pressures urging students to worry about weight and to diet for weight loss, it is imperative that they learn about the role of hunger, the workings of the internal hunger regulatory system, and why weight loss *as a goal* is likely to contribute to the very problems they hope to avoid.

Because teachers are vulnerable to pressures promoting weight loss as an effective goal, it is important to review here the more *effective* goal to be taught to students. The following statement from the Introduction is reprinted here for this purpose:

> **Reclaiming health as a goal**
> As the thin-ideal and the drive to be thin have become normative values, the concept of "health" as a core value has been gradually lost or reconstructed. Instead of strength, stamina, flexibility, vitality, and vigor (including metabolic fitness and nutritional soundness), a more slender or lean appearance is routinely viewed as the objective. This value shift has been accepted even if the means to achieve a reduced size defy principles of health, biological diversity, and internal hunger regulation. The disappearance of both hardiness and heartiness as key values undermines the welfare and well-being of our population. The *Healthy Body Image* curriculum teaches that 1) health is a primary goal that should not be sacrificed, and 2) the lifestyle and attitudinal choices conducive to achieving physical health and well-being at any size.

TEACH FOR THESE OUTCOMES

Students will know:

- There are predictable results when any of the five basic needs are not satisfied.
- Hunger is the signal for one of these needs and can be trusted to regulate how much to eat.
- There are predictable consequences when hunger is not satisfied.
- "Dieting" or restricting hunger to lose weight will probably result in weight loss at first, but weight that is lost will almost always be regained, often with added pounds.
- To allow the internal hunger regulatory system to do its job, each person should satisfy hunger completely with wholesome food according to his or her own internal hunger cues.

Student attitudes will be:

- You can lose weight by "dieting" for a while, but you will be fighting against your nature the whole time.
- I am the best judge of when I am hungry and when I am full.
- If I am tempted to go on a diet to lose weight, I will think twice, remembering that my body needs enough wholesome food to keep me nourished and energized, and my hunger satisfied.
- A good way to avoid overeating is to always eat enough!
- For confidence that my weight is healthy at every size, I will eat when I'm hungry and stop when I'm full, choosing plenty of wholesome food from all five food groups.

CONCEPTS NEEDED TO TEACH THIS LESSON

Regarding basic needs and need deprivation:

- People have basic needs that are central to life: the need for sleep, water, air, food, and warmth. These needs drive for satisfaction. While needs may be temporarily repressed, the intensity of a drive increases with time and the degree to which the need is unsatisfied. When need deprivation has been either extreme or sustained for an extended time, the drive will be toward overcompensation when the opportunity arises.
- The laws of need deprivation are universally predictable and reliable.

Regarding hunger and hunger deprivation:

- Food is needed for life. Hunger is the physical cue for this basic need.
- Normal eating entails:
    1. eating when hungry, stopping when full.
    2. eating according to internal cues until you experience a sense of satiation.
    3. eating what you like, while exercising enough direction over food selection to provide for nutrition and calorie needs.
- As with all basic needs, when hunger is not satisfied completely, there is a compelling drive for satisfaction. The degree and length of time hunger is unsatisfied affects the intensity of the drive. Hunger may be voluntarily repressed temporarily, but it is normal for hunger to become ravenous when food is then freely allowed.
- In contrast to normal eating, "dieting" usually means eating according to externally prescribed plans or criteria limiting when, how much, and/or what to eat for the specific purpose of weight loss rather than according to internal hunger cues for health and well-being.
- Classic studies of calorie or food restriction occurred in the late 1940s. These studies have been repeated in recent years, measuring the results of "restrained" eating patterns that are common to today's typical "weight-loss diets." The following consequences of hunger deprivation are now considered to be reliable and predictable results of "dieting":
    1. obsession and pre-occupation with food.
    2. depression, irritability, and other emotional disturbances; social withdrawal.
    3. ravenous hunger, with compulsive and/or binge eating when dieting is stopped (compensatory overeating).
    4. fear of not getting enough persists even when eating can occur freely, resulting in continued compulsive eating.
    5. a drop in basal rate of metabolism combined with compulsive eating results in weight gain.
- Hunger is a built-in mechanism that can be trusted to regulate eating. Studies show:
    1. given the ready availability of a wide variety of nutritious, appealing foods, people will eat in a healthy, positive manner over time.
    2. hunger does not require (and may resist or be undermined by) "control."

- In a culture that considers any amount of fatness to be abnormal or unnatural, many have become confused about hunger, defining it as a "problem" and viewing it as something to "control." The following offer some explanations for this mistaken conclusion:
    1. The belief that dieting is an effective weight-loss strategy leads people to eat according to external prescriptions for weight loss rather than internal hunger cues. When the effects of food deprivation are experienced, hunger, rather than hunger deprivation, is defined as the "problem."
    2. Mass marketing of high-energy, low-nutrient taste treats as if these were "the way to eat" has been very effective in persuading adults and children to expect food with "entertainment value." Food is increasingly viewed as recreation *in and of itself.* When the motive for eating is "fun" or diversion, hunger may be blamed for both poor nutrition and unhealthy weight gain—even when hunger is frequently over-ridden in decisions about eating these foods.
    3. Hunger cannot necessarily be trusted to regulate eating when food options are not generally wholesome or appealing and are not presented at regular intervals. Studies show that, when an imbalance of highly-flavored, low-nutrient foods are routinely offered as an option for satisfying hunger, problems with selection may occur. Children will have a hard time selecting a balanced variety of foods if they are not provided with the means to do so. Given this, educating adults about the importance of nutritious food options is critical.
- Dieting is common in our culture because:
    1. Many believe any amount of fatness is bad and do not know that dieting is counterproductive to lasting weight loss or maintenance.
    2. Dieting results in weight loss until the effects of food deprivation take effect. This seductive and temporary result reinforces the myth that dieting works and that the dieter is to blame for lacking will power.
    3. Mass marketing promotes both the thin-ideal and dieting, sending the message that both are realistic and that dieting (rather than wholesome eating) is the alternative to an excess of "treats."
- Most weight lost through dieting is regained, along with additional pounds. With time and recurrent dieting, significant weight gain and even obesity may result.

CRITICAL CONCEPTS

In the face of current media messages promoting diets for weight loss, the objectives for this lesson are critical. It is recommended that concepts be presented experientially, following the Suggested Lesson Script.

VOCABULARY

- deprived
- dehydration

LESSON PREPARATION AND MATERIALS

Materials:	**Preparation:**
▪ Copy 7-A and 7-B for overhead projection, if desired. ▪ Copy 7-C for each student for classroom use and Home Education. ▪ 1 narrow drinking straw per student.	▪ Read the *Suggested Lesson Script.* ▪ Familiarize yourself with 7-B. ▪ Plan to send 7-C for Home Education.

LESSON SUMMARY

Part I: Discovering Need Deprivation

- IDENTIFY: People (and all mammals) have basic physical needs.
- DISCOVER: There are universal, predictable consequences of need deprivation.

Part II: The Diet Dilemma

- DISCOVER: There are universal, predictable consequences of dieting.
- CONCLUDE: Dieting for weight loss is a "losing battle."
- ADD: *Body Image Building Block.*
- ASSIGN HOME EDUCATION.

SUGGESTED LESSON SCRIPT

PART ONE: DISCOVERING NEED DEPRIVATION

1. **EXPLAIN:** Everyone has basic needs that must be met in order to live.

   ASK: Who can name the basic needs? (Water, air, food, sleep, warmth)

   TELL: These needs are so strong that we are *driven* to satisfy them. We cannot stop ourselves from trying to satisfy them, even if we try, at least not for long. In fact, there are *very predictable things that happen* if we do not satisfy our needs.

2. **DEMONSTRATE: Sleep deprivation.**

   ASK: For example, think about how many hours you need to sleep at night to be well rested. What happens when you don't get enough sleep one night? (There are mild consequences, such as a little sleepiness and difficulty focusing.)

What if every day for one week you were awakened three hours earlier than you are used to? How would you feel? What if you missed three hours of sleep *every night* for one whole month? (Take answers until you have revealed the following four consequences.)

- You would be persistently thinking about sleep and the desire to sleep.
- It would be hard to concentrate on anything else.
- You would be craving sleep.
- You would be unhappy, crabby, and uncomfortable.

AFFIRM your student's wisdom: (They already know what to predict when sleep needs aren't met.)

ASK: After all of this lost sleep, what would happen if you finally were allowed to sleep as long as you wanted? Would you sleep your average number of hours?

(Affirm that they would not. They would sleep several *extra* hours to make up for the lost sleep, and few would think they were "oversleeping." They would want to "catch up" on their sleep, and, in fact, it might take two to three weeks to get fully back on track. Many teens do this every weekend!)

DEFINE: If you did not get as much sleep as you needed, we would say you were "sleep deprived." When a person is sleep deprived, they can expect the following:

- They will think about and crave sleep, have a hard time focusing or concentrating, be crabby and self-centered, and, when sleep is finally possible, they will want to catch up on that missed sleep. They will want to sleep a long time, until satisfied that they have had enough sleep for them. *Has this ever happened to you?*

3. **DEMONSTRATE: Dehydration.**

ASK: What happens if you are thirsty, but you cannot have a drink right away? (Thirst will be a mild distraction.)

What if it's worse than this? What if someone tells you that, no matter how thirsty you are, you can only have half the liquid you want for a whole week? (Take answers until you have revealed the following consequences.)

- You would be persistently thinking about water or liquids
- It would be hard to concentrate on anything else
- You would be craving a drink; extremely thirsty
- You would be unhappy, short tempered, crabby, and uncomfortable

DEFINE: If a person is not allowed to drink as much as he or she wants, they become *dehydrated.*

ASK: If you were dehydrated but finally could drink as much as you wanted, someone might ask, "Why are you drinking so much?" How would you answer?

EMPHASIZE: With dehydration we could expect a person to gulp large quantities of liquid when it became available.

PART TWO: THE DIET DILEMMA

1. **ASK:** Do you think the same thing would happen if you did not get enough air to breathe? Let's find out!

2. **EXPERIENTIAL ACTIVITY—The Air Diet**

> **Caution:** Use judgment before instructing students with asthma or other lung disorders to participate in this activity. In addition, after reading the introduction below, inform children before proceeding that they may discontinue the activity if they become frightened or anxious about getting enough air. This should not occur for the vast majority of students but could occur for individuals who are, in general, very anxious.

INTRODUCE THE AIR DIET: (Present the following in a tongue-in-cheek manner.)
I think all of you have been breathing entirely too much, and could benefit from a little "air diet." You know the latest style is to have a bluish tone to your skin, and your cheeks are just too rosy. Since oxygen is what gives your cheeks that rosy glow, I think you would *definitely* be better-looking if you cut back on your air so your face coloring will be more drab. Of course, you will need some air to live. But surely you could cut back. And won't it be worth it to have the "right look?"

Instructions:

- *Distribute one narrow drinking straw to each student. Ask students to plug their noses, close their mouths, and breathe entirely through the straw. Laughing is not allowed since it may allow for a gulp of air! However, if students "cheat" (go "off" their air diet), you can playfully tease them: "What's the matter? Don't you have any will power?" While they are on their "air diet," you might read a short current-event item or poem. If students are not attending to your reading, use this opportunity to playfully chide them that they seem to be thinking more about their breathing than learning.*
- *Decide ahead of time whether or not your class may need some movement to experience a "hunger" for more oxygen. If so, the activity could be done in a gym, and students could walk or engage in another moderate activity while on their air diet.*

- *This experiment may be done without straws if students merely plug one nostril, close their mouths, and breathe through the remaining nostril. However, the nasal passage is generally larger than a narrow straw, and gaining the proper effect may take longer.*
- *Continue the "air diet" until students experience the expected consequences of need deprivation. With precise attention to this timing, tell students that they may now "go off" their air diets. If you like, join them for the final minute or so of the "diet" so that you can dramatically demonstrate taking your own big gulps of air when external restrictions are lifted. As they (and you) are gasping for air, ask them why this "overbreathing" is occurring?*
- *Process the experiment, asking questions to help students note all of the expected consequences of need deprivation.*
    - *What were you thinking about when you were on your air diet?*
    - *Were you able to focus on the story I was reading?*
    - *How did you feel when your air was limited?*
    - *How did you feel when you could breathe freely?*
    - *Emphasize that most students naturally gasped for big gulps of air before resuming their normal breathing. Why is this?*

3. **INTRODUCE:** (Overhead 7-A) When our drive for satisfaction of any of the five basic needs is not fully met, we can expect these things to happen every time:
    - We are persistently thinking about what is missing (sleep, water, air, warmth, food).
    - It is hard to concentrate or stay focused on anything else.
    - There is a powerful craving to satisfy the need.
    - Until satisfied, the craving is very uncomfortable. We become crabby and/or self-centered. It is hard to be concerned with others' needs.
    - When the need is finally met, *more* than a normal amount is needed to make up for what was missing.

4. **DISCUSS THE DIET DILEMMA:**

    DISCUSS: Based on what we have learned, what can we predict will happen on a diet that restricts food intake for weight loss? (Use Overhead 7-B. Students may fill in the blanks on HANDOUT 7-B as the concepts are discussed.)

KEY FOR OVERHEAD 7-B and HANDOUT 7-C

1. A dieter is almost constantly thinking about **food**.
2. When dieting, it is hard to **concentrate** on or think about anything else.
3. There is a **powerful** craving for **food**, especially fast-energy foods like sweets and high-fat foods.

4. Not satisfying hunger is very **uncomfortable**. It is not surprising dieters may feel **crabby** and may think most about **their own** needs.
5. A **huge** hunger is felt when a dieter stops dieting. This makes a dieter feel he or she cannot get enough food. It is normal to expect to rapidly eat a very **large** amount of food when going off a diet—far **more** than a normal amount. Dieters may not know they are full until they feel "stuffed."
6. The longer a diet lasts and the more times a person diets, the **more** overeating, or "stuffing," occurs after the diet. **Dieting** is one of the most common causes of overeating.
7. After losing weight on a diet, most people **regain** the weight plus **added** pounds.
8. The more people diet, the harder it is to tell when they are full and when they are still **hungry**. Then they may always **feel** hungry, even if they are not. If they stop dieting long enough, they may get back their normal hunger sensor.

5. **REVIEW the Namuh:** Remember the Namuh ". . . did so much dieting and so much overeating to make up for it that many of them overate themselves right into larger and larger sizes—because that's what happens of course—just the opposite of what they were trying to do! The thinner they tried to be, the fatter they got!"

   ASK: The Namuh decided they were "too hungry." Do you think the Namuh were too hungry?"

   ASK: What was wrong with the Namuh thinking? (Hunger was *not* the problem. Believing they could successfully diet was the problem.)

6. **DIET SUMMARY:** *Many* diets work at first. People lose weight for a while. But because of the "gulping" of food when people go off a diet, diets almost always fail in the end. Diets are known to:
   - Cause an obsession and preoccupation with food, and create *too much* hunger. This is uncomfortable and leads to overeating.
   - Slow metabolism. The less food is eaten, the slower it is burned. This is one of the body's ways of trying to protect itself from starving to death.
   - Fail. Weight that is lost is usually gained back, often with added pounds. This is why people who diet, often diet over and over. Dieting is a "losing battle!"

Students may ask: ***If diets for weight loss do not work, why do people diet?***

- There is so much pressure to be very slim to be attractive, many people think they *need* to be thin*ner* (realistically or not) to be acceptable or happy. Sometimes even those who are lean feel they should weight even less! People who are naturally fatter or who are thin but want to be unnaturally thin may turn to dieting when wholesome eating does not result in a body they (or others) believe to be "slim enough."

- These days, there are many warnings that suggest practically everyone must lose weight to be healthy. Many people have become fearful that eating well and being active will not be enough to discover the healthy weight that is right for them.
- With all of the food "treats" that are available, many people believe the only alternative to eating a lot of these foods is to restrict their eating entirely and go on a "diet." This is an "all or nothing" approach to eating that is common among people who diet.
- Since dieting may result in weight loss for a while, it is easy to believe it could work in the long run. People have not understood that dieting backfires in the end and that there are better ways to find a healthy weight.
- Diet advertisements try to convince us that "their" diet will work even though all others have failed! Diet ads can be very convincing for people who really want to lose weight.

  (If there is time, copy a diet advertisement onto an overhead transparency and practice critical thinking skills, using the tools learned in Lesson 7.)

7. **ADD:** The *Body Image Building Block* for Lesson 7 from I-D to the student's models.

8. **ASSIGN HOME EDUCATION:** Send HANDOUT 7-C and the Home Education slip to be signed and returned.

7-A OVERHEAD

When basic needs for life are not fully met, you can expect the following:

1. You will be constantly thinking about what is missing: sleep, water, air, food, warmth.

2. It will be hard to concentrate or think about anything else.

3. There will be a powerful craving (drive) to satisfy the need (tiredness, thirst, hunger, etc.)

4. Until satisfied, the craving will be very uncomfortable. You may become crabby and self-centered. It will be hard to think about anyone else's needs.

5. When the need is finally met, more than a normal amount will be needed in order to feel satisfied.

7-B OVERHEAD

CONSEQUENCES OF DIETING

1. A dieter is almost constantly thinking about FOOD.
2. When dieting, it is hard to CONCENTRATE on or think about anything else.
3. There is a POWERFUL craving for FOOD, especially fast-energy foods like sweets and high-fat foods.
4. Not satisfying hunger is very UNCOMFORTABLE. It is not surprising that dieters may feel CRABBY and may think most about THEIR OWN needs.
5. A HUGE hunger is felt when a dieter stops dieting. This makes a dieter feel he or she cannot get enough food. It is normal to expect to rapidly eat a LARGE amount of food when going off a diet—far MORE than a normal amount. Dieters may not know they are full until they feel "STUFFED."
6. The longer and more often a dieter diets, the MORE overeating occurs. DIETING is one of the most common causes of overeating.
7. After losing weight on a diet, most people REGAIN the weight plus ADDED pounds.
8. The more people diet, the harder it is to tell when they are full and when they are still HUNGRY. They may always FEEL HUNGRY even if they are not. If they stop dieting long enough, they may get back their normal hunger sensor.

7-C DIETING FOR WEIGHT LOSS CAN CAUSE BIG PROBLEMS

Many believe that eating less than they are hungry for is good for losing weight. But food is a *basic need*. When basic needs are not fully satisfied, here's what you can expect:

1. You will be constantly thinking about what is missing (sleep, water, air, warmth, food).
2. It will be hard to concentrate or think about anything else.
3. There will be a powerful craving to satisfy the need.
4. Until satisfied, the craving will be very uncomfortable. You may become crabby or self-centered. It will be hard to think about others' needs.
5. When you can finally satisfy the need, *more* than a normal amount will be needed for complete satisfaction.

Water, air, food, sleep, and warmth satisfy basic needs.

You can expect these consequences if you restrict your hunger to lose weight:

1) A dieter is almost constantly thinking about ______________________________.

2) When dieting, it is hard to ______________________________ on or think about anything else.

3) There is a______________________________ craving for ______________________________, especially fast-energy foods like sweets and high-fat foods.

4) Not satisfying hunger is very ______________________________. It is not surprising dieters may have ______________________________ patience, feel ______________________________, and may be thinking most about______________________________ ______________________________ needs.

5) A ______________________________hunger is felt when a dieter stops dieting. This makes a dieter feel he or she cannot get enough food. It is normal to expect to rapidly eat a very ______________________________ amount of food when going off a diet—far ______________________________ than a normal amount. Dieters may not know they are full until they feel "______________________________."

6) The longer and more often a dieter diets, the ______________________________ overeating, or "stuffing," occurs. ______________________________ is one of the most common causes of overeating.

7) After losing weight on a diet, most people ______________________________ the weight plus ______________________________ pounds.

8) The more people diet, the harder it is to tell when they are full and when they are still hungry. They may always ______________________________ ______________________________ even if they are not. If they stop dieting long enough, they may get back their normal ______________________________ sensor.

When you need a drink, it's hard to think! Can you concentrate when your lunch is late?	***Dieting to lose weight is not a good idea. To find the natural weight that's best for you, eat well and be active for fun and fitness.***

LESSON 8

EATING WELL FOR CONFIDENCE IN A HEALTHY WEIGHT

Eat for Nutrition, Energy, Satisfaction of Hunger, and Enjoyment

Body Image Building Block:

Satisfy hunger completely with enough wholesome food at regular meals and snacks.

LESSON OBJECTIVES

Students will learn that eating well is half of the behavioral equation for health and a healthy body image in most individuals. Students will learn:

- Combined with physical fitness, eating well completes the equation for health at every size.
- What it means to *eat well.* This includes individual ownership about what is "enough," the purpose and value of nutrition-dense foods, and the place for high-energy/low-nutrient treats.
- Incentives to choose a variety of nutrient-dense foods as the basis for their eating lifestyles.

BACKGROUND

Author's note: The following background material is more extensive than for other lessons in this curriculum for two reasons: 1) Confusion about eating has become widespread in the American culture. Teachers are not immune to this. 2) Information explaining significant changes in the Dietary Guidelines released in January 2005 is included.

With reasonable care, children's bodies can be counted on to grow into diverse sizes, shapes, and weights that are healthy and right for them. But what is reasonable care? Wholesome eating and physical fitness are needed for confidence that this growth is happening as it was intended.

Eating well is a pleasure for most people. It means choosing and enjoying a variety of foods that taste good, provide sufficient energy, and satisfy nutritional needs. It also means tuning *in* to know when we are hungry, what we want to eat, and when we have had enough. Eating well need not be confusing, anxiety-provoking, or conflict-laden. It requires some thoughtfulness and effort but is a part of life that can flow easily and naturally for those who have access to a variety of wholesome food and a basic respect for nutrition. At the same time, eating well can be unbelievably difficult for those who lack good food, do not value balanced nutrition, or have become anxious in their relationship to food.

Many Americans do not eat well. The results include nutrition deficits that may affect health, and/or eating compulsions that leave people afraid, angry, or otherwise out of control around food. Sometimes the results are extreme, contributing to restrictive and compulsive eating disorders, cardiovascular disease, type-two diabetes, hypertension, osteoporosis, and some cancers. The goal of this lesson is to teach students to feel good about eating well, to know how to make healthy choices to carry out that intention, and to maintain responsibility for their own hunger despite unhealthy cultural pressures to the contrary. Ideally, this could be expressed as, "I am the best authority on when I'm hungry and when I'm full. I make a reasonable effort to eat a variety of wholesome foods to satisfy my hunger and nutrition needs on a routine basis." Eating well maintains body esteem in its purest form.

A word about responsibility: It is not right to expect even nutrition-wise children to assume responsibility for healthy eating on their own. Kids rely on adults to provide food and cannot become competent eaters without a good supply of wholesome, appealing food from which they can choose that is presented at regular, reliable intervals.

Unfortunately many adults do not understand their job is to consistently supply the food needed to avoid eating problems, and to model eating well. Those who lack financial resources face additional challenges. Because of this, in teaching young students about food selection, it is important to remember we are giving them information they may or may not be able to use right now, depending on the food that is provided for them. This lesson aims to motivate students to maintain ownership of their hunger while actively seeking a variety of healthy foods as the basis for their eating. But children cannot do their job unless adults first do theirs. Adults, including those in school systems, must be prepared to make choices about the nutritional contribution of the foods they provide, as well as to be role models. As you present this lesson, have students consider how their home and school environments encourage or impede the goal of eating well.

This lesson addresses eating well in general but also attempts to respond to four concerns that commonly interfere with wholesome eating patterns in American culture:

1. INADEQUATE ATTENTION TO NUTRITION NEEDS

Today's children and adults too often satisfy hunger with an imbalance of high-energy/low-nutrient foods, depleting the drive to eat before nutrition needs are met. Given the abundant, seductively advertised, read-to-go, inexpensive supply of yummy-but-low-nutrient foods in our culture, it is easy to understand why many people assume that a full stomach, affordable price, and stimulating taste are what matter. Many people either do not know or regularly rationalize and discount the fact that there are nutritional differences in foods that will fill us up. Unfortunately, few children, and not enough adults, understand the dilemma associated with this: *If health is highly valued, enough restraint in food selection is needed to maintain hunger for a variety of nutrient-dense foods that are known to promote physical well-being.*

It is neither accurate nor helpful to categorize foods as "good" or "bad." What is useful is to recognize that *different foods serve different purposes.* In light of this, with today's vast array of food options and torrent of advertisements pushing certain types of foods much more than others, it is important to consider what we value most when it comes to eating choices.

All foods provide energy. Foods that provide energy *and* that are rich in fiber and nutrients are essential for building and maintaining strong bodies. Foods that provide energy with little or no nutrient value serve another purpose—primarily they are eaten for pleasure or enjoyment as well as entertainment. Eating just for the good taste of it is a delightful part of life for most people. However, since health is so important and hunger is finite, health demands that the *greater portion* of hunger be spent on foods that have high-nutrient value. Children are able to understand this approach is not about "good foods/bad foods" but instead is about a mindful use of resources. Viewing hunger as a limited resource is like teaching a child that, in order to save for a bike, he or she will need to limit the number of smaller toys purchasd. To be a good athlete, student, musician, or to be physically, fit he or she will need to make decisions about allocation of free-time. Just as today's children learn that playing with a friend is not good or bad but serves a different function than, say, doing homework, petting the dog, or reading a book, so too do different foods serve different purposes. To promote health, they will need to save enough of their hunger for foods that are nutrient-dense.

Eating for Emotional Hunger

Educators have raised concerns about "emotionally hungry" children, who may use the satisfying capacity of food to make up for or dissociate from emotional pain. Some have specifically asked for a lesson that addresses "emotional eating." As stated in the preface, some children are more "emotionally hungry" than a child should ever have to be, and these kids will be "hungry" in ways that are beyond the scope of these lessons. Despite this, do not be afraid to encourage them to eat well. Your words can be potent as you express concern, not that they are *eating too much,* but that they are not getting enough of what they need.

2. MISGUIDED MOTIVATION FOR EATING WELL

Many believe that the *main* reason to eat well (or to not eat) is to achieve or maintain a particular weight. This myth holds despite the fact that eating behaviors *may or may not* influence weight as much as people would like to think. In reality, many fat people eat relatively little, while many thin people "eat like horses." More to the point, since quantity says nothing about quality, either person may be well nourished or poorly nourished. On the other hand, there is a lot of evidence that, on the whole, Americans with both large and small appetites do not eat *what they need*. When "weight control" is the primary purpose of eating well, nutritional health suffers in the following ways:

- Inundated with media messages urging them to "Lose weight fast!" many rationalize unbalanced and even bizarre diets in the belief that calories avoided are more important than nutrients needed. Or, alternately, people feel driven to overload on "forbidden" foods—again neglecting nutrition—as they brace for the next diet. Studies have shown that alternating high-calorie/low-nutrient foods with restrictive dieting has become a "normal" eating pattern for many Americans. It is a predominant eating style for many adolescent girls.
- Individuals who tire of pressures and failed attempts to achieve "the right weight," often react against pressures to "lose weight" by developing defiant or complacent eating styles that are not known for balanced nutrition: "Don't tell me what or how much to eat," or "I'll never be thin, so what difference does it make what I eat?"
- With the current emphasis on improving nutrition to reduce overweight, many people who are naturally slim see little reason to eat well. When the goal is size (versus health), the nutritional status of the entire population suffers.

3. FAULTY EQUATIONS RELATED TO WEIGHT "CONTROL"

Concern about the rising rate of fatness has resulted in an emphasis on "weight control" as a goal. In 1998 the U.S. Surgeon General stated that giving up this goal would result in a "don't worry, be flabby" mentality. Even recommendations accompanying the new USDA *My Pyramid* appear to suggest that hunger can be discounted in order to manipulate weight—dismissing the many complex factors not in our control that influence fatness and thinness. Statements such as, "Monitor your body weight to see if you need to adjust your calorie intake," without reference to "always satisfy hunger fully with a variety of wholesome foods" are a naive invitation to engage in the diet mentality. Emphasis on calorie prescriptions has backfired, contributing to:

- A population that systematically forgets about innate size diversity and endorses weightist attitudes.
- An epidemic of formula-based, calorie-reduction diets with dismal and counterproductive long-term effects.
- Widespread complacency and defiance about nutrition and fitness when these do not result in the desired size and shape.
- A population of fearful, conflicted eaters who lack confidence in finding a healthy weight that's right for each of them.

Children can be taught a more effective eating equation. Children can and should be taught that *health at any size* is the primary objective of wholesome lifestyle choices. The same applies to the adults who want to set good examples. Motivation for a healthy lifestyle should not be to eliminate size diversity but to experience competency and trust in choices that maintain integrity, health, and well-being.

4. CONFUSION ABOUT HOW TO EAT WELL

Eating well means satisfying hunger completely with enough varied, wholesome, good-tasting food at regular intervals. When eating well occurs, "overeating" and unstable or unbalanced eating are unlikely. Unfortunately, when people learn to fear that eating will make them fat, and fatness means undesirability, trusting internal hunger may feel like shooting themselves out of a cannon. At the same time, the definition of "wholesome" is increasingly a mystery. Confusion about how to eat well prevails.

- Eating "enough" to satisfy hunger is frequently equated with "overeating" if the resulting weight does not produce the desired slimness.
- "Overeating" is often inappropriately labeled. Even self-diagnosed "overeaters" rarely eat "too much"—that is, *more quantity* of food than the recommended daily servings for all the food groups. It is far more likely that not *enough* servings of varied foods are chosen from all food groups, as hunger is satiated with choices from only one or two groups or from food high in fats and sugar. Unfortunately, the prescribed "solution" is often to "eat less" (restrict hunger) rather than to *eat better*.
- Unstable or unbalanced eating is common. Erratic, busy schedules, exhaustion, and lack of access to or understanding of good-tasting, nutrient-dense foods can make eating well seem an insurmountable effort.
- Eating well does not mean following rigid rules. Rules that aim to control eating are the cause of most disordered eating. In contrast, *guidelines* for eating are about what works and what doesn't to get the end result we want: healthy, happy, well-nourished children and adults who enjoy eating as an important part of life. This requires an approach that includes forethought and some planning to provide for nutritional needs but that is flexible and based on trust rather than a rigid "diet plan." Eating well includes choosing foods that satisfy our nutritional requirements most of the time but eating for fun or entertainment on occasion, as well. Studies show that, when individuals have permission to eat until they are satisfied and have a good supply of wholesome food provided at regularly spaced intervals, they will eat well naturally.

It is important to note that in an ideal world children would probably not need this instruction to insure their health. Given a variety of hearty foods in a predominantly wholesome food environment, children have repeatedly shown they will eat when they are hungry and stop when they are full, choosing foods that provide balanced nutrition without conflict or anxiety. Unfortunately, this is not the environment in which most of today's children develop. Instead, kids must learn from an early age to navigate in a sea of affordable, ready-to-eat, taste-stimulating foods packaged and promoted specifically to lure them into overvaluing and craving it. At the same time, children hear a never-ending stream of messages about the size and shape their bodies should be and how to achieve this through manipulation (restriction) of food and exercise. In light of this contamination, children cannot be expected to maintain body esteem and competency as eaters without guidance.

Other concerns contribute to confusion about eating well. It is a common assumption that, if weight is within the "normal" range, nutrition must be adequate. Unless there are other extenuating circumstances, eating habits and activity levels are rarely questioned for the generally lean, allowing poor nutrition to go undetected. This is of particular concern for developing children. On the other hand, health professionals at all levels routinely and automatically diagnosis "overweight" based on external measures rather than assessing lifestyle choices. Fatter-bodied, active, fit individuals who may eat very well are routinely told to "lose weight" without an assessment of their actual lifestyle. In both cases, healthy choices are discouraged when eating habits are inferred from size.

TEACH FOR THESE OUTCOMES

Students will know:

- Bodies regularly need a variety of nutritious foods from *all* the food groups.
- Foods are not "good" or "bad" but serve different purposes. Some foods are packed full of the nutrients, fiber, and energy that the body needs, and some foods provide energy and fun but little nourishment. It's important to know the difference.
- If hunger is spent by eating from one or two food groups, there may not be enough left for a balance of foods from other groups.
- When we fill up with low-nutrient taste-treats, there may not be enough hunger left for nutritious food.
- Mass marketing influences our culture's eating habits.
- Eating well is one of the two behaviors I can choose for confidence that my weight is healthy.
- Eating well requires *active* choices.

Student attitudes will be:

- Everybody is different. Only I can know for sure when I am hungry and when I am full.
- Eating well is an important value.
- I hope the adults in my life will provide me with a variety of wholesome food to choose from.
- It's important to listen to my hunger and satisfy my appetite with a variety of nutritious foods that I enjoy.
- I eat "entertainment foods" for fun, but my priority is to eat a balance of foods that give my body all the nutrients it needs.
- I eat well and am active (see Lesson 10), so I am confident this is a healthy weight for me.

CONCEPTS NEEDED TO TEACH THIS LESSON

- In the past 40 years a profusion of weight-control and diet plans for weight loss have come to coexist with an abundance of mouth-watering, high-energy/low-nutrient foods cleverly marketed at low cost. In light of this, an increasing number of people make food choices for the primary purpose of "weight control" or, alternately, for the primary purpose of entertainment or diversion. As a result, the value of eating well for health and well-being has diminished. Many well-intentioned people are confused about how to correct this problem.

- It is unfortunate that weight- or size-management has become a driving force, since there are so many factors *outside of our control* that *limit* healthy manipulation of weight or BMI. **It is important to recognize that *weight* is not a *behavior*, and, as such, it is not in our power to choose.** On the other hand, two behavioral options *influence* weight (within limits), and most certainly influence health:
  - Eating
  - Physical Activity

  Given this, it is important for young students to learn to value eating well and being active *for the purpose of health*, while learning to accept the many diverse, healthy sizes and shapes that result. This is a shift from current, normative beliefs suggesting that the purpose and goal of healthy choices is to lose weight or maintain a slim appearance.

- Eating well means:
  - Deciding for yourself how much is "enough" food to satisfy hunger.
  - Routinely selecting a balanced variety of foods from the five basic food groups to satisfy hunger and to provide the necessary nutrients and energy for growth, healing, and maintenance.
  - Eating what you like, including some flavor favorites that may provide primarily energy (with little nutrition), as long as these do not routinely diminish hunger needed for good nutrition.
  - Eating at regular intervals to avoid both eating constantly and excessive hunger.

- Most concerns about becoming "overweight" or "underweight" can be resolved by:
  - Habitually eating enough varied, nutrient-dense foods from all food groups to satisfy hunger.
  - Limiting sedentary entertainment and routinely engaging in vigorous activity.
  - Trusting that a *well-nourished and metabolically fit body* may be healthy at any size.

- Consequences occur when a *balance* of foods from all five food groups is not routinely available. Since hunger drives eating to satiation, larger amounts of food will be eaten from one or two food groups if these are what is handy.

- Because of its intense flavor, low-cost, ready availability, and promotion through mass marketing, low-nutrient/high-fat/high-sugar foods have become very appealing to most people. Easy access to these food options can make balanced eating more difficult, as their selection crowds out hunger needed for high-nutrient foods.

- Mass marketing of food:
  - Was not common prior to 40 years ago.
  - Has resulted in a proliferation of easy and stimulating-to-eat, widely available, cheap, high-energy/low nutrient foods.
  - Presents low-nutrient foods as if they fulfill the same function as nutrient-dense foods; i.e., as if these are "the way to eat."
  - Presents images of low-nutrient foods that appeal to or exploit social or emotional needs (i.e., the wish to belong, be "cool," have fun, relax, be "treated," etc.).

- Key recommendations of the new USDA Dietary Guidelines released in January, 2005 include:
  - Variety—Eat foods from all food groups and subgroups.
  - Proportionality—Eat more of some foods (whole grains, fruits, vegetables, low-fat milk products) and less of others (foods high in saturated or trans-fats, added sugars, cholesterol, and salt).
  - Moderation—Eat when hungry and stop when full. Satisfy hunger with foods that are "nutrient dense" (with little or no solid fats or added sugars).
  - Activity—Be physically active every day.

- Key concepts for each food group include:
  - Grains—Make at least half of total grains eaten whole grains.
  - Vegetables—Eat the recommended amount and choose a variety each day.
  - Fruit—Eat the recommended amount and choose a variety each day.
  - Milk, yogurt, and cheese—Consume three cups of skimmed or 1% milk, or an equivalent amount of yogurt or cheese per day. Consume other calcium-rich foods if milk products are not used.
  - Meat or beans—Make choices that are low-fat or lean when selecting meats and poultry.

- Fats—Choose most fats from monounsaturated and polyunsaturated fats, such as fish, nuts, seeds, and vegetable oils.
- Sugar—Limit foods with added sugar.
- Salt—Choose and prepare foods with less salt.

CRITICAL CONCEPTS

The concepts presented in this lesson teach skills that are important for eating competency. The lesson focuses on behavior and is not intended to replace curricula on *nutrition.* In field tests, teachers reported that the food journal activity, *Do You Eat Enough?* was extremely effective in helping children to personally examine their eating habits. It is essential that teachers remain sensitive to the fact that children cannot make wholesome eating choices unless options for doing so are made available to them by adults.

VOCABULARY

- priority
- dilemma
- contradiction
- calorie
- nutrition

LESSON PREPARATION AND MATERIALS

Materials:	**Preparation:**
▪ Copy 8-B for use with the Activity and for Home Education. ▪ Copy 8-C for each student for each day they will record *Do You Eat Enough?* ▪ Copy 8-D for each student to graph his or her results of 8-B. ▪ Copy 8-E if electing to do the optional activity.	▪ Read the *Suggested Lesson Script.* ▪ Become familiar with 8-C—*Do You Eat Enough?* If desired, use it to record your own food intake for one day, and copy onto an overhead transparency, for use as an example.

LESSON SUMMARY

- DISCUSS: The primary purpose of eating; how and what to eat.
- REVIEW: 8-A—*My Pyramid,* and 8-B—*Food Guidelines: Do You Eat Enough?* based on the USDA Food Guidelines.
- INFORM: Differences between whole and refined grains.
- ASSIGN HOMEWORK ACTIVITY: 8-C—*Do You Eat Enough?* to examine food selection over five days.

- GRAPH AND DISCUSS: 8-D—*Do You Eat Enough?*
- OPTIONAL: 8-E—*Does Advertising Affect What You Choose to Eat?*
- ADD: *Body Image Building Block.*
- ASSIGN HOME EDUCATION.

SUGGESTED LESSON SCRIPT

1. **TELL:** We have learned it is important to satisfy hunger.

2. **ASK:** What are your favorite foods for satisfying hunger?

   If you could eat your favorite foods morning, noon, and night, what you would eat? *(Have fun with this. Encourage students to imagine days filled only with their favorites. Many students will imagine only "treats," but some might dream of only fruit or bread for three meals a day. Other students will be in tune with their natural appetites and know their bodies would hunger for a variety of foods.)*

   ASK: Would this be a good way to eat regularly? Why not?

   NOTE: Students may comment that if their choices were all high-fat and/or sugary treats, they would get fat. If they do:

   - ***Emphasize*:** This could make some people fatter than they were meant to be. But that would depend on the person and his or her metabolism.
   - ***Review:*** Some fatter people eat very few treats. Some very thin people eat treats all the time, and still don't get fat—even if they are couch potatoes!

   ASK: Why not eat only one or two of your favorite foods morning, noon, and night? As long as you satisfy your hunger, what difference does it make? Aren't all foods the same?

   TELL: Not all foods serve the *same purpose* in our bodies.

   ***Different foods serve different purposes*:**

   - **All foods have flavor**. This flavor may make them more or less appealing in our mouths. Some foods have a very intense flavor; some medium, while others may be very bland.
   - **All foods contain energy (calories) to keep us going**. Some foods contain a lot of energy in just a few bites, while others contain very even in a whole bowlful.

- **Not all foods contain nutrients.** Some foods contain many essential nutrients and fiber that are needed to build bodies and keep them strong. Other foods contain very few nutrients or none at all.
- **Nutritious foods contain different nutrients from one another.** Vegetables, grains, fruits, dairy foods, and protein foods, such as meat, provide a wide variety of nutrients and fiber that the body needs for health.

3. **DISCUSS: What is the primary purpose of eating?**
    - To satisfy our hunger—so we can think about other things! (It is surprising how many dieters have learned to deny and/or discount this reason.)
    - To get all of the nutrients our bodies need—to be as healthy as possible.
    - To gain energy to do all the things we want to do.
    - To enjoy! It feels good to quiet our hunger drive, and most people like the good taste and pleasure of sharing food with family and friends.

ASK: How do we know *how to eat* for health? "How to eat" has become an important question in modern times.

TELL: In today's world, we have a *very wide variety* of foods to choose from—more choices than anyone could have imagined 50 years ago. In addition to many new and different foods, food is plentiful in Western cultures, with a lot of it ready-to-eat by simply opening a bag or dropping coins in a vending machine. For the first time in history it is possible for most people (adults at least) to satisfy hunger by eating pretty much *whatever and whenever* they wish with little effort. In fact, we are regularly *encouraged* to do this by advertisements promoting snacks or drinks, urging us to eat here or there or to grab something quick to munch along the way without regard to nutrition needs. Unfortunately, there is a problem with this approach to eating.

- ***One way to understand this problem is to think of hunger as being like money.***

    Most people have a limited amount of money. If a person with limited money wanted to save for something that had *great value* to him or her (like a bike, a car, a trip, or a house), that person would need to save a sizable portion of his or her allowance or earnings for this purpose. If instead they spent most of their money on trinkets or games, they would not end up with enough money for the more important item.

    Like money, most of us have a limited amount of hunger. Given this, if we value health, it is important to learn to "spend" our hunger (satisfy it) on foods that promote it. If we eat only our flavor-favorites or "whatever/whenever," how can we be sure to have hunger for all the nutrients our body needs?

It is important to save *most* of our hunger for regular meals and snacks that provide the nutrients needed by our body.

ASK: How do we know *what to eat*?

TELL: When people "listen" to their bodies, most find they get hungry for the variety of foods that are needed to grow and stay strong: whole grains, fruits, vegetables, meats and other protein foods, and dairy foods or other foods high in calcium.

Unfortunately, in today's world, a lot of "noise" may make it hard to "tune in" to natural hunger. Colorful and entertaining advertisements try to tempt us with mouth-watering pictures and messages about what and when to eat. *(Ask students for examples.)* In addition, many new foods with highly concentrated flavors have been created in recent years. Many of these contain a lot of energy but few nutrients. Once we have sampled the intense flavor of sugary treats and deep-fried snacks, we remember it! Sometimes the memory of these flavors makes it hard to get in touch with what our bodies require to maintain health. When this happens, we may need a reminder about the balance of nutrients needed for good health.

TELL: The U.S. government has provided us with guidelines that remind us what our bodies need for a balance of nutrients every day.

SHOW: Overhead 8-A—*My Pyramid* This symbol has replaced the former Food Guide Pyramid. This Pyramid serves as a reminder to make wise food-choices from *all* the food groups and to be physically active for fitness and fun every day. *(We will talk about fitness in Lesson 9.)*

If your class has previously learned about the Food Guide Pyramid, you may wish to tell them this graphic was updated in April 2005, based on the revised 2005 U.S. Dietary Guidelines. For further information, see www.health.gov/dietaryguideline.

You may wish to point out that this pyramid contains no serving amounts. Instead, the relative proportion of foods that should be eaten is shown by the different widths of the bands. This is because everybody is different, and the quantities of food needed vary as well, depending on many factors. However, the 2005 Dietary Guidelines still recommends the minimum daily requirements essential for the health of growing children and adults. In addition, daily physical activity is recommended as the counterpart of wholesome eating.

PRESENT: 8-B—*Food Guidelines; Do You Eat Enough?* Review the information it contains. Important information regarding the distinction between whole grains and refined grains is included in the reference box on page 137.

4. **INTRODUCE THE ACTIVITY: 8-C— *Do You Eat Enough?***

For this activity, you will consider whether you are eating enough of what your body needs to be well-nourished. You will be using this chart to record what you eat during one whole day. You will record what you eat each day for up to five days. At the end of that time, you will be graphing your results. Then you will have an idea whether there are foods you need to eat more or less of to satisfy both your hunger and your health needs.

Guiding Students in the *Do You Eat Enough?* Activity

- Help students understand servings in an uncomplicated way. The last thing you want is for students to become obsessive about measuring serving sizes. Encourage students to count one piece of bread, an average bowl of cereal, a scoop of rice, a small pile of pasta, one fruit, medium piles of veggies, a glass of milk, a piece of chicken, the amount of tuna it takes to cover a piece of bread, etc., as one serving. Unless students report eating very large or small portions, then "some" is good enough.

- At the same time, there may be students in your class who might happily eat half a chicken or only one bite. Provide a little direction to understand such portions as more or less than one serving. This should be offered as information only and without any suggestion of judgment. For example, "If one serving of chicken is about the size of a deck of cards, then how many servings do you think there are in a half-chicken?" "If a serving of rice is about the size of my fist, do you think one teaspoon of rice contains the nutrients of one serving?"

- Inform students that counting servings and recording food intake is not something they need to do in everyday life. It is only helpful to occasionally check to be sure they have developed the habit of eating *enough* varied foods from all five food groups. Very few people overeat on a regular basis if they are eating the *minimum* from all categories as a rule. Hunger satiation should be the cue for when they have eaten enough.

- Help students categorize foods. For example, some will not know that ice cream is a combination food that should be listed both in the fat/sugar and dairy food categories. Spaghetti with red sauce and meatballs contains grain (pasta), vegetable (tomato sauce), and meat (meatballs). Foods that are deep-fried are listed as fats as well as whatever other category applies. Potatoes, while high in carbohydrates, are still vegetables.

- Allow students to have time after lunch to record their intake for the previous 24 hours.

- Students may tend to record only major feedings. Urge them to *stretch* their memories, especially to recall tidbits of candy or raw vegetables, after-school snacks, hand-held fruits, beverages, etc. that were consumed "on the run." Encourage regular meals and snacks versus a grazing approach.

- There is no minimum for added fats and sugars because these are "add-ons." They taste very good to most people and provide energy. But because they lack nutrients, we say they provide "empty" calories. We enjoy these as spreads or dressings or in treats, but suggest they be limited to insure a balance of nutrition. Some fat is essential to health, but since it is already built into many foods, added amounts are generally not required.

- Consider asking parents to join students in doing this activity.

5. **GRAPHING 8-D—*Do You Eat Enough?* AND DISCUSSING THE ACTIVITY**

   After recording is completed, ask students to graph their daily food-group totals by transferring the number in their "count" column on 8-C to the 8-D graph. This will give them an important visual picture to see at a glance if they eat enough nutritious food in an average day.

   ASK:

   - Our bodies need the minimum in each food group most days. Are you eating enough? If so, congratulations! Your body thanks you!
   - If not, how can you make room for what you need?

   TELL: If you are eating a balanced *variety of food from the five main food groups* on most days, you can be confident you are eating for health and a healthy weight for you.

6. **CONSIDER:** If time allows, consider 8-E—*Does Advertising Affect What You Eat?*

7. **ADD the *Body Image Building Block*** for Lesson 8 from I-D to the student models.

8. **ASSIGN HOME EDUCATION:** Send 8-A, 8-B, and 8-C along with the Home Education slip for home discussion. On the back of 8-B have students write whether they "ate enough" and, if not, what they will try to do to correct this. If possible, try to entice families to do this activity with their students.

Choosing Whole versus Refined Grains

It is not necessary for elementary school students to learn detail about the vitamins, minerals and fiber that are contained in foods. However, scientists have recently learned about important differences in foods that contain whole grain, versus foods that are made primarily from refined grains. Many adults are still on the learning curve regarding this, making it important for children to hear this information reinforced outside the home.

For years USDA Dietary Guidelines have advised us to choose grains as the foundation of what we eat. The new, 2005 Dietary Guidelines recommend we chose *whole* grains more often versus those that are refined. Since many are not accustomed to whole grains, making the switch may take some adjustment. This may come easier if the reasons for the change are better understood.

When whole, natural grains are processed and refined, the nutrient-rich outer bran and inner germ are removed, leaving a pure carbohydrate food that contains energy (calories) but that is stripped of all 22 of its vitamins and minerals, all its fiber, and one-quarter of its protein. Besides losing nutritional value, with less substance these refined grains are digested and absorbed into the bloodstream very quickly, causing a spike in blood sugar and, in turn, insulin as the body attempts to restore balance. Among other effects, this fluctuation in blood sugar can trigger a compensatory craving for more food, even though more energy is not yet needed. It turns out that a diet based primarily on highly processed and refined carbohydrates may contribute to nutrition deficits and metabolic problems such as type-two diabetes. In contrast, whole grains are full of nutrients, high in fiber, and protective against many medical problems, and are digested and metabolized more slowly, providing a longer feeling of fullness. For these reasons, it is recommended that *at least* half of grains chosen be whole grains.

The lack of distinction between refined and unrefined carbohydrates in the recent "low-carb" craze has been detrimental and has added to confusion about healthy eating. Educators should take the lead in teaching students to resist the hype that urges people to avoid "carbs." Instead, students should learn that there is a difference between refined carbohydrates that provide energy (calories) with little fiber or nutrient value (such as sugar) and whole grains, which provide the foundation for wholesome eating.

How do we know if a food contains primarily whole or refined grains? Read the label. For wheat products, such as bread, pasta, and some cereals, the word "whole" must precede the word "wheat" on the label. Many breads are labeled "wheat" or "enriched wheat"* and tinted a caramel color. Don't be fooled. The label must list "whole wheat" as the first ingredient. Look for other whole grains, such as oats, barley, rye, brown rice, etc, with these listed prominently and first on the label.

**Note: In the early part of the 20th century, when the federal government recognized the loss in nutrients resulting from refined grains, laws were passed requiring that manufacturers "enrich" their products by putting back four vitamins (niacin, riboflavin, thiamin, folic acid) and one mineral (iron) after the milling process was completed. Many cereals and other foods are now "fortified." Even so, the fiber is lost, and the nutritional value remains limited compared to whole grains.*

8-A

My Pyramid

STEPS TO A HEALTHIER YOU

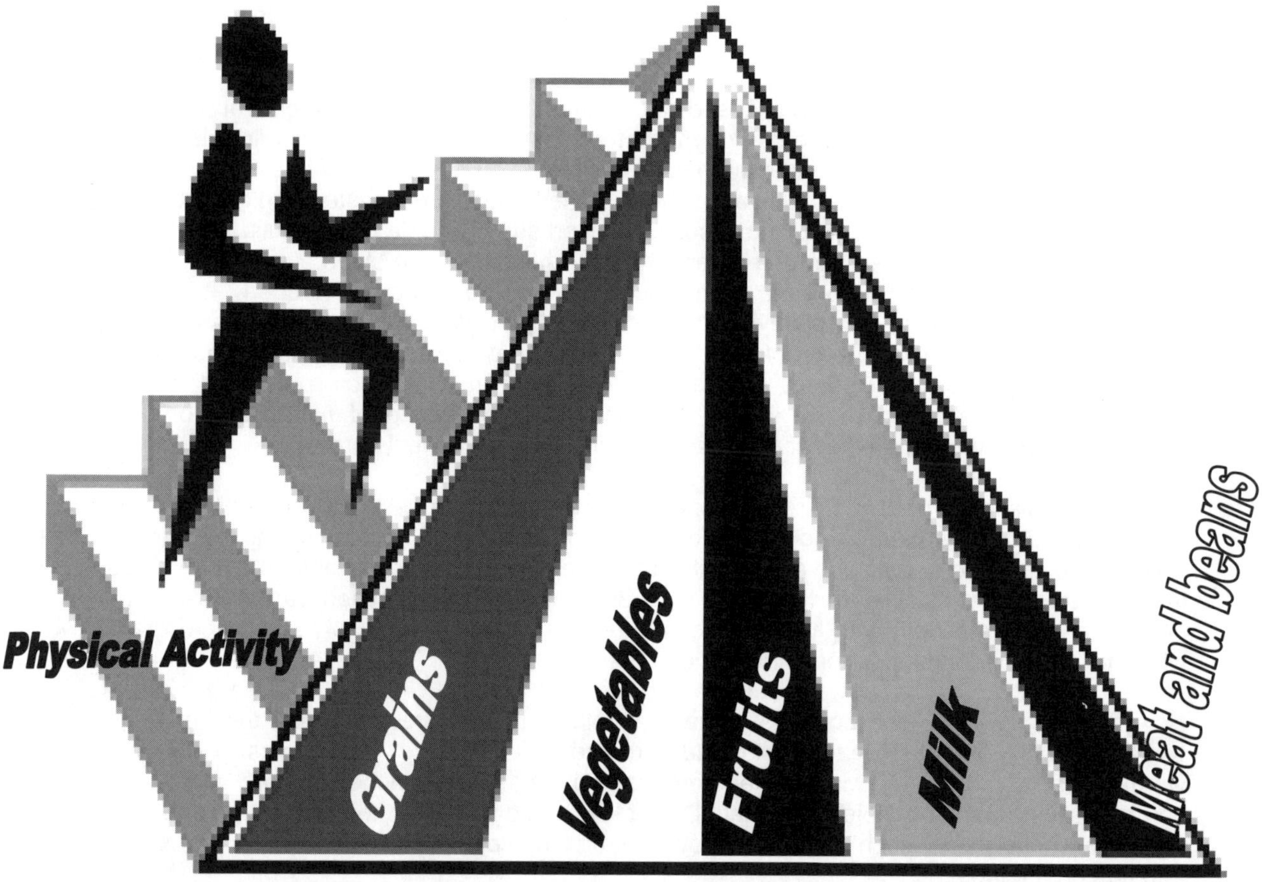

8-B

Food Guidelines—DO YOU EAT ENOUGH?

FOOD GROUP	DO YOU EAT ENOUGH FOR HEALTH?
GREAT GRAINS Build your body with great grains from the earth. Make at least half of your choices *whole* grains, like *whole wheat* bread, pasta, and cereal, and brown and wild rice. Don't be fooled by caramel-colored "wheat" bread or cereal. Whole oats, barley, buckwheat, bulgur, corn, wheat, and rye are all examples of whole grains.	**EAT at least 5-6 servings of grain a day. Make half or more of these *whole* grains.** A serving is 1 average slice of bread, 1/2 bagel, 1 cup of flaked cereal, or ½ cup of pasta or rice. Most people need more than one serving of grain in a meal to satisfy hunger and to get in enough grain in a day.
VERY VARIED VEGETABLES Eat veggies raw or cooked, fresh or frozen, canned or any other way you like to get a variety of types and colors every day. Dark green, orange, brown, red, white, or yellow—choose a variety of colors to get all the different nutrients these provide.	**EAT at least 4 servings of vegetables a day.** A serving is about the size of ½ cup. Eat 2 or more cups of different vegetables each day.
FRUIT FOR FUN Eat fruit fresh, whole or cut up, canned or cooked. Mix it into yoghurt, put it on your cereal, make a smoothie, or freeze it into popsicles. Choose 2-3 different fruits every day just for the health of it.	**EAT at least 3 servings of fruit a day.** A serving is about the size of ½ cup. Eat 1½ or more cups of different fruits each day.
MILK, YOGURT AND CHEESE, AND OTHER CALCIUM-RICH FOODS Your bones need a lot of calcium to grow strong. Choose low-fat milk, yogurt, cheese, and ice cream. If you cannot drink dairy products, choose calcium-fortified foods, soy-based foods, and some fish.	**DRINK 3 glasses of skimmed or 1% milk a day, or an equal amount of other calcium-rich foods.**
MEAT AND BEANS FOR LEAN PROTEIN Eat protein to build strong muscles. Choose chicken, turkey, lean beef, pork, or lamb without visible fat. Choose more low-fat lunch meats than those with a greasy feel, like salami. Peanut butter and eggs are also rich in protein.	**EAT low-fat meat, brown beans, peanut butter, eggs, tofu, or other high-protein foods at least once or twice a day.**
FATS FROM PLANTS AND FISH Fats are essential for health. However, we now know that fats that come from animals, like butter and fat that is hidden in cheese, meat, and cream, can contribute to heart problems. Fats that come from vegetables, nuts, or fish do not cause the same health concerns.	Many foods have fat built into them. Therefore, *added* fats are not required for most people. However, fats carry the flavor in foods and make them very satisfying. Use butter, mayonnaise, salad dressings, or oils used for cooking with some restraint for the taste, hunger satisfaction, and enjoyment they provide. Eat deep-fried foods occasionally rather than as a rule.
SUGAR Sugar is a fun food. Almost everyone enjoys its sweetness. But sugar contains calories without nutrients. Satisfy hunger with nutritious food before too much is spent on sweet treats.	No added sugar is needed for health.

8-C

Do You Eat Enough? Daily Food Record ©

DIRECTIONS: Use a new copy of this page for each day that you record what you eat. At the end of each day, count the number of servings that you have eaten from each food group and write that number in the "count" column. When you have records for up to 5 days, record your results on 8-D—the *Do You Eat Enough?* graph. The graph will show you whether you are giving your body enough of the nutrients it needs.

MEAL ⇨ **FOOD GROUP** ⇩	**BREAKFAST**	**LUNCH**	**DINNER**	**SNACKS:** Morning Afternoon Evening	**COUNT**
GRAIN (note which are whole grains Cereal, rice, pasta, breads, wild rice, grits, tortillas, cous cous, popcorn, pancakes, waffles, etc.					
VEGETABLES Corn, peas, beans, potatoes, carrots, broccoli, beets, parsnips, lettuce, tomatoes, peppers, avocados, mushrooms, sprouts, etc.					
FRUIT Apples, bananas, oranges, melons, grapes, pineapple, peaches, pears, berries, mangos, etc.					
MILK/CALCIUM Low-fat milk, cheese, ice cream, yogurt (if these are made with cream and sugar, count also as fat/sugar), other calcium-rich foods.					
MEAT AND BEANS Fish, meats, eggs, tofu, nuts, peanut butter, brown beans, and other legumes.					
ADDED FAT/ SUGAR Butter, oil, margarine, mayonnaise, cream, cheese, cream, sugar, all foods combined with fats & sugars so most of their energy comes from the fat and/or sugar.					
WATER (Count the number of times you take a drink.)					

8-D *Do You Eat Enough?* Graph Daily Food Intake

- **Mark the number of servings you ate each day from each food group.**
- **Reach to touch the gray for the minimum each day!**

GRAINS—At least 5-6 servings per day. Try to make more than half of your choices *whole* grains.

Servings	1	2	3	4	5	6	7	8	9
Day 1									
Day 2									
Day 3									
Day 4									
Day 5									

1. Do you eat enough from each food group?

VEGETABLES—4 or more servings per day

Servings	1	2	3	4	5	6	7	8	9
Day 1									
Day 2									
Day 3									
Day 4									
Day 5									

2. If not, how can you make room for what you need?

FRUITS—3 or more servings per day

Servings	1	2	3	4	5	6	7	8	9
Day 1									
Day 2									
Day 3									
Day 4									
Day 5									

MILK, OR CALCIUM-RICH FOODS—3 glasses per day or the equivalent

Servings	1	2	3	4	5	6	7	8	9
Day 1									
Day 2									
Day 3									
Day 4									
Day 5									

MEAT AND BROWN BEANS OR LEGUMES—Once or twice per day

Servings	1	2	3	4	5	6	7	8	9
Day 1									
Day 2									
Day 3									
Day 4									
Day 5									

ADDED FATS AND SUGAR—No portions needed; enjoy in limited amounts.

Servings	1	2	3	4	5	6	7	8	9
Day 1									
Day 2									
Day 3									
Day 4									
Day 5									

Water fulfills a basic need. On average, how many drinks did you have each day? ______

8-E

In my neighborhood, stores that sell treats are everywhere.
When I see the signs, I always think, "Let's stop and get some!" (Second-grade student)

Draw an advertisement urging people to eat a variety of wholesome foods. What "story" will your advertisement tell?

Does advertising affect what you choose to eat?

LESSON 9

PHYSICAL ACTIVITY FOR CONFIDENCE IN A HEALTHY WEIGHT

Be Active for Lifelong Fitness, Strength, Enjoyment, and Balance

Body Image Building Block:

It's important not to sit too much in our free time. Being active is one of the best things we can do for our health and self-confidence.

LESSON OBJECTIVES

This lesson teaches that physical activity is the second half of the equation for confidence in a healthy weight at every size. Students will learn:

- Physical activity pairs with eating well for health at every size.
- Incentives to limit sedentary entertainment and pursue more active amusement or recreation during free time.
- To examine their daily activity choices as these relate to health and well-being.

BACKGROUND

The benefits of physical activity are indisputable. Given adequate nutrition, metabolic fitness is the single-most potent antidote known for prevention of disease and injury at every stage of life. Physical strength, flexibility, and stamina keep doors open for a wide array of satisfying activities well into old age. A proven stress reliever, activity improves sleep quality, balances a hearty enjoyment of food, and reduces depression.

Active people consistently rate their lives as more interesting and fun than those who are more sedentary. They measure higher on self esteem inventories and lower on negative body image scales. Among adolescent girls, those who are physically active have the highest self esteem scores. Being active appears to boost confidence in physical competence and encourages appreciation for bodies for reasons other than appearance.

Longitudinal studies show that many health risks associated with higher weights may be more accurately attributed to a lack of fitness. In fact, fatter people who are fit are significantly healthier than leaner people who are not fit. Given the benefits, clearly children of every size and age should be taught to *value* activity and fitness and make it a priority. Unfortunately, there is a dramatic decline in participation of girls in sports and other vigorous physical activities following entry into middle school.

Generally sedentary lifestyles have increased among Americans in the past two decades. The assumption that children get enough exercise simply by "being kids" is no longer valid. While the decline in physical activity relates to many factors beyond the scope of this lesson, three areas of concern will be addressed in this lesson:

1) DEFAULT SEDENTARY LIFESTYLES

Because significant movement is no longer an essential part of daily life for most people, reaping its benefits requires an active *choice* in use of free time. A dramatic increase in sedentary entertainment options has made this choice more difficult. Even those who describe fitness as an important personal value admit that, after fulfilling their work/study obligations, they routinely are enticed to choose captivating passive options over those requiring movement for recreation and relaxation. Engaging sedentary entertainment is available at the turn of a switch and requires little effort or expense in return for hours of amusement. Boredom rarely has the chance to stimulate more energetic options. Unfortunately, few understand the health and wellness cost associated with pairing sedentary work and school time with sedentary free time.

2) MISPLACED MOTIVATION

Despite the health, social, and emotional benefits of physical activity, many teens and adults believe that the only reason to exercise is to lose weight or to be competitive at sports.

Physical activity is a critical part of the equation for confidence in a healthy weight. Unfortunately, many people feel being active is not worth it if they "only" achieve a healthy, strong body versus weight loss or a desired size.

> *"I exercised five days a week for three months and didn't lose any weight. I thought, 'What's the point?'"*

Many sedentary people are naturally thin, and many active people are naturally fat. Choosing to be physically active may or may not result in a prescribed weight change, but it has been shown to reliably result in significant improvement in metabolic health, mental health, and overall health risks, regardless of size. Additional benefits include improved energy, confidence in physical competence and strength, greater likelihood of social inclusion, and sheer enjoyment. Finally, people *of any size* who are physically fit can be confident that they are taking charge of what they can to achieve a healthy weight.

3) MISUNDERSTANDING THE EQUATION FOR AN ACTIVE LIFESTYLE

Media messages that encourage an "all or nothing" mentality regarding exercise are self-defeating. "No pain, no gain" is an extreme on a continuum, and the perception that only tedious, aerobic workouts at a gym are beneficial leads many adults to abandon all efforts. Children and adults need to know that aerobic activity provides important benefits, but movement of *any* kind makes a difference. Recent studies have shown that an overall reduction in sedentary lifestyle may have more significant health benefits than intermittent aerobic activity. In addition, when sedentary entertainment is limited, boredom and the drive for diversion are likely to compel movement without the need for monumental doses of "will power" or "discipline."

Each child should be helped from an early age to discover movement options that are enjoyable for him or her and to understand that making time for these on a daily basis is a priority. This is not different than teaching children to understand the value of making daily time for wholesome eating, hygiene, sleep, homework, chores, playtime, family time, "down" time, etc.

Many adolescents say they dropped out of sports or other activities they enjoyed in grade school because pressures to compete took the fun out of it. Children and adults need encouragement to be active in ways that leave them feeling successfulS and that can be an ongoing, enjoyable part of their lives. This means success cannot be measured by the same standards of performance used for more physically pre-disposed individuals.

TEACH FOR THESE OUTCOMES:

Students will know:

- Being physically active and eating well are the two most important contributors to health and wellness within their control.
- A physically active life is one-half of the formula for a healthy weight, regardless of size.
- Being active includes many movement options and is not limited to an "aerobic work-out" or "sports."
- Physical activity requires making a choice, since so much of daily life is otherwise sedentary.
- In today's world, most people, thin or fat, will not be fit unless they make fitness and health a clear priority.

Student attitudes will be:

- I make it a point to be physically active every day.
- Even if TV or quiet games are fun, too much of these can crowd out the time I need to get my body moving.
- It is important for everyone to be physically active every day.
- My body can do a lot of things.
- I am regularly active and eat well, so I am confident of my weight, my strength, and my stamina.

CONCEPTS NEEDED TO TEACH THIS LESSON

- In the past, most people were physically active in the course of day-to-day life. Today's lifestyles are different and often require significant sedentary time. As a result, if active choices are not made to limit elective sedentary options and to look for opportunities that include movement, inactivity occurs by default.

  There are many physical, social, and emotional benefits to gain from physical activity.

  Physically it:

  - Strengthens the heart and other muscles and the skeletal system, and improves respiratory and circulatory function.
  - Improves agility, flexibility, balance, and speed.
  - Increases metabolism, thereby helping to balance a robust appetite with energy expenditure for a healthy weight.
  - Improves sleep.
  - Maximizes the internal regulation of body chemistry for stress relief and reduced depression.

  Emotionally it:

  - Improves self-confidence from physical competence, skill, and strength.
  - Adds to a broader sense of identity: "I am a person who is physically active and fit."
  - Increases appreciation of the body unrelated to appearance.
  - Provides an outlet for and distraction from tension.
  - Can offer a fun or pleasant pastime.
  - Challenges stagnation by offering goals for self-improvement or maintenance.

  Socially it:

  - Provides options for balanced interests (as emphasized in Lesson 2).
  - Provides opportunities for engagement or interaction with people.

- A lifestyle that is too sedentary may promote the opposite of these physical, emotional and social benefits.

- Regular aerobic activity is highly beneficial, but any movement helps to balance an otherwise sedentary lifestyle. Activities that build on personal interests are less dependent on "discipline" and are most likely to become part of a person's identity and therefore lifestyle: "I am a gardener, hiker, runner, woodworker, person who takes the stairs, dancer, nature lover," etc.

- Fitness *cannot* be assumed based on body size, weight, or BMI. We should expect participation by people with diverse levels of physical abilities, talents, and weights.

- Levels of interest in physical activity may naturally range from "born" athletes who "need" to move, to persons who find movement to be truly an effort. Social learning may encourage or discourage this innate level of interest but will probably not change it. Nonetheless, fitness as a value should be encouraged for all, just as, for example, education is valued and even mandatory while varying levels of interest and skill are accepted.

- It is safe to feel confident of a healthy weight when lifestyle behaviors routinely include wholesome eating and activities leading to metabolic fitness.

CRITICAL CONCEPTS

Students should be clear that physical activity is a vital part of the equation for confidence in a healthy weight, regardless of size. Just as eating well is vital *for both slim and fat children,* movement and fitness are, too. The *Activity Diary* that is part of this lesson has helped children gain insight into their daily activity choices.

VOCABULARY

- lifestyle
- sedentary
- fitness

LESSON PREPARATION AND MATERIALS

<table>
<tr>
<td>

Materials:

- Make an overhead of HANDOUT 9-A.
- For Activity 1: Also make overheads of 9-B or 9-D (read and choose which you prefer to use) as an example of a finished activity record. As an alternative, make an overhead of your own record (9-C or 9-E) for this purpose.
- Copy 9-C or 9-E for each student for each day they will keep a record of their activity.
- If you ask parents to keep an activity record with students, make extra copies of 9-C or 9-E.

</td>
<td>

Preparation:

- Read the *Suggested Lesson Script.*
- Become familiar with the *Guided Imagery.*
- Chose Activity 1 or Activity 2.
- For Activity 1:
  - Chose between the 9-C—*Activity Diary* and the 9-E—*Activity Pyramid.* Decide the number of days to run this activity.
  - If you prefer, complete your own 9-C or 9-E to show as an example.
- For Activity 2: Read the preparations needed for this activity. Consider inviting your physical education teacher to participate.

</td>
</tr>
</table>

LESSON SUMMARY:

- EXPLAIN: Lifestyles have changed. People are now more sedentary by default.
- READ: Guided imagery: *A Lifestyle Change for a Wild Cat.*
- DETERMINE: The outcomes of a too-sedentary lifestyle.
- PERSONALIZE: The options for developing confidence in optimal health and weight.
- DISCUSS: Three myths related to physical activity.
- INTRODUCE AND ASSIGN: Activity 1 or Activity 2 or both.
- DISCUSS: The *Activity Diary* or *Activity Pyramid.*
- ADD: *Body Image Building Block.*
- ASSIGN HOME EDUCATION.

SUGGESTED LESSON SCRIPT

PART 1: WHY BOTHER TO HAVE AN ACTIVE LIFESTYLE?

1. **IMAGINE:** Imagine I adopted a strong, frisky puppy. I liked the puppy so much, I did not want to take any chances that it might be hurt or might hurt itself in any way. To keep it safe, I never let him run around inside or out. In my home, I protected my puppy by keeping him in a nice, cushioned pen, carpeted all around, just large enough for him to grow and walk around a bit and for me to sit or stand beside him. I always made sure my dog had enough good food, fresh water, and several soft toys to chew on; and several times per day I would go into the pen to pet, brush, and hug him, and to keep him company. Two or three times a day I would take him on a leash for a nice, slow walk around the block. But to keep him from straining himself or getting hurt, I never let him run and jump around.

   Imagine that after two years of owning my dog, I decided to move to the country. Once there, I realized it was safe for the dog to run outside in the lush, grassy countryside around my new home. I opened the pen and called for the dog to run with me out across the field and up a big hill.

   ASK: What do you think the dog would do?

   TAKE ANSWERS, REVEALING THIS: The dog would not run! Or, if he ran, it would not be long before his legs became wobbly! He would quickly stop, panting hard, his heart pounding.

ASK: Why? (Even if we fed the dog for good energy, he would need to actually *use* his leg, heart, and lung muscles, or they would become very, very weak.)

TELL: The same is true with our bodies. In Lesson 8 we talked about feeding our bodies the nutrients they need. Today we are going to talk about moving our bodies so that they remain strong and healthy, *inside and out*.

2. **EXPLAIN: Lifestyles have changed**

- Not long ago people (including children) had to do a lot of physical activity just to live. They had to work with their bodies every day to get around, to work, to keep up their homes, to stay clean, to eat, and to play. (Ask students for examples.)
- Not long ago people did not think about "needing to get exercise." But in modern times, we have many machines that help us do our work that did not exist 40 or so years ago. (Ask students for examples.)
- In addition, we now have many new ways to use our free time that involve sitting. (Ask students for examples.) As a result, today people spend more time *sitting* than humans ever have. We are more *sedentary*. Since consequences occur as a result, it is very important that everyone learn and understand what happens when humans and mammals of all kinds are too sedentary.

3. **READ the following *Guided Imagery—A Lifestyle Change for a Wildcat***

Read slowly, allowing time for imaginations to work.

PART I: Have you ever wondered what it would be like to be an animal? Use your imagination to see what you can learn from an animal about our activity level affects us. Rest your elbows on your desk or knees, close your eyes, and put your hands over them. Keep them closed, stay in this position, and relax while you listen and imagine.

You are a wild cat. You can be a tiger with a large, striped body, stalking through tall grass, muscles ready to pounce on your supper.You can be a cheetah—the fastest animal in the whole world. Or, you can be a mountain lion, balancing on ledges and leaping across wide rocky crevices without fear. Decide which you will be: a powerful tiger, lightening-speed cheetah, leaping mountain lion?

After deciding which cat you are, take a few moments to get into that cat's skin. Imagine becoming the cat. Feel your cat body. Imagine yourself moving freely in the wild. Feel your muscles as you walk, run, or leap, moving through your wild world looking for food and water, pushed to be on the move by the instinct to hunt. You are strong and have to survive based on that strength and speed. You are ready to protect and care for yourself and your family with power of your healthy body, and you feel confident in your physical being.

Your daily life is balanced. You rest, you play actively with your cat family, and you follow your hunger drive and instincts to prowl and hunt for food and water. Your life is a rhythm of rest, play, hunt, and feed. You must be on the move every day to survive, but you have no trouble with this because you are strong and ready for whatever comes your way. *How do you feel about yourself?*

PART II: Now, change the scene. You are still a wild cat, and you have been born with the same strong and muscular body. But in this scene you have been born into a zoo. You and your cat family spend your days together, but you have never known the wild. You have never known what it is to run long distances through tall grass or to have to leap from rock to rock to chase down your food. Your life exists entirely within a space about the size of this classroom.

You play with your family, and there are rocks to climb. But when you wrestle or run, only a few bounds bring you to a fence that stops you. When you are hungry, instinct makes you look for food—but you never have to look far because food is brought right to you at the same time every day—ready to eat. You have no real use for your great strength. Very little physical effort is needed. You feel thirsty, and water is there, a few steps away. You walk slowly around your cage. Life is very, very easy—but you feel a little restless. You don't know why. Something drives you to pace back and forth along the fenced wall. Mostly you eat and sleep, eat and sleep, eat and sleep, and watch.

Pay attention to how you feel as this cat in the zoo. In particular, how does your body feel? How do your muscles feel? As you grow older, you spend less time pacing and more and more time resting or sleeping. There's not much reason to move, your needs are so well taken care of. When you are hungry, you eat. But your body doesn't use all the food you eat. Without use, your muscles are not as strong. The less you do, the less you feel like doing. You watch the world go by. How do you feel?

DISCUSS the imagery after each segment. Points to be made include:

- There is a range of activity that is innately optimal for a species. Quality of life is best when that level is met.
- Cats born in the zoo are not aware their lifestyle was not optimal. They did not know what was missing. While they had no way to know this, their sedentary lives rendered them less healthy physically, emotionally, and socially than they would have been in the wild where they would have been compelled to *move* by unmet needs.
- Similarly, people who have only known sedentary lives often do not know what they have lost and how their lack of physical fitness affects them.

ASK: We have talked about a puppy and about a wild cat in the zoo. What are some of the things that happen when human bodies are too inactive or sedentary?

CONVEY THE FOLLOWING: Muscles that are not well used (which includes the big muscles of your legs and arms but also the *internal* muscles, such as the heart and lungs) become weak. When this happens, our heart must work much harder to circulate the blood that keeps the rest of our body working properly. As a result, risks for many diseases increase, and our ability to participate fully in life is diminished.

ASK: We can't see our heart and lungs. How can a person know if he or she is exercising these muscles?

ANSWER: We know we are exercising the muscles of our heart and lungs when we move our arms and legs until we are breathing hard and our heart is pumping faster than normal. In this way we exercise these internal muscles that we never see.

DEMONSTRATION: *Have students count their resting pulse and count the number of breathes they take in 15 seconds at their desks before this activity begins.*

Ask students to stand by their desks and run or hop in place while moving their arms up and down rhythmically above their hearts until they begin to feel they are breathing hard and that their hearts are pumping. For some students this will happen very quickly, and for others it may take a few minutes. The more physically fit one is, the longer this takes in most cases. The main purpose of this activity is to consciously experience the point at which the heart and lungs begin to do some work.

Students should count their pulse and rate of breathing again and note the difference. Wait about two to three minutes and repeat these measures to note the return to their base level.

TELL: You can see it is easy to tell when we are exercising our heart and lungs.

4. **ASK:** Are there similarities between what happened to the zoo cats and what has happened to people in our culture in the past 40 years? What are they?

   (NOTE: If students mention that a sedentary lifestyles will make you fat, emphasize the following: Too much sitting may contribute to fatness, depending on the person. But some very thin people are "couch potatoes" and still don't get fat—even if they don't eat very well!)

TELL: Modern conveniences make it possible for us, like the zoo cats, to go through a whole day of school, work, and free time without doing much the physical activity that our bodies need to keep them strong, fit, and healthy. Too much sitting makes us sluggish. In addition, it is harder to make full use of the energy in the food we eat if we are not active.

CONCLUDE: The zoo cats did not have a choice, but you do. You can decide to be active every day throughout your life.

PART TWO: TAKING ACTION FOR FITNESS AND STRENGTH

1. **ASK**: What do we mean by movement? (Allow students to name activities that would be movement. Write answers on the board. Students may need help to broaden their thinking about all types of movement.)

   TELL: There are so many activities that can be considered movement! It seems that as long as we are not sitting completely still, we are moving. However, this can range from almost no movement to a lot. Can we put these activities into different categories? (Use Overhead 10-A to discuss these categories of movement: 1) Passive sitting, 2) Active sitting, 3) Normal movement, 4) Vigorous movement, 5) Aerobic Movement.)

   DISCUSS: What is the difference between these categories? Can you give examples of things you do in your own life that are examples for each of these categories? (Help students define the categories, using Overhead 10-A as a guide.)

2. **DISCUSS MYTHS ABOUT PHYSICAL ACTIVITY:**

   - **Myth #1: "No pain, no gain." (Explain if necessary.)**

     Fact: Studies have shown that simply *not sitting so much* helps for fitness, health, and finding your natural weight range. While getting your heart pumping every day is the best kind of exercise, too much sitting is the *biggest* problem.

     Personalize: Are there times when you could choose to do something that gets you moving rather than keeps you sitting?

   - **Myth #2: Physical activity is for people who are athletic.**

     Fact: Sure. And everyone else. You can help your health and be most confident in your weight if you are on the move with several things you like to do every day. That could include a fast-moving sport, but **what else could it include?** (standing on heads, playing jacks, a pillow fight, walking the dog, building a fort, rollerblading, cooking dinner versus buying ready to eat food, swinging, playing drums, etc.)

   - **Myth #3: Fatter people cannot be physically active.**

     Fact: What if we said, "People who aren't talented at math cannot learn to add and subtract," "People who are short cannot learn to play basketball," "People with fair skin can't go out in the sun," "People who are heavy or fatter cannot be physically active?"

Fact: Everyone can be physically active.You cannot assume someone is or is not in shape by how fat or thin he or she looks.

Some people who are very thin will not be fit at all. Some people who are fat may be more fit than you will ever be! You cannot tell how people eat by how they look, and you cannot tell how active they are, either.

What you *can* trust is, if *you* are:

a) filling up on plenty of good, nutritious food,

b) getting plenty of activity just about every day,

c) then you are doing your part to find a healthy weight that is right for you.

Don't let weight stop you from being active.

3. **ASSIGN ACTIVITY: Choose from Options 1 or 2.**

4. **ADD the *Body Image Building Block*** for Lesson 9 from I-D to the students' models.

5. **ASSIGN HOME EDUCATION:** Send the completed 9-C or 9-E Activities home as well as the Home Education slips.

How to respond if children are victims of size prejudice

Children are sometimes harassed or put down based on size, especially when they participate in vigorous activities. Prejudice about weight, height, or shape is wrong. It is usually based on ignorance, but, regardless of the reason, weightist attitudes can have long-term damaging effects. Whether students are fat or thin, help them to understand these facts:

- It shows intelligence for everyone to be physically active.
- Weightism is a form of prejudice. It is usually based on ignorance (versus merely meanness), but it is wrong, nonetheless.
- Anyone who is the target of prejudice will feel hurt, sad, and probably angry. In any case, that individual is completely justified in wanting it to stop. It is reasonable to expect adults will ensure that hurtful behaviors are stopped when these are observed or reported.
- Adults should respond to size prejudice with the same immediate, clear, zero-tolerance response that would be used with any type of harassment or prejudicial treatment.

If a child is the target of prejudice based on size, give this advice:

- Don't let it stop you from being physically active.
- Look for friends who will support you in feeling good about being active.
- Tell a teacher or other adult who understands that put-downs of any kind are wrong, and expect them to intervene to prevent further instances.

ACTIVITY—OPTION 1

Display Overhead 9-D as a guide and example for students. Distribute HANDOUT 9-E for students to record their activities for one day. Ask students to complete one *Activity Pyramid* for each day they continue the activity.

When students have kept a record of their activity for a few days, use the following set of questions for discussion.

DISCUSSION QUESTIONS:

- Did you get plenty of everyday movement most days (walking, taking the stairs, playing outside, or active play indoors)?
- Did you move vigorously for at least 30 minutes most days?
- Did you have extended (30-minute) aerobic activity most days?
- Were you surprised at the amount of sedentary time in your days?
- Do you think you're getting enough physical activity?
- If not, how can you fit more activity into your life? (Hint: Can you turn some of your sedentary entertainment time into more active fun?)

Emphasize the importance of consciously considering their daily free-time choices in order to attain a balance. Since so much of our day is spent in involuntary, sedentary school or work time, this usually requires looking for opportunities to move. For example, walking when distances are reasonable (instead of asking for a ride), taking stairs when possible, walking or running with the dog rather than letting him run in a pen, biking to chat with a neighbor rather than calling, etc. Vigorous or aerobic movement options will often have to be purposefully planned. At the same time, these can and should be intrinsically enjoyable when interests are combined with movement. Make the point that activity does not mean drudgingly going to the gym. Creative thinking about combining personal interests with movement is the key to lifelong fitness.

If time allows, repeat the activity for more days or a whole week. Encourage students to set a reasonable goal for themselves and use what they have learned to include enough physical activity in their daily lives.

ACTIVITY—OPTION 2

SET-UP FOR THIS ACTIVITY:

This activity is best done in a gym, a large, spacious room, or outside. The area should be set up into five stations, each with a sign indicating one of the five levels of physical activity (see table below). Each station should be supplied with a generous variety of equipment befitting activities for that category. You may have students bring in equipment on the day of the lesson to increase the options available.

STATIONS	EXAMPLES OF EQUIPMENT NEEDED
Passive sitting	Personal CD or tape players, stories or music on CDs, tapes or videos, crossword puzzles or other quiet, one-person games, books, computers, etc.
Active sitting	Large poster boards and colored markers, other art materials requiring use of upper body while sitting, action-figure toys or dolls, board games, etc.
Normal movement	Walking track, blackboard and chalk (standing), dress-up clothes (appropriate for both boys and girls), materials to make a sandwich, broom for sweeping, etc.
Vigorous movement	Track for skipping, cartwheels, or other large-muscle tricks, basketballs, soccer balls, a climbing area, free weights, bicycle, stilts, pogo stick, swing set, teeter-totter, climbing equipment or jungle gym, etc. These activities may be intermittent versus sustained.
Aerobic movement	Jump rope, running track, timed obstacle course, dance area with up-tempo music, hula-hoops, trampoline, etc. Activities should be done for a sustained time.

STATE: We have learned about all the many types of movement that exist. Now let's try moving at all the different levels.

Divide students evenly into five groups, and assign each group to one of the five different activity stations that you have previously set up with equipment. When you say, "Go," students should choose one activity in their station and do it without interruption until you say, "Stop" (perhaps five minutes). If you see that students stop their chosen activities before the time is up, encourage them to continue. Have students note their reactions while doing the activities. Do they enjoy them, or become tired or bored? Tell them you will discuss their reactions with them after the time is up.

After five to seven minutes, have students move to the next station, until all students have sampled activities at all five levels. When finished, have students come together to discuss their experiences.

ASK:

- How did you feel about the different activity levels?
- What did you like/not like? Why?
- Who stopped or wanted to stop before the time was up? Why?

Allow students to choose a station to which they would like to return. Let students revisit their choices for a few more minutes. If too many students choose the same station or activity within that station, you will have to device a system to allow students to have their turns.

ASK:

- Who enjoyed the activity they chose? Why?
- Who did not enjoy their activity? Why not?
- Who chose an activity at level 4 or 5? Level 1 or 2? Why did you choose that activity?
- Ask each student to name five level 4 or 5 activities that they enjoy or think they would enjoy (whether or not those options were available in your stations).

For students who cannot name any level 4 or 5 activities that they enjoy, ask them what type of movement they do enjoy. Do they like playing in teams or alone? Do they like competition or the quiet of nature and exploring? Do they like music? Too often people limit themselves unnecessarily. Encourage students to think about and experiment with activities until they discover options that will help to keep them strong and fit.

9-A OVERHEAD

CATEGORIES OF MOVEMENT

1. **Passive sitting**—Awake but sitting with both upper and lower body still. EX: Watching a video, reading, thinking, writing a letter, talking quietly, playing a hand-held game, or using a computer.

2. **Active sitting**—Sitting but with the upper body busy. EX: Doing artwork, playing cards, eating, enjoying lively conversation, or playing a more active game in which your upper body is moving.

3. **Normal movement**—Everyday movement on your feet. EX: Walking normally, doing chores, playing on your feet, going shopping, walking to school or the corner store, rehearsing a play.

4. **Vigorous movement**—On the go at a faster pace. EX: Walking fast, playing a start-stop running game, climbing trees, playing in the water, or riding a bike. This kind of movement includes a rise in heartbeat and breathing but either for short bursts of time or for sa moderate rise that is sustained for a longer time.

5. **Aerobic movement**—Working large muscles so the heart is beating rapidly for an extended time (15 to 30 minutes or more). EX: Dancing fast, swimming hard, aerobic walking, soccer or another running sport, skiing, rollerblading, or biking at a fast pace.

9-B OVERHEAD

Sample Activity Diary

	Sedentary	Active sitting	Movement	Vigorous	Aerobic
Before school		Played with cat: 15 min. Ate breakfast: 15 min. Rode bus: 15 min.	Showered: 15 min. Got dressed: 15 min.	Played & did handstands at bus stop: 15 min.	
School-day morning	Read and listened: 1/2 hr.	Worked at desk: 1 hr.	Library: 30 min. Walking: 15 min.	Phys. ed. warm-up: 15 min.	Phys. ed. running games: 15 min.
Lunch period		Ate lunch and talked with friends: 30 min.	Talked on playground: 15 min.	Played keep-away: 15 min.	
School-day after-noon	Read and listened, saw video: 1-1/4 hr.	Wrote a test: 30 min. Worked in small group: 30 min.	Choir practice: (standing) 30 min. Walked: 15 min.	Spelling "bee"—(standing & nervous): 15 min.	
After school until dinner	TV: 1 hr.	Rode bus: 15 min. Homework: 30 min.	Walked dog: 15 min.	Warmed up for soccer and on sidelines: 30 min.	Played soccer: 35 min.
Dinner and until bed	Computer game: 30 min. Read: 15 min.	Dinner: 30 min. Played cards: 15 min. Talked on phone: 15 min. Piano: 30 min.	Walked dog: 15 min. Did dishes: 15 min. Played with sister: 30 min.		
TOTALS:	*2 hours, 30 min.*	*5 hours, 30 min.*	*3 hours, 15 min.*	*1 hour, 30 min.*	*35 min.*

9-C

HOW MUCH ARE YOU ACTIVE? HOW MUCH DO YOU SIT?

Directions: Record your activity for at least two days using the following key. Use a separate Activity Diary for each day. "Guestimate" the time to the nearest 15 minutes.

Sedentary activity: Sitting very still, absorbed and focused: TV, computer games, reading, etc.
Active sitting: Sitting but busy: writing, artwork, playing cards, eating, etc.
Normal movement: Up and moving: normal walking, building an indoor fort, doing dishes, shopping
Vigorous movement: On the go: swinging, climbing, hide & seek, playing catch, heavy chores, etc.
Aerobic activity: Any activity that makes your heart race for several minutes or more without stopping.

	Sedentary	Active sitting	Movement	Vigorous	Aerobic
Before school					
School-day morning					
Lunch period					
School-day afternoon					
After school until dinner					
Dinner and until bed					
TOTALS:					

9-D ACTIVITY PYRAMID

How will you use your free time?

Sedentary:
Sitting with little movement.

Limit when possible

Active sitting:
Sitting but with upper body movement.

Do a little less

Vigorous movement:
Examples: Fast walking, playing in water, swinging, hide & seek, playing catch, heavy chores, karate, riding bike, etc.

Do a lot or regularly

Heart-pumping movement:
Examples: Fast dancing, long-distance running or swimming, aerobic walking, playing soccer, jumping rope, tag with the dog, skiing, skating, or biking fast, etc.

Do more. Do 30 minutes every day in 10 minute or longer intervals.

Everyday chores and activities on your feet:
Walking to school, building a fort, shopping, taking the stairs, playing outside, walking the dog, making the bed, helping a neighbor, rehearsing a play, painting a wall, giving a speech, sweeping the floor, baby-sitting, etc.

Do plenty every day.

9-E ACTIVITY PYRAMID

How will you use your free time?

Sedentary:

Limit when possible

Active sitting:

Do a little less

Vigorous movement:

Do a lot or regularly

Heart-pumping movement:

Do more. Do 30 minutes every day in 10 minute or longer intervals.

Everyday chores and activities on your feet:

Do plenty every day.

LESSON 10

COMPARED TO WHOM?

Selecting a Standard for Choosing Role Models

Body Image Building Block:
Choose role models you admire for things deep inside and who make you feel good about who you are.

LESSON OBJECTIVES

Students will consider how fads and fashions may sway their choice of role models, and learn what to consider in choosing healthy role models. Children will:

- Gain confidence in identifying their own needs, wants, interests, preferences, and talents, even if these differ from what appeals to others.
- Understand the difference between preferences and judgments.
- Use critical thinking to determine when fads and fashions can be fun or positive and when they become limiting or even destructive.
- Examine their current role models and consider how they will choose future role models.

BACKGROUND

Adolescents face tremendous conflicts as they begin to define themselves as young men and women. The looming possibility of increasing freedom and separation from parental figures brings eager excitement to pubescent children but also an acute sense of vulnerability. Wanting free will but still needing support and reassurance, preteens and young adolescents naturally transfer dependency needs to peers. Being accepted and included thus becomes critical. To minimize the risk of being left out, most adolescents become keenly aware of pressures to follow group norms in order to "fit in."

Individuals have historically used fads and fashions to make a statement and identify those who are "members" of their circles. But adolescents pressured by today's image-oriented culture feel that inclusion increasingly demands a unified "look." The criteria for acceptability have become ever more stringent. It is not so much who they are as who they can *appear* to be that matters. At this precarious time, many adolescents feel forced to choose between who they are and trying to fit in.

Girls: It is bad enough to worry unduly about looks, but in recent decades, we have seen a dissociative crisis in many girls that is marked by their belief that they have to risk even their health to have relationships. The statement, "Looks are everything," is widely accepted as a condition for inclusion, and the idea that girls must be thin and "look good" at any cost is often taken literally. In light of this, girls begin at an early age to look for role models who reflect "what it takes"—those who will provide desperately wanted cues about what will be favorably received, rather than role models who personify their true selves. This perceived need to bury the authentic self in favor of creating the "correct" image to present to the world takes a tragic toll on the self-esteem of adolescent girls.

Boys: Boys increasingly struggle to learn "what it takes," although the standards and options for males appear to be more flexible and the risks less extreme. In addition, boys may be less likely to take it out on themselves if they don't have the tall, lean, and buff build that is presented as "normal" in mass media advertising and entertainment. While statistics show that more boys than ever feel dissatisfied with their body sizes and shapes, males are still more likely than girls to maintain perspective—accepting the limits to their control over appearance and remembering that looks are only one aspect of who they are—not the sum total. Rather than trying to make themselves over at any cost, boys commonly redirect their energy to arenas in which they can succeed. Despite this, a growing number of boys succumb to pressures and attempt unhealthy body make-overs through excessive exercise, dieting, costly body-building products, and dangerous steroid use.

Defining group norms is developmentally normal for preteens and adolescents. But when external messages push norms based on "the way to look and act to win popularity," it is not hard to understand how adolescents opt to lose themselves rather than risk categorical dismissal. Statistics tell us only the most resilient and courageous do not succumb to these pressures.

In light of pressures facing boys and girls today, our challenge is to help young students maintain integrity, stay connected to themselves, and make choices that will enhance their health and well being. Children can be helped to think critically about toxic judgments before they are consumed by them. But this cannot occur if adults—their primary role models—are silent. When, in the face of powerful cultural forces, adults feel overwhelmed and helpless, it becomes necessary to step back to see how we, too, have been caught and desensitized to the status quo. Sometimes a question from a simple children's story can help: What if the Ugly Duckling had stayed with the ducks? Unfortunately, this is the common choice today, with many adults and young people learning to compare themselves without question to a standard that was never realistic for them in the first place and feeling ugly as a result.

Whether we are able to stop the ducks or any others from unfair and harsh judgments, we know instinctually what to say to the swan and to our young students: *"Be who you are, and find those with whom you can grow into all you can be."* This message is the heart of Lesson 10 and this curriculum.

TEACH FOR THESE OUTCOMES

Students will know:

- How to discern preferences and judgments.
- Fads and fashions can be fun and encourage connections, or hurtful and encourage exclusion.
- In making comparisons, the standard used must be very carefully chosen.
- How to chose positive, realistic role models with deeper qualities that make us feel good about who we are.

Student attitudes will be:

- I know what I like.
- My idea of what's cool and someone else's idea may be different.
- I can stay true to what I like and who I am even if others don't think it's cool.
- People are different. This doesn't mean they are better or worse.
- You have to be who you are on the inside, even if others don't understand.
- If I feel bad about myself when I compare myself to someone, I've probably chosen the wrong role model.
- It can help to have role models you admire for qualities that are deep inside.
- I will look for friends with whom I feel good.

CONCEPTS NEEDED TO TEACH THIS LESSON

- The essence of a person is the *authentic self*. If the authentic self is buried, the result is a repressed or potentially dissociated personality, and optimal growth is diminished.
- *Judgments* reflect right and wrong, good and bad. *Preferences* come out of the authentic self and reflect natural diversity.
- Needing connection and a sense of interdependency are signs of health and normalcy. Humans need relationships and are enriched by a sense of "belonging" within a community. Given this need, if expression of the authentic self is negatively judged (or seems at risk of judgment), the true self may be hidden in hopes of securing relationships.
- Adolescents are at particular risk. Because of this unique and vulnerable transition stage, when identification is gradually transferred from primary caregivers to others, acceptance by others becomes critical. If "what's cool" is perceived as a criterion for acceptance by others, then *having* "what's cool" naturally becomes vital. When adolescents are unsure if they are "cool enough," fear of judgment increases, and relationships are perceived to be at risk. Adolescents may very well try to suppress their true selves in order to appear to "have what it takes" to be included.

- When honest preferences are suppressed long enough, they may become repressed, or lost from conscious awareness. Individuals may sacrifice the ability to know or do what pleases or displeases them for the sake of "acceptability." This loss puts the individual at risk for other unhealthy choices.
- Mass media has become instrumental in culture-wide promotion of a narrow set of criteria defining "what's cool" or acceptable. Mass media directly targets youth as a market with money to spend, delivering messages that stress the need to meet these criteria in order to be perceived as desirable.
- Children can be supported in maintaining integrity and autonomy by lessons teaching them critical thinking skills and what to consider in choosing healthy role models.
- Adults can influence children to have a stake in choosing healthy role models by identifying toxic social environments and media messages, and intervening *before* children become desensitized.

CRITICAL CONCEPTS

This lesson provides skills for choosing healthy, realistic role models. Since choosing role models is a major task of adolescence, these are critical skills.

VOCABULARY

- role model

LESSON PREPARATION AND MATERIALS

Materials:	**Preparation:**
▪ Copy an overhead of HANDOUTS 10-A for discussion. ▪ Copy 10-B and 10-C.	▪ Read the *Suggested Lesson Script.* ▪ Obtain the story of *The Ugly Duckling* by Hans Christian Anderson. Many versions may be found on the Internet.

LESSON SUMMARY

- READ: *The Ugly Duckling.*
- EXPERIENCE & DEFINE: Judgments versus preferences.
- CONSIDER: Fads and fashions can be fun, or they can be limiting or destructive.
- DISCERN: What helped the Ugly Duckling get through his painful time?
- RECOGNIZE: It makes a difference who or what you compare yourself or others to.
- ACTIVITY: 10-B—*Who Will You Choose as Your Role Models?*

- ASSIGN: 10-C—*When You or Someone You Know Felt Like the Ugly Duckling*
- ADD: *Body Image Building Block.*
- ASSIGN HOME EDUCATION.

SUGGESTED LESSON SCRIPT

1. **INTRODUCE:** *The Ugly Duckling* is a familiar story, and it has an important message. As you listen to this story, think about these questions:

> *Show overhead 10-A or list these questions on the blackboard:*
>
> A. What if the swan had stayed with the ducks?
>
> B. If one choice is "good," are other choices "bad?"
>
> C. We all like things that are "cool." Are there times when what is considered to be "cool" is not right for everyone?
>
> D. Does it matter to what or to whom we compare ourselves?
>
> - If apples compared themselves to oranges, how would they feel about being apples?
> - The Namuh compared themselves to tall, thin, unusually beautiful models. How did this affect them?
>
> E. How can the experience of the Ugly Duckling help you in your life?

READ: *The Ugly Duckling*

2. **DISCUSSION OF QUESTIONS**: (Refer to Overhead 10-A or the blackboard.)

A) What if the swan had stayed with the ducks?

DISCUSS: This conversation should help students consider the negative effect of comparing oneself to a standard that is not realistic in the first place and feeling awful as a result. The swan was wise to pay attention to the pain this was causing him and to make a courageous decision to look for another option.

B) If one choice is "good," are other choices "bad"?

- What if someone said his or her favorite color or song was different than yours? (Most will feel fine about this.)
- What if someone said your favorite:
  - Color was ugly?
  - Activity was boring?
  - Clothes were not cool?
  - Hair style was not "in"?
  - Food was "yucky"?
  - Friend was a "nerd"?
- What if a whole group of kids said these things?

CLARIFY: These are judgments, and they do not feel good.

Judgments conclude something is "good" or "bad." Judgments say this way is "right" and that is "wrong." Judgments say this is "cool" and that is "not cool." Judgments are all or nothing, black or white.

ASK: Who has felt that something about you was judged? How did that feel?

- Did you feel a little like the Ugly Duckling must have felt? Why? Why not?
- Did your experience change how you felt about yourself? (Or how you felt about an item you liked, your idea or wish?) Why? Why not?

C) We all like things that are "cool."

> ***Example***: If the latest cool thing to do is to wear the school colors every Friday, anyone can be part of that fad if they want to join in. If they don't, that's OK too. Most fads come and go. They're fun. They don't hurt anyone. They make life interesting.

ASK: Are there times when what is considered to be cool isn't right for everyone?

TELL: When what is cool becomes a judgment, this can hurt.

DISCUSS: What if "what's cool" doesn't work or fit for you? What if, like the Ugly Duckling, you cannot go along and still be true to who you are?

> ***Example***: You don't like the latest fad; you're not good at it; you don't believe in it; it means acting or looking a certain way that just isn't your style or way of doing things, etc.

EMPHASIZE: This is a problem that happens to everyone at some time. It is important to stay true to yourself.

D) Does it matter to what or whom we compare ourselves?

- If apples compared themselves to oranges, how would they feel about being apples?
- The Namuh compared themselves to tall, thin, unusually beautiful models. How did this affect them?
- When the swan compared himself to the ducks, he felt ugly.

DEFINE: Role models are people we admire and look up to. We see qualities in our role models that we would like to develop in ourselves.

Everyone has role models (whether we know it or not). As we have seen, when we compare ourselves to a person we have chosen as a role models, it can either help or hurt us.

- It is important to choose role models that provide a standard against which we can feel good about ourselves.
- It is important to choose role models that reflect qualities that we value deep inside—not merely surface traits.
- It is important to think about the qualities we value the most and choose role models that will help us be the best you that we can be.

E) How can the experience of the Ugly Duckling help us in our lives?

Include these points in your discussion: (Points are also listed at the bottom of Handout 11-C)

What helped the Ugly Duckling when he could not be cool with the ducks?

- He did not keep trying to be something he wasn't. When the ducks did not appreciate him, he decided he could not stay with them. Even though he felt awful, he realized he would be better off leaving them behind. At the same time, he did not give up. He looked for another place to belong.
- Even though they were not a perfect fit, the swan found caring companions along the way. When he met those who did not have his best interests at heart, he moved on again.
- Finally he saw some creatures who touched him very deeply inside.

- He realized what had touched him was what he shared in common with these creatures. In the end, because he followed his own heart, he discovered the beauty he shared with his fellow swans. He felt good about himself.
- He accepted that he could not change the ducks' judgment, but he knew that they were wrong about him. He believed in himself.

3. **ACTIVITIES:** Follow the directions for one or both of the following activities:

   10-B—*Who Will You Chose as Your Role Models?*

   10-C—*When You or Someone You Know Felt Like the Ugly Duckling*

4. **ADD** the *Body Image Building Block* for Lesson 10 from I-D to student's models.

5. **DISCUSS and ADD** the final *Body Image Building Block* from I-D to students' models.

Body Image Building Block:

It helps to support each other in having a healthy body image, in eating well, and in being active.

6. **ASSIGN HOME EDUCATION**: Have students discuss Handouts 10-B and/or 10-C at home and return the Home Education slip.

Optional Activity—Influencing School Policy

Does your school have a policy prohibiting size discrimination? If not, would your students like to present a proposal to the school board or administration asking for a policy to promote health at every size and mandate zero-tolerance for size discrimination? Students could develop their arguments based on concepts learned throughout the *Healthy Body Image* curriculum and ask for a hearing to present their case.

10-A Overhead

WHAT DO YOU THINK?

A. What if the swan had stayed with the ducks?

B. If one choice is "*good,*" are other choices "*bad*"?

C. We all like things that are "cool." Are there times when what is considered to be cool isn't right for everyone?

D. Does it matter to what or to whom we compare ourselves?

- If apples compared themselves to oranges, how would they feel about being apples?
- The Namuh compared themselves to tall, thin, unusually beautiful models. How did this affect them?

E. How can the experience of the *Ugly Duckling* help you in your life?

10-B WHO WILL YOU CHOOSE FOR YOUR ROLE MODELS?

1. People we admire often become our role models. Think of two people you admire and might choose as role models. At least one should be someone you know personally. The other may be someone you do not know but have read or heard a lot about.
   - *You should know more than one quality about your role model. For example, you may admire a famous athlete, but if you only know he or she is a great athlete, and nothing more, that would not be enough.*

2. List at least five qualities about each of these people that you admire and would like to develop in yourself. If you cannot think of five, choose a different person for your role model.
   - *Consider deeper qualities in your role model, not merely what you see on the surface. For example, what type of person he or she is, what does he or she believe in and how does he or she act?*
   - *If you were to try to be like the role models you have chosen, would you feel healthy and stronger, or would you feel mismatched, like the Ugly Duckling?*

Name of your role model:	**Name of your role model**
______________________	______________________
Five qualities you admire in this person:	**Five qualities you admire in this person:**
______________________	______________________
______________________	______________________
______________________	______________________
______________________	______________________
______________________	______________________
______________________	______________________
______________________	______________________
______________________	______________________
______________________	______________________
______________________	______________________
______________________	______________________
______________________	______________________
______________________	______________________
______________________	______________________
______________________	______________________

10-C **Adults may also answer the following question and share their responses with students.**

Draw a picture or write about a time when you or someone you know felt like the Ugly Duckling

Just about everyone has felt like the *Ugly Duckling* sometime. Think of a real-life example of this from your own or someone else's life. Then draw a picture or write about this. How did you or the person cope with this? What ideas do you have now about what might have helped?

Remember what helped the Ugly Duckling? The same things could help you:

- He did not keep trying to be something he was not meant to be.
- He did not keep trying with those who would not appreciate him.
- He did not give up. He knew he needed to belong somewhere.
- He let caring companions help him along the way.
- When he met those who did not have his best interests at heart, he moved on.
- He paid attention to what had touched him in a good way *deep inside.*
- He found others with whom he naturally shared things in common and saw their beauty in himself.
- He recognized he could not change the ducks, but he knew they were wrong about him.
- He realized he could feel good about himself.

APPENDIX

Table of Contents

A *Whole-School* Approach to a Healthy Body Image, Eating, Nutrition, Fitness, and Weight

Most educators know that there is a check-list of signs and symptoms for dangerous eating and weight-management problems (such as eating disorders) that calls for an active response. Unfortunately, few are attuned to the fact that most of the primary risk factors for these serious problems are considered perfectly "normal" in the environment in which today's children grow up. Negative body image, fear of fatness, restrictive dieting for weight loss, and complacency about health habits are an everyday part of life for most girls and boys. Students either experience these problems themselves or are quite literally surrounded by peers and adults who do. This is not a benign environment. While lesson plans such as this one can have a positive prevention effect, the need for support from the social context within which students spend their days is essential for long-term change. For this to take place, health and healthy body image principles, such as those included in this curriculum, should be taught not only to students but to school administrators, teachers, coaches, support staff, and parents. In turn, a micro-environment can be created within which students are supported.

A *whole-school approach* has been encouraged by notable prevention specialists for the past decade or more. As summarized by Michael Levine, experts agree that:

> *"...increases in individual resistance to negative influences must be supported and facilitated by active changes in the systems that define the lives of (students) in general... Programs...need to change the people—including adults...and the social systems that influence and regulate the lives of children."*

A systemic approach to body image, eating, nutrition, fitness, and weight concerns may be dismissed because it is a big undertaking as well as potentially "controversial." However, anecdotal experiences of schools that have taken on this goal, as well as the published work of Niva Piran (in particular), demonstrate that it is, indeed, possible and effective. When schools undertake to change the *overall climate* in regard to attitudes about body image, weight, and lifestyle habits, students are supported, not only conceptually, but through the common knowledge, values, language, and actions of the community.

The creation of a *whole-school* environment within which students feel safe, respected, nurtured, and encouraged to grow and develop with appreciation and respect for their diverse physical bodies is entirely compatible with the policies already in place at most, if not all, schools. It does, however, require an additional commitment to consciousness-raising for adults about the intense pressures faced by students regarding appearance, the clash between their biology and cultural expectations, the dangers of restrictive dieting for weight loss, and the challenges of wholesome eating and active lifestyles in today's world.

In addition to heightened awareness of these problems, new models for promoting realistic body image attitudes and healthy lifestyle habits, such as the *Model for Healthy Body Image*, should be shared by the entire community. In addition, opportunities to name and discuss pressures that students feel, as well as channels for activism and advocacy within the system, should be provided. Empirical evidence suggests that environments that encourage a student's "voice" in response to challenges to healthy body esteem help to prevent destructive responses, such as disordered eating. For example, such environments help students to convert negative personal indictments, such as "I am fat and disgusting," into words describing the source of their feelings: "There is so much pressure to look and be a certain way to be accepted. It makes me feel afraid and out of control."

Promotion of health versus a "war on obesity"

Many physicians, health organizations, educators, and parents are concerned about the health risks that have been associated with overweight and obesity. In turn, schools across the country are feeling pressured to join the battle against fat. Before taking action, it is essential that schools inform themselves about the problems associated with a response that does not take into account the *entire spectrum* of body image, eating, nutrition, fitness, and weight concerns. As readers of this manuals are aware, not only does a focus on weight loss not solve the problem, it routinely contributes to it.

Prevention specialists recommend an alternative paradigm—a perspective to successfully and simultaneously address the concerns of 1) those wishing to prevent and reverse unhealthy overweight and obesity, 2) those concerned with eating and dieting disorders, 3) those concerned with prejudicial and unjust "weightist" attitudes, and 4) those simply concerned with health. This approach urges policy makers, educators, and lay people alike to reframe the issue as one of health promotion versus one of size and weight. This argument turns the "plan of attack" from one that is essentially negative and pejorative (i.e., focused on the "bad" behavior people should stop doing—as in "stop eating so much candy," "stop watching so much TV"—which provokes shame or resistance) into one that is positive, respectful, and universally feasible. Rather than waging a *war on obesity,* prevention experts recommend that we teach *what to do for health* as a far more effective strategy that is consistent with principles of learning and motivation.

Within micro-environments such as whole-school communities, children and adults can learn and mutually support constructive values, attitudes, and behaviors that actually work. Imagine an environment in which the norm is to 1) maintain perspective on the importance of appearance, 2) accept innate diversity in body size and shape, 3) develop an identity based on inner strengths, 4) eat more nutritious food regardless of weight, 5) be active for fun, fitness, and sociability regardless of size, and 6) appreciate and enjoy strength, vitality, and stamina.

A whole-school approach

In the face of conflicting pressures, schools are urged to incorporate programs and policies that promote principles of health for all, without discrimination. Once a suitable model has been chosen, such as that taught by this *Healthy Body Image* curriculum, it will be helpful for schools to develop a *whole-school approach* to encourage a supportive environment for students within the wider culture. To guide administrators, teachers, and parents, an outline adapted from the work of Niva Piran is presented on the following page.

Guidance for Developing a *Whole-School Approach** to Healthy Body Image, Eating, Fitness, and Weight

Administration

- Move beyond ambivalence.
- Assume responsibility for and commit to challenging an unhealthy status quo, even if it is culturally "normal."
- Discern health promotion models that consider the entire spectrum of body image and health concerns.
- Develop a systematic approach for eliminating unhealthy norms. Administer policies toward that end.
- Communicate new norms to students, parents, and families and to the wider community.

Teachers

- Examine your own experiences, knowledge base, prejudices, and attitudes about body size, eating, fitness, and weight.
- Learn about the developmental challenges children face within the context of social pressures and prejudices about size.
- Network and seek validation for initiatives to transform student's experiences, knowledge, and competencies.
- Seek curricular support for this work. Integrate body image lessons into existing curricula (science, health, and social studies).
- Model a healthy lifestyle, including body acceptance, a non-dieting pproach, positive eating behaviors, and physical fitness, regardless of size.
- Educate yourself about signs of and referral resources for weight/shape concerns.
- Actively create and reinforce class norms supporting health and healthy body image.
- Empower students and student "voice."
- Step in when sub-threshold signs and symptoms become apparent (i.e., overt display of negative body image, restrictive dieting, inadequate attention to nutrition needs, etc.).

Parents:

- Do self-exploration. Examine your own experiences, knowledge, prejudices, and attitudes about body size and eating.
- Learn about the developmental challenges children face within the context of social pressures and prejudices.
- Actively talk to children about adverse pressures (unhealthy media messages, teasing, etc.).
- Educate children about normal developmental changes expected with puberty, and genetic diversity of body size and shape.
- Model a healthy lifestyle, including body acceptance, a non-dieting approach, positive eating behaviors, physical fitness, etc.
- Educate yourself about signs of and referral resources for weight/shape concerns.
- Step in when sub-threshold signs and symptoms become apparent (i.e., overt display of negative body image, restrictive dieting, inadequate attention to nutrition needs, etc.).

* Adapted from the work of Niva Piran, Ph.D., University of Toronto

To parents and caregivers from the author of the *Healthy Body Image* curriculum.

Your child is about to begin a series of lessons called *Healthy Body Image: Teaching Kids to Eat and Love Their Bodies, Too!* This unit is designed to promote healthy body image, eating, nutrition, fitness, and weight related knowledge, attitudes, and behaviors.

Following is the mission statement for the *Healthy Body Image* curriculum:

- To empower boys and girls to form a foundation for positive body esteem based on recognition of what they can and cannot control in regard to body size and shape.
- To prepare and empower boys and girls to resist unhealthy and unrealistic cultural pressures regarding body image, eating, nutrition, fitness, and weight.
- To inspire boys and girls to develop a stake in wholesome eating and physical fitness.

Just about everyone today is affected by many confusing and conflicting messages about size, shape, weight, eating, fitness, and health. I hope you, as a parent, welcome this opportunity for your child to receive clear, realistic, age-appropriate lessons that will help him or her to:

- develop an identity based on inner strengths, not on appearance.
- gain historical perspective on today's body image attitudes.
- understand normal weight gain during puberty.
- respect genetic diversity of size and shape.
- become aware of the dangers and counterproductive effects of dieting for weight loss.
- think critically about media messages.
- become motivated to eat well and stay fit for health at every size.

A companion book for parents is now available, entitled *Real Kids Come in All Sizes: Ten Essential Lessons to Build Your Child's Body Esteem,* by Kathy Kater. This book provides the same lessons that your child will be learning in the classroom in an easy-to-read guide for parents at home. You will find it at major book stores, or may order it by phone from the National Eating Disorders Association (206-382-3587) or on-line at www.nationaleatingdisorders.org.

Many of the *Healthy Body Image* lessons contain handouts for students to take home. It will be helpful if you read and discuss these with your child. It's possible some adults may find these healthy-body image lessons to be challenging due to their own body image demons. If this is true for you, do not feel that you are alone. Many adults have learned to struggle with body image, eating, nutrition, fitness, and weight. In light of this, if you can embrace these positive lessons for yourself, I hope you will. If not, take heart in knowing you can reinforce a healthier and easier path for your child.

Kathy J. Kater

STAFF DEVELOPMENT AND COMMUNITY EDUCATION OPTIONS

The lessons in this curriculum guide are designed to be self-instructive for teachers. However, concepts may be challenging in light of prevalent cultural norms about size, shape, weight, eating, nutrition, and fitness, and schools may wish to consider additional training options for staff and/or the wider school community.

The author of the *Healthy Body Image* curriculum, is available on a limited basis as a staff trainer, workshop leader, or speaker. A variety of opportunities are possible, ranging from a ninety-minute community education event to half or full days of in-service training for teachers.

Contact information:

Kathy Kater, LICSW
2497 7th Avenue East, Suite 109
North St. Paul, MN 55109

Website: *www.bodyimagehealth.org*

Telephone: 651-770-2693 Email: kathykater@isd.net

COMPANION BOOK FOR PARENTS AND AUXILIARY EDUCATORS

Real Kids Come in All Sizes

Ten Essential Lessons to Build Your Child's Body Esteem

By Kathy Kater

(Broadway Books/Random House, 2004)

\$14.00 U.S. \$21.00 Canada

Real Kids Come in All Sizes was written in response to the need for parents and other supporting adults to learn the same healthy body image concepts that students were learning in the classroom. This 250-page book is an easy-to-read, friendly guide that helps parents to provide a supportive environment for boys and girls at home, and auxiliary school staff to reinforce the *Healthy Body Image* lessons school-wide.

You will find *Real Kids Come in All Sizes* in major bookstores, or you may order it from the address below:

National Eating Disorders Association

603 Stewart Street, Suite 803

Seattle, WA 98101

Telephone: 206-382-3587 Website: www.NationalEatingDisorders.org

ABOUT THE AUTHOR

Kathy Kater is a psychotherapist who has treated body image, eating and weight concerns for 27 years. Frustrated that progress in understanding these problems had not been matched by effective prevention, she authored *Healthy Body Image: Teaching Kids to Eat and Love Their Bodies Too!* when her own daughter was about to enter 4th grade. This comprehensive prevention curriculum, first published in 1998 by the National Eating Disorder Association, is among the first of its kind to demonstrate significant, measurable improvement in weight related attitudes in pubescent children. *Healthy Body Image* has been recommended by the U.S. Department of Health, Office of Women's Health in their *BodyWise* information packet for educators, and is used in schools all across the country. This fully revised edition updates the empirical basis for these lessons, responds to scientific, social and cultural changes in the past 6 years, and integrates the experience of seasoned teachers who have taught these lessons.

In response to requests from educators and parents, Kathy Kater wrote *Real Kids Come in All Sizes: Ten Essential Lessons to Build Your Child's Body Esteem*, published in 2004 by Broadway Books/Random House.

Kater is an internationally recognized speaker on promotion of healthy body image, eating, nutrition, fitness, and weight. She has been a featured guest on Public Television and Radio, and is regularly interviewed as an expert consultant by nationally distributed magazines and newspapers. For more information, go to www.bodyimagehealth.org.

RECOMMENDED READING FOR STAFF, PARENTS, AND CHILDREN

Books for adults

Real Kids Come in All Sizes: Ten Essential Lessons to Build Your Child's Body Esteem, by Kathy Kater. A companion book to the *Healthy Body Image* curriculum provides the same lessons students receive in the classroom as an easy-to-read guide for parents.

Can't Buy My Love: How Advertising Changes the Way We Think and Feel, by Jean Kilbourne. An important book on the power and purpose of mass media.

Afraid to Eat: Children and Teens in Weight Crisis, by Frances M. Berg. A well-researched book that challenges how the American culture promotes unhealthy eating and body image attitudes.

Underage and Overweight, Frances M. Berg. Guide for parents who want their children to lead healthy, active lives at every size.

How To Say It to Girls, by Nancy Gruver. A guide to talking with daughters.

A Very Hungry Girl: How I Filled Up on Life…and How You Can, Too!, by Jessica Weiner. A powerful story of rebuilding body integrity and esteem.

The Body Myth: Adult Women and the Pressures to be Perfect, by Margo Maine and Joe Kelly. Discusses how the culturally generated drive to be thin can become a dangerous addiction.

The Body Project, by Joan Jacobs Brumberg. Chronicles the change in body image attitudes in women over the past 100 years through the diaries of girls.

Body Wars: Making Peace with Women's Bodies, by Margo Maine. An activist's guide for those who want to fight the forces that pressure women to feel uncomfortable in their own bodies.

Big Fat Lies: The Truth About Your Weight and Your Health, by Glen Gaesser. Summarizes the medical research on body-size diversity and the expected failure of dieting for weight loss. Written for lay audiences.

How to Get Your Child to Eat—But Not Too Much, by Ellyn Satter. A no-nonsense approach to feeding kids well without power struggles.

The Secrets of Feeding a Healthy Family, by Ellyn Satter, Helps adults establish a positive feeding relationship with children.

Preventing Childhood Eating Problems, by Jane Hirschmann and Lela Zaphiropoulos. Based on evidence that children will naturally self-regulate their eating if rigid rules are not imposed.

The Rules of "Normal" Eating, by Karen Koenig. A practical guide for a healthy relationship with food clears up the confusion about "eating right."

Intuitive Eating, by Evelyn Tribole. Helps readers equate feeling good with health, not weight loss.

Am I Hungry? What To Do When Diets Don't Work, by Michelle May. Provides tools to understand hunger, with sound recommendations about nutrition and fitness.

Bodylove, by Rita Freedman. Affirms every person's right to live comfortably in her own body.

Self-Esteem Comes in All Sizes, by Carol Johnson. Upbeat book on loving yourself and taking care of your health at any size.

Dads and Daughters: How to Inspire, Understand, and Support Your Daughter When She's Growing Up So Fast, by Joe Kelly. Help for Dads in relating to their developing daughters.

Father Hunger: Father's, Daughters, and the Pursuit of Thinness, by Margo Maine. Explains the emptiness and resulting food and body image disorders experienced by women with distant or emotionally absent fathers.

Reviving Ophelia, by Mary Pipher. An eye-opening book on the everyday dangers of growing up young and female in America.

Am I Fat? Helping Young Children Accept Differences in Body Size, by Joanne Ikeda and Priscilla Naworski.

The What's Happening to My Body? For Girls and *The What's Happening to My Body? For Boys*, Lynda Madaras. Good information about pubescent changes.

The Adonis Complex, by Harrison G. Pope, Jr. Discusses male body obsession.

Moving Away From Diets, by Karin Kratina, R.D. Help for adults and parents in breaking the diet mentality.

The Skinny on Fat, by Shana Vogel.

Body Thieves: Help Girls Reclaim Their Natural Bodies and Become Physically Active, by Sondra Friedman. Offers girls the right messages in today's cultural environment.

When Women Stop Hating Their Bodies, by Jane Hirschmann.

Books for adults about eating disorders in children and teens

Helping Your Child Overcome an Eating Disorder, by Bethany Teachman.

When Your Child Has an Eating Disorder, by Abigail Natenshon.

Help Your Teenager Beat an Eating Disorder, by James Lock and Daniel Le Grange.

Surviving an Eating Disorder; Perspectives and Strategies for Family & Friends, by Michelle Siegel and Judith Brisman.

The Parent's Guide to Childhood Eating Disorders, by Marcia Herrin and Nancy Matsumoto.

Eating Disorders: A Parent's Guide, by Rachel Bryant-Waugh and Bryan Lask.

Over It: A Teen's Guide to Getting Beyond Obsessions with Food and Weight, by Carol Emery Normandi and Laurelee Roark. For mature middle schoolers and high school students.

Videos for adults and teens (Use discretion for young audiences.)

Behind Closed Doors: Available at a nominal cost from www.remudaranch.com. Dramatically demonstrates how unrealistic images are purposefully created by advertisers to develop a sense of insecurity to promote sales.

Killing Us Softly 3: Available from the Media Education Foundation, www.mediaed.org. Describes how the image of women in advertising has changed in the past 20 years.

Books for children

Fiction

Shapesville, by J. Andrew Mills and Rebecca Osborn.

Full Mouse, Empty Mouse, by Dina Zeckhausen

I Like Me! by Nancy Carlson

Liking Myself, by Pat Palmer

Charlie the Caterpillar, by Dom Deluise

Wish I were a Butterfly, by James Howe

The Missing Piece, by Shel Silverstein

A Porcupine Named Fluffy, by Helen Lester

Beanpole, by Barbara Park

King Midas and His Golden Touch, Greek mythology

Leo the Late Bloomer, by Robert Kraus

Seven Blind Mice, by Ed Young

Star Bellied Sneeches, by Dr. Seuss

Oh, the Places You'll Go! by Dr. Seuss

The Ugly Duckling, by Hans Christian Anderson

The Berenstain Bears and Too Much TV, by Jan and Stan Berenstain

The Berenstain Bears and Too Much Junk Food, by Jan and Stan Berenstain

Little Two Eyes, by Brothers Grimm

William's Doll, by Zolotow

The Lovables in the Kingdom of Self-Esteem, by Diane Loomans

Nell's Quilt, by Susan Terris

Blubber, by Judy Blume

Tales of A Fourth Grade Nothing, by Judy Blume

One Fat Summer, by Robert Lipsyte

Heads You Win, Tails I Lose, by Isabelle Holland

The Pig-Out Blues, by Jan Greenberg

Belinda's Bouquet, by Leslea Newman & Alyson Wonderland (Available from NAAFA 916-558-6880.)

Are You Too Fat, Ginny? by Karin Jasper (Available from NAAFA 916-558-6880.)

Nothing's Fair in Fifth Grade, by Barthe DeClements

Non-fiction for children

Girl Zone Body Talk: The Straight Facts on Fitness, Nutrition & Feeling Great About Yourself, by Ann Douglas & Julie Douglas

Girl Power in the Mirror: A Book About Girls, Their Bodies, and Themselves, by Helen Courdes

Real Gorgeous: The Truth About Body and Beauty, by Kaz Cooke

Children Just Like Me: A Unique Celebration of Children Around the World, by B. & A. Kindersley

People, by Peter Spier

New Moon: The Magazine for Girls, available at news stands or from New Moon Publishing, P. O. Box 3587, Duluth, MN 55803-3587.

Am I Fat? Helping Young Children Accept Differences in Body Size, Joanne Ikeda & Priscilla Naworski

What Do You Stand For? A Kid's Guide to Building Character, by Barbara Lewis

Good Answers to Tough Questions About Weight Problems and Eating Disorders, by Joy Berry

Websites and organizations

Dads and Daughters: www.dadsanddaughters.org — Provides tools for fathers to strengthen relationships with their daughters and to transform messages that value young women more for how they look than who they are.

Gurze Books: www.bulimia.com — Specializes in eating disorder resources and education.

Measured Outcomes Using The *Healthy Body Image* Curriculum

Two published studies have reported the results of the *Healthy Body Image* curriculum in fourth- through sixth-grade classrooms. Abstracts of these reports are included here along with references for the full article.

1. ***An Elementary School Project for Developing Healthy Body Image and Reducing Risk Factors for Unhealthy and Disordered Eating,* by Kathy Kater, John Rohwer, and Michael P. Levine; Eating Disorders: Journal of Treatment and Prevention; Wtr. 1998, Vol. 8:1: 3-16.**

   Negative body image and disordered eating patterns are prevalent among American adolescents, especially girls. Because attitudes are extremely difficult to change once they are established, researchers have proposed that prevention programs that aim to challenge prevalent cultural norms contributing to these problems be developed for older elementary-age children whose body image attitudes are not yet intractable. This article describes the short-term outcomes of a new school-based curriculum model for developing healthy body images and preventing disordered eating with 222 fourth and sixth grade boys and girls. Preliminary results indicate the curriculum positively influenced knowledge, attitudes, and intentions related to body image, the limits to control of body size and shape, the hazards of weight-loss dieting, and unrealistic media images. While existing prevention curricula aimed at adolescents has had little positive impact, the promising effect of this model appears related to 1) the targeted age-range, 2) the experiential pedagogy, 3) the emphasis on identity development from diverse sources that reflect competency and interests rather than image, and 4) critical thinking regarding the clash between cultural values and human biology. "Booster" lessons to reinforce these primary prevention concepts should follow as children progress through the transitional middle school years.

2. ***Evaluation of an Upper Elementary School Program to Prevent Body Image, Eating and Weight Concerns*, by Kathy Kater, John Rohwer, and Karen Londre; Journal of School Health; May 2002, Vol. 72:5: 199-204.**

   Preparing young students to resist the socio-cultural pressures that contribute to body image and eating problems in American culture poses a monumental challenge. This project determined whether the 11-lesson *Healthy Body Image: Teaching Kids to Eat and Love Their Bodies Too!* curriculum would have a positive effect when presented to upper elementary–age children. A controlled study with 415 test students measured changes from pre-test to post-test related to: 1) body image, 2) knowledge about the biology of size, shape, and restricted hunger, or dieting, 3) body-size prejudice, 4) media images, 5) self-image; and 6) lifestyle behaviors. Boys and girls who completed the curriculum showed significant or notable improvement compared to a control group not exposed to the curriculum. Results suggest it is possible to provide children with a knowledge base to use as they face increasing pressures about appearance, weight, and eating in the critical middle school years.

REFERENCES

In an effort to provide some categorization but eliminate repetition, references are listed only once under one of the headings below. However, since all references are included for their relevance to body image and weight related attitudes as well as eating and fitness behaviors, many contain material pertinent to several categories. For example, most references under #3) The effects of weight loss diets, are part of # 2) Etiology of disordered eating, as are references under # 4) Social learning theory and cultural context. Even so, the rough groupings seemed preferable to no subdivision at all.

1) Developmental perspectives

Brumberg, J. (1997). *The Body Project: An Intimate History of American Girls.* New York: Random House.

Emmons, L. (1994). Predisposing factors differentiating adolescent dieters and non-dieters. *Journal of the American Dietetic Association, 94,* 725-731.

Ewell, F., Smith., S., Karmel, M. P., & Hart, D. (1996). The sense of self and its development: A framework for understanding eating disorders. In L. Smolak, M. Levine, & R. Striegel-Moore, (Eds.), *The Developmental Psychopathology of Eating Disorders: Implications for Research, Prevention, and Treatment* (pp. 107-134) NJ: Lawrence Erlbaum Associates.

Fabian, L, & Thompson, J. K. (1989). Body image and eating in young females. *International Journal of Eating Disorders,* 8:63-74.

Field, A., Camargo, C., Taylor, C. B., et al. (1999). Overweight, weight concerns, and bulimic behaviours among girls and boys. Journal for the *American Academy for Child Adolescent Psychiatry* 38:754-60.

Fisher, J., and Birch, L. (2000). Parents' restrictive feeding practices are associated with young girls' negative self-evaluation of eating. *Journal of the American Dietetic Association,* 100:1341–346.

Gilligan, C. (1982). *In a Different Voice: Psychological Theory and Women's Development.* Cambridge, MA: Harvard University Press.

Graber, J., Bastiani, A., & Brooks-Gunn, J. (1999). The role of parents in the emergence, maintenance, and prevention of eating problems and disorders. In Piran, N., Levine, M., & Steiner-Adair, C. (Eds.), *Preventing Eating Disorders: A Handbook of Interventions and Special Challenges,* Taylor and Francis..

Hamilton, J. C., Falconer, J. J., & Greenberg, M. D. (1992). The relationship between self-consciousness and dietary restraint. *Journal of Social and Clinical Psychology,* 11:158-166.

Killen, J., Hayward, C., Litt, I., Hammer, L., Wilson, D., Miner, B., Taylor, C., Varady, A., & Shisslak, C. (1992). Is puberty a risk factor for eating disorders? *American Journal of Diseases of Children,* 146:323-325.

Killen, J., Hayward, C., Wilson, D., Taylor, C., Hammer, L., Litt, I., Simmonds, B., & Haydel, F. (1994). Factors associated with eating disorder symptoms in a community sample of 6th and 7th grade girls. *International Journal of Eating Disorders,* 15:357-367.

Levine, M. P., & Smolak, L. (2002). Body image development in adolescence. In T. F. Cash & T. Pruzinsky (Eds.), *Body Images: A Handbook of Theory, Research, and Clinical Practice* (pp. 74-82). New York: Guilford Publications.

Mendelson, B., & White, D. (1985). Development of self-body-esteem in overweight youngsters. *Developmental Psychology,* 21:90-96.

Murnen, S., Smolak, L., Hill, J., & Good, L. (2003). Thin, sexy women and strong, muscular men: Grade-school children's response to objectified images of women and men. *Sex Roles,* 49:427-437.

Nichter, M., & Nichter, M. (1991). Hype and weight. *Medical Anthropology,* 13:249-284.

Nichter, M., & Vuckovic, N. (1994). Fat talk: Body image among adolescent girls. In N. Sault (Ed.), *Many Mirrors: Body Image and Social Relations* (pp. 109-131). New Brunswick, NJ: Rutgers University Press.

Orenstein, P. (1994). *School Girls: Young Women,Self-Esteem, and the Confidence Gap.* New York: Doubleday.

Rosen, K. (1996). The principles of developmental psychopathology: Illustration from the study of eating disorders. In S. Scarr, (1992), Developmental theories for the 1990s: Development and individual differences. *Child Development,* 63:1-19.

Rosenberg, M. (1979). *Conceiving the Self.* New York: Basic Books.

Smolak, L. (2005). Gender and eating problems. In D. Bell, S. Foster, & E. Mash (Eds.), *Handbook of Emotional and BehavioralProblems in Girls* (pp. 463-488). New York: Kluwer Academic/Plenum Publishers.

Smolak, L. (2002). Body image in children. In T. Cash & T. Pruzinsky (Eds.), *Body Images: A Handbook of Theory, Research, and Clinical Practice* (pp. 65-73). NY: Guilford.

Smolak, L., & Levine, M. P. (1996). Adolescents—Transitions and the development of eating problems. In L. Smolak, M. P. Levine, & R. H. Striegel-Moore (Eds.), *The Developmental Psychopathology of Eating Disorders: Implications for Research, Prevention, and Treatment*, (pp. 207-234). Mahwah, NJ: Erlbaum.

Smolak, L., Levine, M. P., & Shermer, F. ((1999). Parental input and weight concerns among elementary school children. *International Journal of Eating Disorders*, 25:263-71.

Smolak, L., Levine, M. P., & Streigel-Moore, R. (1996). In L. Smolak, M. P. Levine, & R. Striegel-Moore (Eds.), *The Developmental Psychopathology of Eating Disorders: Implications for Research, Prevention, and Treatment*. Mahwah, NJ: Erlbaum.

Smolak, L. & Striegel-Moore, R. (1996). The implications of developmental research for eating disorders. In L. Smolak, M. P. Levine, & R. Striegel-Moore (Eds.), *The Developmental Psychopathology of Eating Disorders: Implications for Research, Prevention, and Treatment*, (pp. 183-204). Mahwah, NJ: Erlbaum.

Stice, E., Agras, W. S., & Hammer, L. D. (1999). Risk factors for emergence of childhood eating disturbances. *International Journal of Eating Disorders*, 25:375-387.

Striegel-Moore, R., & Marcus, M. (1995). Eating disorders in women: Current issues and debates. In A. Stanton & S. Gallant (Eds.), *Women's Health* (pp. 445-490). Washington, DC: American Psychological Association.

Thompson, J. K. & Smolak, L. (Eds.) (2001). *Body Image, Eating Disorders, and Obesity in Youth: Theory, Assessment, Treatment, and Prevention*. Washington, DC: American Psychological Association.

Tobin-Richards, M. H., Boxer, A. M., & Petersen, A. C. (1983). The psychological significance of pubertal change: Sex differences in perceptions of self during early adolescence. In J. Brooks-Gunn & A. C. Petersen (Eds.), *Girls at Puberty* (pp. 127-154). New York: Plenum.

Tolman, D. L., & Debold, E. (1994). Conflicts of body image: Female adolescents, desire and the no-body body. In P. Fallon, M. A. Katzman, & S. C. Wooley (Eds.), *Feminist Perspectives on Eating Disorders* (pp. 301-317). New York: Guilford.

Wadden, T., Brown, G., Foster, G., & Linowitz, J. (1991). Salience of weight-related worries in adolescent males and females. *International Journal of Eating Disorders*, 10:407-414.

Wood, K. C., Becker, J. A., & Thompson, J. K. (1996). Body image dissatisfaction in preadolescent children. *Journal of Applied Developmental Psychology*, 17:85-100.

Zerbe, K. (1993). *The Body Betrayed*. Washington, DC: American Psychiatric Press.

2) Etiology of disordered eating

Attie, I., & Brooks-Gunn, J. (1992). Developmental issues in the study of eating problems. In J. H. Crowther, D. L. Tennenbaum, S. E. Hobfoll, & M. A. P. Stephens (Eds.), *The Etiology of Bulimia Nervosa: The Individual and Familial Context* (pp. 35-58). Washington, DC: Hemisphere.

Blundell, J. E., & Hill, A. J. (1993). Binge eating: Psychobiological mechanisms. In C. G. Fairburn & G. T. Wilson (Eds.), *Binge Eating: Nature, Assessment, and Treatment* (pp. 206-226). New York: Guilford.

Brooks-Gunn, J., Attie, I., Burrow, C., Rosso, J., & Warren, M. (1989). The impact of puberty on body and eating concerns in athletic and nonathletic contexts. *Journal of Early Adolescence*, 9:269-290.

Bruch, H. (1973). *Eating Disorders: Obesity, Anorexia Nervosa and the Person Within*. New York: Basic Books.

Cafri, G., Thompson, J. K., Ricciardelli, L., McCabe, M., Smolak, L., & Yesalis, C. (2005). Pursuit of the muscular ideal: Physical and psychological consequences and putative risk factors. *Clinical Psychology Review*, 25:215-239.

Cash, T. F. & Prunzinsky (Eds.) (2004). *Body Images: A Handbook of Theory, Research, and Clinical Practice*. New York: Guilford Publications.

Cash, T. F., & Henry, P. E. (1995). Women's body images: The results of a national survey in the USA. *Sex Roles*, 33:19–28,.

Cattarin, J., & Thompson, J. K. (1994). A three-year longitudinal study of body image, eating disturbance, and general psychological functioning in adolescent females. *Eating Disorders: The Journal of Treatment and Prevention*, 2:114-125.

Connors, M. E. (1996). Developmental vulnerabilities for eating disorders. In Smolak, L., Levine, M., & Striegel-Moore, R. (Eds.). *The Developmental Psychopathology of Eating Disorders: Implications for Research, Prevention, and Treatment*, (pp. 285-310). Mahwah, NJ: Erlbaum.

Davison, K. K., Markey, C. N., & Birch, L. L. (2003). Etiology of body dissatisfaction and weight concerns in 5-year-old-girls. *Appetite* 35:143-51.

Fisher, J. & Birch, L. (2000). Parents' restrictive feeding practices are associated with young girls' negative self-evaluation of eating. *Journal of the American Dietetic Association,* 100:1341-346.

Garfinkel, P., Goldbloom, D., Davis, R., Olmstead, M., Garner, D., & Halmi, K. (1992). Body dissatisfaction in bulimia nervosa: Relationship to weight and shape concerns and psychological functioning. *International Journal of Eating Disorders,* 11:321-325.

Graber, J., Brooks-Gunn, J., Paikoff, R., & Warren, M. (1994). Prediction of eating problems: An eight-year study of adolescent girls. *Developmental Psychology,* 30:823-834.

Gralen, S., Levine, M. P., Smolak, L., & Murnen, S. (1990). Dieting and disordered eating during early and middle adolescence: Do the influences remain the same? *International Journal of Eating Disorders,* 9:501-512.

Hill, A. J., & Bhatti, R. (1995). Body shape perception and dieting in preadolescent British Asian Girls: Links with eating disorders. *International Journal of Eating Disorders,* 17:175-183.

Huon, G. F. (1994A). Dieting, binge eating, and some of their correlates among secondary school girls. *International Journal of Eating Disorders,* 15:159-164.

Huon, G.F. (1994B). Towards the prevention of dieting-induced disorders: Modifying negative food- and body-related attitudes. *International Journal of Eating Disorders,* 16:395-399.

Irving, L. M. (1990). Mirror images: Effects of the standard of beauty on the self- and body-esteem of women exhibiting varying levels of bulimic symptoms. *Journal of Social and Clinical Psychology,* 9:230-242.

Killen, J., Taylor, C., Hayward, C., Wilson, D., Hammer, L., Robinson, T., Litt, I., Simmonds, B., Haydel, F., Varady, A., & Kraemer, H. (1994). The pursuit of thinness and the onset of eating disorder symptoms in a community sample of adolescent girls: A three-year prospective analysis. *International Journal of Eating Disorders,* 16:227-238.

Koff, E., & Rierdan, J. (1991). Perceptions of weight and attitudes toward eating in early adolescent girls. *Journal of Adolescent Health,* 12:307-312.

Levine, M. P., & Smolak, L. (1992). Toward a model of the developmental psychopathology of eating disorders: The example of early adolescence. In J. Crowther, D. Tennenbaum, S. Hobfoll, & M. Stephens (Eds.), *The Etiology of Bulimia Nervosa: The Individual and Familial Ccontext* (pp. 59-80). Washington, DC: Hemisphere.

Levine, M. P., Smolak, L., Moodey, A., Shuman, M., & Hessen, L. (1994). Normative developmental challenges and dieting and eating disturbances in middle school girls. *International Journal of Eating Disorders,* 15:11-20.

McKnight Investigators. (2003). Risk factors for the onset of eating disorders in adolescent girls: Results of the McKnight Longitudinal Risk Factor Study. *American Journal of Psychiatry,* 160:248-254.

Neumark-Sztainer, D., Story, M., Toporoff, E., Cassuto, N., Ressnick, M. D., & Blum, R. W. (1996). Psychosocial predictors of binge eating and purging behaviors among adolescents with and without diabetes mellitus. *Journal of Adolescent Health,* 19:289–296.

Pike, D. M. (1995). Bulimic symptomatology in high school girls: Toward a model of cumulative risk. *Psychology of Women Quarterly,* 19:373-396.

Pumariega, A. J. (1986). Acculturation and eating attitudes in adolescent girls: A comparative and correlational study. *Journal of the American Academy of Child Psychiatry,* 25:276-279.

Rodin, J., Silberstein, L., Striegel-Moore, R. (1985). Women and weight: A normative discontent. In T. Sonderegger (Ed.), *Nebraska Symposium on Motivation: Vol. 32. Psychology and gende,* (pp. 267-308). Lincoln, NE: University of Nebraska Press.

Rodin, J., Striegel-Moore, R. H., & Silberstein, L. R. (1990). Vulnerability and resilience in the age of eating disorders: Risk and protective factors for bulimia nervosa. In J. Rolf, A. S. Masten, D. Cicchetti, K. H. Nuechterlein, & S. Weintraub (Eds.), *Risk and Protective Factors in the Development of Psychopathology* (pp. 361-383). New York: Cambridge University Press.

Rodriquez-Tome, H., Bariaud, F., Zardi, M., Delmas, C., & Szlagyi, P. (1993). The effects of pubertal changes on body image and relations with peers of the opposite sex in adolescence. *Journal of Adolescence,* 16:421-438.

Rosenblum, G. D., & Lewis, M. (1999). The relations among body image, physical attractiveness, and body mass in adolescence. *Child Development* 70:50–64.

Shisslak, C. M, Crago, M., McKnigh,t K. M., Estes, L. S., Gray, N., & Parnaby, O. G. (1998). Potential risk factors associated with weight control behaviors in elementary and middle school girls. *Journal of Psychosomatic Research,* 44:301-313.

Smolak, L., & Levine, M. P. (1996). Adolescent transitions and the development of eating problems. In L. Smolak, M. Levine, & R. Striegel-Moore (Eds.). *The Developmental Psychopathology of Eating Disorders: Implications for Research, Prevention, and Treatment* (pp. 207-235). Mahwah, NJ: Erlbaum.

Smolak, L., & Striegel-Moore, R. (1996). The implications of developmental research for eating disorders In L. Smolak, M. Levine, & R. Striegel-Moore (Eds.). *The Developmental Psychopathology of Eating Disorders:*

Implications for Research, Prevention, and Treatment (p. 183-204). Mahwah, NJ: Erlbaum.

Smolak, L. (1996). Methodological implications of a developmental psychopathology approach to the study of eating problems. In L. Smolak, M. Levine, & R. Striegel-Moore (Eds.). *The Developmental Psychopathology of Eating Disorders: Implications for Research, Prevention, and Treatment* (pp. 31-56). Mahwah, NJ: Erlbaum.

Smolak, L., & Levine, M. (1994A). Critical issues in the developmental psychopathology of eating disorders. In L. Alexander & D. Lumsden (Eds.), *Understanding Eating Disorders* (pp. 37-60). Washington, DC: Taylor & Francis.

Smolak, L., Levine, M. P., & Gralen, S. J. (1993). The impact of puberty and dating on eating problems among middle school girls. *Journal of Youth and Adolescence,* 22:355-368.

Stice, E., Agras, W. S., & Hammer, L. D. (1999). Risk factors for emergence of childhood eating disturbances. *International Journal of Eating Disorders*, 25:375-387.

Striegel-Moore, R. (1993). Etiology of binge eating: A developmental perspective. In C. Fairburn & G. T. Wilson (Eds.), *Binge Eating: Nature, Assessment, andTtreatment* (pp. 144-172). New York: Guilford.

Stirling, L, and Yeomans, M. (2004). Effect of exposure to a forbidden food on eating in restrained and unrestrained women. *Eating Disorders*, 35:1.

Thelen, M. H., Lawrence, C. M., & Powell, A. L. (l992). Body image, weight control, and eating disorders among children. In J. H. Crowther, D. L. Tennebaum, S. E. Hobfoll & M. A. Stephens (Eds.), *The Etiology of Bulimia Nervosa: The Individual and Familial Context* (81-101). Washington, DC: Hemisphere.

Thompson, J. K., & Smolak, L., (Eds.). (2001) *Body Image, Eating Disorders, and Obesity in Youth.* Washington, DC: American Psychological Association.

Wilson, G. T., Nonas, C. A., & Rosenblum, G. D. (1993). Assessment of binge eating in obese patients. *International Journal of Eating Disorders,* 13:25-33.

Yankovski, S. (1993). Binge eating disorder: Current knowledge and future directions. *Obesity Research,* 1:306-318.

3) The effects of weight-loss diets

Anderson, J., Konz, E., & Jenkins, D. (2000). Health advantages and disadvantages of weight-reducing diets: A computer analysis and critical review. *Journal of the American College of Nutrition* 19:578-590.

Anderson, A. (1994). The last word. *Eating Disorders* 2:1, 81-82.

Berg, F. (1995). Health risks of weight loss. Hettinger, ND: Healthy Weight Journal Publishing Network.

Berg, F. (July/August 1992). Harmful weight loss practices among adolescents. *Healthy Weight Journal,* 69-72.

Bowers, M., The last word. *Eating Disorders*, 1:4, 375-377.

Brownell, D., & Rodin, J. (1994). The dieting maelstrom: Is it possible and advisable to lose weight? *American Psychologist,* 49:781-791.

Crisp, A. H., Hsu, L. K. G., & Harding, B. (1980). The starving hoarder and voracious spender: Stealing in anorexia nervosa. *Journal of Psychosomatic Research,* 24:225-231.

Coakley, E. N., Rimm, E. B., Colditz, B., Kawachi, I., & Willett, W. (1998). Predictors of weight change in men: Results from the health professionals follow-up study. *International Journal of Obesity Related Metabolic Disorders*, 22:89-86.

Fantino, M., & Cabanac, M. (1980). Body weight regulation with a proportional hoarding response in the rat. *Physiology and Behavior*, 24:939-942.

Garner, D., & Wooley, S. (1991). Confronting the failure of behavioral and dietary treatments for obesity. *Clinical Psychology Review,* 11:729-780.

Grodstein, R., Levine, R., Troy, L., Spencer, T., Colditz, G., & Stampfer, M. (1996). Predictors of weight gain over two years among a population of working adults: The Healthy Worker Project. *International Journal of Obesity and Related Metabolic Disorders,* 181:145-154.

Heatherton, T., & Polivey, J. (1992). Chronic dieting and eating disorders: A spiral model. In J. Crowther, D. Tennenbaum, S. Hobfoll, & M. Stephens (Eds.), *The Etiology of Bulimia Nervosa: The Individual and Familial Context*, (133-156). Washington, DC: Hemisphere.

Hill, A. (1993). Pre-adolescent dieting: Implications for eating disorders. *International Review of Psychiatry,* 5:87-100.

Horn, J., & Anderson, K. (1993). Who in America is trying to lose weight? *Annuals of International Medicine,* 119:672 – 676.

Hewing, R., Liebermeister, H., Daweke, F., Gries, F., & Gruneklee, D. (1973). Weight regain after low calorie diet: long term pattern of blood sugar, syrup lipids, ketone bodies and serum insulin levels. *Diabetalogia* 9:197-202.

Keys, A., Brozek, J., Henschel, A., Mickelsen, O., & Taylor, H. L. (1950). The Biology of Human Starvation (2 vols.). Minneapolis: University of Minnesota Press.

Korkeila, M., Rissan, M., Kaprio, J., Sorensen, T., and Koskenvuo, M (1999). Weight-loss attempts and risk of major weight gain: A prospective study in Finnish adults. *American Journal of Clinical Nutrition* 70:965-975.

Lowe, M. R. (1993). The effects of dieting on eating behavior: A three-factor model. *Psychological Bulletin,* 114:100-121.

Mauer, M., Harris, R., and Bartness, T. (2001). The regulation of total body fat: Lessons learned from lipectomy studies. *Neuroscience Biobehavioral Review,* 25:15-28.

Miller, W. C. (March 1997). The history of dieting and its effectiveness, *Healthy Weight Journal,* 28-29.

National Task Force on the Prevention and Treatment of Obesity. (1994). Weight cycling. *Journal of the American Medical Association* 272:1196-1202.

Omichinski, L. (1996). Teens & diets - No Weigh. *Healthy Weight Journal,* 10:49-52.

Platte, P., Wurmser, H., Wade, S. E., Mecheril, A., & Pirke, K. M. (1996). Resting metabolic rate and diet-induced thermogenesis in restrained and unrestrained eaters. *International Journal of Eating Disorders,* 20:33-41.

Polivy, J. (1996). Psychological consequences of food restriction. *Journal of American Dietetic Association,* 96:589-592.

Polivy, J., Zeitlin, S. B., Herman, C. P., & Beal, A. L. (1994). Food restriction and binge eating: A study of former prisoners of war. *Journal of Abnormal Psychology,* 103:409-411.

Polivy, J. & Herman, C. P. (1985). Dieting and bingeing: A causal analysis. *American Psychologist,* 40:193-201.

Polivy, J. & Herman, C.P. (1987) Diagnosis and treatment of normal eating. *Journal of Consulting and Clinical Psychology,* 55:635-644.

Ruderman, A. J. (1986). Dietary restraint: A theoretical and empirical review. *Psychological Bulletin,* 99:247-262.

Russell, C. (May 1993). High cost of shedding pounds. *Washington Post Health News.*

Sea, M., Fong, W., Huang, Y., & Chen, Z. (2000). Weight cycling-induced alternation in fatty acid metabolism. *American Journal of Physiology—Regulator, Integrative & Comparative Physiology,* 279:R1145-R1155.

Story, M., Rosenwinkel, K., Himes, J. H., Resnick, M., Harris, L. J., & Blum, R. W. (1991). Demographic and risk factors associated with chronic dieting in adolescents. *American Journal of Diseases of Children,* 145:994-998.

Williamson, D., Serdula, M., Anda, R., Levy, A., & Byers, R. (1992). Weight loss attempts in adults: Goals, duration, and rate of weight loss. *American Journal of Public Health* 82:1251-1257.

4) Social learning theory and cultural context

Becker, A. (1996). Culture, media and eating disorders. *Harvard Review of Psychiatry,* 1:163-167.

Berg, F. (1997). *Afraid To Eat.* Hettinger, ND: Healthy Weight Publishing Network.

Bordo, S. (1993). *Unbearable Weight: Feminism, Western Culture, and the Body.* Berkeley: University of California Press.

Brumberg, J. (1988). *Fasting Girls: The Emergence of Anorexia Nervosa as a Modern Disease.* Cambridge, MA, Plume Publications.

Crandall, C. S. (1994). Prejudice against fat people: Ideology and self-interest. *Journal of Personality and Social Psychology,* 66:882-894.

Czajka-Narins, D., & Parham, E., (1990). Fear of fat: Attitudes toward obesity: The thinning of America. *Nutrition Today,* 26-32.

Fallon, P., Katzman. M., Wooley, S. (1994). *Feminist Perspectives on Eating Disorders.* New York: Guilford Press.

Field, A. E., Camargo, C. A. J., Taylor, C. B., Berkey, C. S., Roberts, S. B., & Colditz, G. A. (2001). Peer, parent, and media influences on the development of weight concerns and frequent dieting among preadolescent and adolescent girls and boys. *Pediatrics,* 107:54-60.

Field, A. E., Camargo, C. A., Taylor, C. B., Berkey, C. S., Colditz, G. A. (1999). Relation of peer and media influences to the development of purging behaviors among preadolescent and adolescent girls. *Archives of Pediatric Adolescent Medicine,* 153:1184-9.

Fredrickson, B., & Roberts, T. (1997). Objectification theory: Towards understanding women's lived experiences and mental health. *Psychology of Women Quarterly,* 21:173-206.

Garner, D.M. (1997). Psychoeducational principles in the treatment of eating disorders. In D. M. Garner & P. E. Garfinkel (Eds), *Handbook for Treatment of Eating Disorders* (pp. 145-177). New York: Guilford Press.

Garner, D. M., Garfinkel, P. E., Schwartz, D., & Thompson, M. (1980). Cultural expectations of thinness in women. *Psychological Reports,* 47:483-491.

Groesz, L. M., Levine, M. P., & Murnen, S. K. (2002). The effect of experimental presentation of thin media images on body satisfaction: A meta-analytic review. *International Journal of Eating Disorders,* 31:1-16.

Guillen, E. O., & Barr, S. I. Nutrition, dieting, and fitness messages in a magazine for adolescent women, 1970-90. *Journal of Adolescent Health,* 15:464-72.

Gustafson-Larson, A., & Terry, R. (1992). Weight-related behaviors and concerns of fourth-grade children. *Journal of the American Dietetic Association,* 22:818-822.

Heinberg L. J., & Thompson, J. K. (1995). Body image and televised images of thinness and attractiveness: A controlled laboratory investigation. *Journal of Social and Clinical Psychology*, 14:325-38.

Katzmarzyk, P.T., Davis, C. (2001). Thinness and body shape of *Playboy* centerfolds from 1978 to 1998. *International Journal of Obesity Related Metabolic Disorders*, 25:590-592.

Kilbourne, J. (2000). *Can't Buy My Love; How Advertising Changes the Way We Think and Feel.* New York: Free Press.

Labre M. P. (2002). Adolescent boys and the muscular male body ideal. *Journal of Adolescent Health*, 20:233-42.

Leit, R. A., Pope, H. G., & Gray, J. J. (2001). Cultural expectations of muscularity in men: The evolution of *Playgirl* centerfolds. *International Journal of Eating Disorders,,* 29: 90: 8-10.

Levine, M. P., Piran, N., & Stoddard, C. (1999). Mission more probable: Media literacy, activism, and advocacy in the prevention of eating disorders. In N. Piran, fM. P. Levine, & C. Steiner-Adair (Eds.), *Preventing Eating Disorders: A Handbook of Interventions and Special Challenges* (pp. 3-25). Philadelphia: Brunner/Mazel.

Levine, M. P., Smolak, L., & Hayden, H. (1994). The relation of sociocultural factors to eating attitudes and behaviors among middle school girls. *Journal of Early Adolescence,* 14:471-490.

Markus, H., Hamill, R., & Sentis, K. (1987). Thinking fat: Self-schemas for body weight and the processing of weight relevant information. *Journal of Applied Social Psychology,* 17:50-71.

Meltzoff, A. N. (1990). Foundations for developing a concept of self: The role of imitation in relating self to other and the value of social mirroring, social modeling, and self practice in infancy. In D. Cicchetti & M. Beeghly (Eds.), *The Self in Transition: Infancy to Childhood* (pp. 139-164). Chicago: University of Chicago Press.

Nasser, M., Katzman, M., & Gordon, R. (2001) *Eating Disorders and Cultures in Transition.* New York: Taylor & Francis.

Perry, C. L., Baranowski, T., & Parcel G. (1990). How individuals' environments and health behaviors interact: Social learning theory. In K. Glanz, F. M. Lewis, & B. Rimer (Eds.), *Health Behavior and Health Education.* San Francisco: Jossey-Bass.

Pipher, M. (1994) *Reviving Ophelia; Saving the Selves of Adolescent Girls.* New York: Ballantine Books, Random House.

Ricciardelli, L. A., & McCabe, M. P. (February 2001). Self-esteem and negative affect as moderators of sociocultural influences on body dissatisfaction, strategies to decrease weight, and strategies to increase muscles among adolescent boys and girls. *Sex roles: A Journal of Research.*

Rothblum, E. D. (1992). The stigma of women's weight: Social and economic realities. *Feminism and Psychology,* 2:61-73.

Smolak, L., & Murnen, S. (2004). Feminist perspectives on eating problems. In J. K. Thompson (Ed.), *Handbook of Eating Disorders and Obesity* (pp. 590-606). New York: Wiley.

Smolak, L., Murnen, S., & Thompson, J. K. (In press). Sociocultural influences and muscle building in adolescent boys. *Psychology of Men and Masculinity.*

Smolak, L., & Striegel-Moore, R. (Ed.), (2002). Body Image. In J. Worrel, *The Encyclopedia of Gender.* New York: Academic Press.

Stice, E. (1994). Review of the evidence for a sociocultural model of bulimia nervosa and an exploration of the mechanisms of action. *Clinical Psychology Review,* 14(7):633-661.

Steiner-Adair, C. (1986). The body politic: Normal female development and the development of eating disorders. *Journal of the American Academy of Psychoanalysis,* 14:95-114.

Striegel-Moore, R. H. (1994). A feminist agenda for psychological research on eating disorders. In P. Fallon, M. Katzman, & S. Wooley (Eds.), *Feminist Perspectives on Eating Disorders* (pp. 438-454). New York: Guilford Press.

Striegel-Moore, R. H., & Kearne-Cooke, A. (1994). Exploring determinants and consequences of parents' attitudes about their children's physical appearances. *International Journal of Eating Disorders,* 15: 377-385.

Streigel-Moore, R. H., & Marcus, M. (1995). Eating disorders in women: Current issues and debates. In A. Stanton & S. Gallant (Eds.), *Women's Health* (p. 445-490). Washington, DC: American Psychological Association.

Striegel-Moore, R. H., McAvay, G., & Rodin, J. (1986). Psychological and behavioral correlates of feeling fat in women. *International Journal of Eating Disorders,* 5:935-949.

Striegel-Moore, R. H., Silberstein, L. H., & Rodin, J. (1993). The social self in bulimia nervosa: Public self-consciousness, social anxiety and perceived fraudulence. *Journal of Abnormal Psychology,* 102:297-303.

Cash, T. F., & Pruzinsky, T. (Eds.) (2004) *Body Images: A Handbook of Theory, Research, and Clinical Practice* (pp. 74-82). New York: Guilford Publications.

Tiggemann, M., Gardiner M., & Slater, A. "I would rather be size 10 than have straight A's": A focus group study of adolescent girls' wish to be thinner. *Journal of Adolescent Health,* 23:645-659.

Yuker, H., & Allison, D. (1994). Obesity: Sociocultural perspective. In L. Alexander-Mott & D. B. Lumsden (Eds.), *Understanding Eating Disorders: Anorexia Nervosa, Bulimia Nervosa, and Obesity* (pp. 243-270). Washington, DC: Taylor & Francis.

5) Media influence

Abramson, E., & Valene, P. (1991). Media use, dietary restraint, bulimia and attitudes toward obesity: A preliminary study. *British Review of Bulimia and Anorexia Nervosa,* 5:73-76.

Gerbner, G., Gross, L., Morgan, M., & Signorielli, N. (1994). Growing up with television: The cultivation perspective. In J. Bryant & D. Zillmann (Eds.), *Media Effects: Advances in Theory and Research* (pp. 17-41). Hillsdale, NJ: Lawrence Erlbaum Associates.

Gonzalez-Lavin, A., & Smolak, L. (1995, March). *Relationships between television and eating problems in middle school girls.* Paper presented at the meeting of the Society for Research in Child Development, Indianapolis, IN.

Harris, R. J. (1994). *A cognitive psychology of mass communication* (2nd ed.). Hillsdale, NJ: Lawrence Erlbaum Associates.

Jasper, K. (1993). Monitoring and responding to media messages. *Eating Disorders,* 1:109-114.

Kilbourne, J. (1994). Still killing us softly: Advertising and the obsession with thinness. In P. Fallon, M. Katzman, & S. Wooley (Eds.), *Feminist Perspectives on Eating Disorders* (pp. 395-419). New York: Guilford.

Levine, M. P., & Smolak, L., (1996). Media as a context for the development of disordered eating. In L. Smolak, M. Levine, & R. Striegel-Moore. (Eds.) *The Developmental Psychopathology of Eating Disorders: Implications for Research, Prevention, and Treatment* (pp. 259-284). Mawhaw, NJ: Lawrence Erlbaum Associates.

Liebert, R. M., & Sprafkin, J. (1988). *The Early Window: Effects of Television on Children and Youth* (3rd ed.). New York: Pergamon.

Martin, M. C., & Kennedy, P. F. (1993). Advertising and social comparison: Consequences for female preadolescents and adolescents. *Psychology & Marketing,* 10:513-530.

Martin, M. C., & Kennedy, P. F. (1994A). The measurement of social comparison to advertising models: A gender gap revealed. In J.A. Costa (ed.), *Gender Issues in Consumer Behavior* (pp. 104-124). Thousand Oaks, CA: Sage.

Martin, M. C., & Kennedy, P. F. (1994B). Social comparison and the beauty of advertising models: The role of motives for comparison. *Advances in Consumer Research,* 21:365-371.

Morris, A. M. & Katzman, D. K, (1995). The impact of the media on eating disorders in children and adolescents. *Pediatrics and Childhood Health:* 8 (5).

Myers, P. N., Jr., & Biocca, F. A. (1992). The elastic body image: The effect of television advertising and programming on body image distortion in young women. *Journal of Communication,* 42:108-133.

Nemeroff, C. J., Stein, R. I., Diehl, N. S., & Smilack, K. M. (1994). From the Cleavers to the Clintons: Role choices and body orientation as reflected in magazine article content. *International Journal of Eating Disorders,* 16:167-176.

Ogletree, S. M., Williams, S. W., Raffeld, P., Mason, B., & Fricke, K. (1990). Female attractiveness and eating disorders: Do children's television commercials play a role? *Sex Roles,* 22:791-797.

Peirce, K. (1990). A feminist theoretical perspective on the socialization of teenage girls through *Seventeen* magazine. *Sex Roles,* 23:491-500.

Rice, R. E., & Atkin, C. (1994). Principles of successful public communication campaigns. In J. Bryant & D. Zillmann (Eds.), *Media Effects: Advances in Theory and Research* (pp. 365-387). Hillsdale, NJ: Lawrence Erlbaum Associates.

Richins, M. L. (1991). Social comparison and idealized images of advertising. *Journal of Consumer Research,* 18:71-83.

Shaw, J., & Waller, G. (1995). The media's impact on body image: Implications for prevention and treatment. *Eating Disorders: The Journal of Treatment & Prevention,* 3:115-123.

Silberstein, B., Perdue, L., Peterson, B., & Kelly, E. (1986). The role of mass media in promoting a thin standard of bodily attractiveness for women. *Sex Roles,* 14:519-532.

Stice, E., Schupak-Neuberg, E., Shaw, H. E., & Stein, R. I. (1994). Relation of media exposure to eating disorder symptomatology: An examination of mediating mechanisms. *Journal of Abnormal Psychology,* 103:836-840.

Stice, E., & Shaw, H. E. (1994). Adverse effects of the media portrayed thin-ideal on women and linkages to bulimic symptomatology. *Journal of Social and Clinical Psychology,* 13:288-308.

Story, M. (1990). Study group report on the impact of television on adolescent nutritional status. *Journal of Adolescent Health Care,* 11:82-85.

Story, M., & Faulkner, P. (1990). The prime time diet: A content analysis on eating behavior and food messages in television program content and commercials. *American Journal of Public Health,* 80:738-740.

Waller, G., Hamilton, K., & Shaw, J. (1992). Media influences on body size estimation in eating disordered and comparison subjects. *British Review of Bulimia and Anorexia Nervosa,* 6:81-87.

Wolf, N. (1991). *The Beauty Myth: How Images of Beauty Are Used Against Women.* New York: Morrow.

6) Cross cultural differences

Abrams, K. K., Allen, L. R., & Gray, J. J. (1993). Disordered eating attitudes and behaviors, psychological adjustment, and ethnic identity: A comparison of black and white female college students. *International Journal of Eating Disorders, 14*, 49-57.

Allan, J. D., Mayo, K., & Michel, Y. (1993). Body size values of white and black women. *Research in Nursing and Health, 16*, 323-333.

Chandler, S. B., Abood, D. A., Lee, D. T., Cleveland, M. Z., & Daly, J. A. (1994). Pathogenic eating attitudes and behaviors and body dissatisfaction differences among black and white college students. *Eating Disorders, 2,* 319-328.

Edwards-Hewitt, T., & Gray, J. (1993), *The prevalence of disordered eating attitudes and behaviors in Black-American and White-American and Caucasian-American college women: Ethnic, regional, class and media differences.* Paper presented at the Annual Meeting of the Eastern Psychological Association.

Edwards-Hewitt, T., & Gray, J. (1993). The prevalence of disordered eating attitudes and behaviors in Black - American and White-American college women: Ethnic, regional, class, and media differences. *Eating Disorders Review, 1,* 41-54.

Emmons, L. (1994). Dieting and purging behavior in black and white high school students. *Journal of the American Dietetic Association, 92,* 306-312.

Ferron, C. (1997). Body image in adolescence in cross-cultural research. *Adolescence, 32,* 735-745.

Harris, S. M. (1994). Racial differences in predictors of college women's body image attitudes. *Women and Health, 21,* 89-104.

Kemper, K. A., Sargent, R. G., Drane, J. W., Valois, R. F., & Hussey, J. W. (1994). Black and white females' perceptions of ideal body size and social norms. *Obesity Research, 2,* 117-126.

Kumanyika, S. K. (1994). Obesity in minority populations: An epidemiological assessment. *Obesity Research, 2* , 166-182.

Kumanyika, S., Wilson, J. F., & Guilford-Davenport, M. (1993). Weight-related attitudes and behaviors of black women. *Journal of the American Dietetic Associations, 93,* 416-422.

Neumark-Sztainer, D., Croll, J., Story, M., Hannan, P. J., French, S. A., & Perry, C. (2002). Ethnic/racial difference in weight-related concerns and behaviors among adolescent girls and boys. *Journal of Psychosomatic Research, 53,* 963-974.

Nichter, M., Vuckovic, N., & Parker, S. (1999). The looking good, feeling good program: A multi-ethnic intervention for healthy body image, nutrition, and physical activity. In N. Piran, M. Levine, & C. Steiner-Adair. (Eds.), *Preventing Eating Disorders: A Handbook of Interventions and Special Challenges.* Philadelphia: Brunner/Mazel.

Parker, S., Nickter, M., Nichter, M., Vuckovic, N., Sims, C., & Ritenbaugh, C. (1995). Body image and weight concerns among African American and white adolescent females: Differences that make a difference. *Human Organization, 54,* 103-114.

Pate, J. E., Pumariega, A. J., Hester, C., & Garner, D. M. (1992). Cross-cultural patterns in eating disorders: A review. *Journal of the American Academy of Child and Adolescent Psychiatry, 31,* 802-809.

Powell, A. D., & Kahn, A. S. (1995). Racial differences in women's desires to be thin. *International Journal of Eating Disorders, 17,* 191-195.

Root, M. P. (1990). Disordered eating in women of color. *Sex Roles, 22,* 525-536.

Rucker, C. E., III, & Cash, T. F. (1992). Body images, body-size perceptions, and eating behaviors among African-American and white college women. *International Journal of Eating Disorders, 12,* 291-300.

Schreiber, G. B., Robins, M., Striegel-Moore, R., Obarzanek, E., Morrison, J. A., & Wright, D. J. (1998). Weight modification efforts reported by black and white preadolescent girls: National Heart, Lung, and Blood Institute Growth and Health Study. *Pediatric,s 98*, 62-70.

Spencer, M. B., & Markstrom-Adams, C. (1990). Identity processes among racial and ethnic minority children in America. *Child Development, 61,* 290-310.

Striegel-Moore, R., Schreiber, G., Pike, K., Wilfley, D., & Rodin, J. (1995). Drive for thinness in black and white preadolescent girls. *International Journal of Eating Disorders, 18,* 59-69.

Striegal, M., & Smolak, L. (2002). The influence of ethnicity on eating disorders in women. In R. Eisler & M. Hersen *(Eds.), Handbook of Gender, Culture, and Health* (227-254). Mahwah, NJ: Erlbaum.

Striegel-Moore, R. & Smolak, L. (2002). Gender, ethnicity, and eating disorders. In C. Fairburn & K. Brownell (Eds.), *Eating Disorders and Obesity: A Comprehensive Handbook (2nd* ed). New York: Guilford.

Striegel-Moore, R. & Smolak, L. (1996). The role of race in the development of eating disorders. In L. Smolak, M. Levine, & R. Striegel-Moore (Eds.), *The Developmental Psychopathology of Eating Disorders: Implications for Research, Prevention, and Treatment* (pp. 259-84). Mahwah, NJ: Erlbaum.

Striegel-Moore, R. H., Wilfley, D. E., Caldwell, M. B., Needham, M. L., & Brownell, D. D. (1996). Weight related attitudes and behaviors of women who diet to lose weight: A comparison of black dieters and white dieters. *Obesity Research* 4: 109-116..

Thompson, B. W. (1992). "A way outa no way": Eating problems among African-American, Latina, and White women. *Gender and Society, 6,* 546-561.

Wilson, D. B., Sargent, R., & Dias, J. (1994). Racial differences in selection of ideal body size by adolescent females. *Obesity Research, 2,* 38-43.

7) Prevention

Body Wise Eating Disorder Information Packet for Middle School Personnel. Office on Women's Health, Educational Services, U.S. Department of Health and Human Services, 1150 Connecticut Avenue, NW, Suite 1100, Washington, DC 20036.

Dryfoos, J. G. (1990). *Adolescents at Risk: Prevalence and Prevention.* New York: Oxford University Press.

Flay, B. R., Ryan, K. B., Best, J. A., Brown, K. S., Kersell, M. W., d'Avernas, J. R., & Zanna, M. P. (1985). Are social psychological smoking prevention programs effective? The Waterloo study. *Journal of Behavioral Medicine, 8,* 37-59.

Friedman, S. (1999). Discussion groups for girls: Decoding the language of fat. In N. Piran, M.Levine, & C. Steiner-Adair (Eds.), *Preventing Eating Disorders: A Handbook of Interventions and Special Challenges.* Philadelphia: Brunner/Mazel.

Garmezy, N., & Masten, A. (1991). The protective role of competence indicators in children at risk. In E. M. Cummings, A. Greene, & K. Karraker (Eds.), *Life-Span Developmental Psychology: Perspectives on Stress and Coping* (pp. 151-174). Hillsdale, NJ: Lawrence Erlbaum Associates.

Gresko, R. B., & Karlsen, A. (1994). The Norwegian program for the primary, secondary and tertiary prevention of eating disorders. *Eating Disorders, 2,* 51-61.

Griffiths, R. A., & Farnill, D. (1996). Primary prevention of dieting disorders: An update. *Journal of Family Studies, 2(2).* 179-191.

Hansen, W. B. (1992). School-based substance abuse prevention: A review of the state of the art in curriculum, 1980-1990. *Health and Education Research, 7,* 403-430.

Huon, G. F., Braganza, C., Brown, L. P., Ritchie, J. E., & Roncolato, W. G. (l998). Reflections of prevention in dieting-induced disorders. *International Journal of Eating Disorders, 23(4)*, 455-458.

Ikeda, J., & Naworski, P. (1992). *Am I fat? Helping young children accept differences in body size.* Santa Cruz: ETR Associates.

Irving, L. (1999). A bolder model of prevention: Science, practice, and activism. In N. Piran, M. P. Levine, & C. Steiner-Adair (Eds.), *Preventing Eating Disorders: A Handbook of Interventions and Special Challenges.* Philadelphia: Brunner/Mazel.

Irving, L., Neumark-Sztainer, D., (2002). Integrating the prevention of eating disorders and obesity: Feasible or futile? *Preventive Medicine, 34,* 299-309.

Kater, K., (2004). *Real Kids Come in All Sizes: Ten Essential Lessons to Build Your Child's Body Esteem.* New York: Broadway Books.

Kater, K. (1998). *Healthy Body Image: Teaching Kids to Eat and Love Their Bodies Too!* (Curriculum guide). Seattle: National Eating Disorders Association.

Kater, K., Rohwer, J., & Levine, M. P. (1998). An elementary school project for developing healthy body image and reducing risk factors for unhealthy and disordered eating. *Eating Disorders: Journal of Treatment and Prevention; Vol 8, No. 1.*

Kater, K., Rohwer, J. & Londre, K. (2002). Evaluation of an upper elementary school program to prevent body image, eating and weight concerns. *Journal of School Health, Vol. 72 (5),* pp. 199-204.

Killen, J. D. (1985). Prevention of adolescent tobacco smoking: The social pressures resistance training approach. *Journal of Child Psychiatry and Psychology, 26,* 7-15.

Killen, J. D. (1996). Development and evaluation of a school-based eating disorder symptoms prevention program. In L. Smolak, M. Levine, & R. Striegel-Moore (Eds.), *The Developmental Psychopathology of Eating Disorders: Implications for Research, Prevention, and Treatment* (pp. 313-340). Mahwah, NJ: Lawrence Erlbaum Associates.

Killen, J. D., Taylor, C. B., Hammer, L. D., Litt, I., Wilson, D. M., Rich, T., Hayward, C., Simmonds, B., Kraemer, H., & Varady, A. (1993). An attempt to modify unhealthful eating attitudes and weight regulation practices of young adolescent girls. *International Journal of Eating Disorders, 13,* 369-384.

Levine, M. P. (1998). Prevention of eating disorders, eating problems and negative body image. In R. Lemberg (Ed.), *Controlling Eating Disorders with Facts, Advise, and Resources.* (2nd ed.). Phoenix: Oryx Press.

Levine, M.P. (2001). Commentary on Varnado-Sullivan et al.'s "Development and implementation of the Body Logic Program for Adolescents: A two-stage prevention program for eating disorders." *Cognitive and Behavioral Practice 8(3).*

Levine, M. P. (2003). Commentary on Wade, Davidson, and O'Dea's preliminary controlled evaluation of a school-based media literacy program and self esteem program for reducing eating disorder risk factors. *International Journal of Eating Disorders*

Levine, M., & Piran, N (1996). Special Prevention Issue. *Eating Disorders: Journal of Treatment and Prevention, 4(4),* 291-384.

Levine, M. P., & Piran, N. (2001).The prevention of eating disorders: Towards a participatory ecology of knowledge, action, and advocacy. In R. Striegel-Moore & L. Smolak (Eds.), *Eating Disorders: Innovative Directions for Research and Practice* (233-253). Washington, DC: American Psychological Association.

Levine, M., & Piran, N. (1999). Reflections, conclusions, and future directions. In N. Piran, M. Levine, & C. Steiner-Adair (Eds.), *Preventing Eating Disorders: A Handbook of Interventions and Special Challenges.* Philadelphia: Brunner/Mazel.

Levine, M. P., & Piran, N. (2004).The role of body image in the prevention of eating disorders. *Body Image, 1,* 57-70.

Levine, M. P., Piran, N., & Irving, L. (2000). "GO GIRLS!" media literacy, activism, and advocacy project, *Healthy Weight Journal, 14,* 89-90.

Levine, M. P., Piran, N., & Irving, L. (2003). Primary prevention of disordered eating behavior in adolescents. In T. P. Gullotta & M. Bloom (Eds.), *The Encyclopedia of Primary Prevention and Health Promotion* (pp. 423-428). New York: Kluwer Academic/Plenum Publishers.

Levine, M. P., Piran, N., & Steiner-Adair, C. (1999). *Preventing Eating Disorders: A Handbook of Interventions and Special Challenges.* Philadelphia: Brunner/Mazel.

Levine, M. P., & Smolak, L. (1998). Lessons from lessons: An evaluation of an elementary school prevention program. In G. Noordenbos & W. Vandereycken (eds.), *The Prevention of Eating Disorders* (137-172). London: Athlone.

Levine, M. P., & Smolak, L. (2001). Primary prevention of body image disturbance and disordered eating in childhood and adolescence. In J. K. Thompson & L. Smolak (Eds.), *Body Image, Eating Disorders, and Obesity in Youth: Assessment, Prevention, and Treatment* (pp. 237-260). Washington, DC: American Psychological Association.

Levine, M. P., & Smolak, L. (2002). Body image development in adolescence. In T. F. Cash & T. Pruzinsky (Eds.), *Body Images*: A Handbook of Theory, Research, and Clinical Practice (pp. 74-82). New York: Guilford Publications.

Levine, M. P., & Smolak, L. (2002). Ecological and activism approaches to prevention. In T. F. Cash & T. Pruzinsky (Eds.), *Body Images: A Handbook of Theory, Research, and Clinical Practice* (pp. 497-505). New York: Guilford Publications.

Levine, M. P., & Smolak, L. (2005). *The prevention of eating problems and disorders: Theory, research, and practice.* Mahwah, NJ: Lawrence Erlbaum Associates.

Levine, M. P., Smolak, L., & Striegel-Moore, R. (1996). Conclusions, implications, and future directions. In Smolak, L., Levine, M., & Striegel-Moore, R. (Eds.) *The developmental psychopathology of eating disorders: Implications for research, prevention, and treatment.* (399-416) NJ: Lawrence Erlbaum Associates.

Moreno, A. B., & Thelen, M. H. (1993). A preliminary prevention program for eating disorders in a junior high school population. *Journal of Youth and Adolescence, 22,* 109-124.

Neumark-Sztainer, D. (1996). School-based programs for preventing eating disturbances. *Journal of School Health, 66(2),* 64-71.

Neumark-Sztainer, D. (1995). Excessive weight preoccupation: Normative but not harmless. *Nutrition Today, 30(2),* 68-74.

Yager, Z., & O'Dea, J. A. (2005). The role of teachers and other educators in the prevention of eating disorders and child obesity: What are the issues? *Eating Disorders: The Journal of Treatment & Prevention, 13,* 261-278.

Paxton, S. J. (1993). A prevention program for disturbed eating and body dissatisfaction in adolescent girls: A one year follow-up. *Health Education Research, 8,* 43-51.

Perry, C. L., (1990) Conceptualizing community-wide youth health promotion programs. In D. Nutbearn (ed.), *Youth Health Promotion: From Theory in School and Community.* London: Forbes Publishing.

Phelps, L., Dempsey, M., Sapia, J., and Nelson, L. (1999). The efficacy of a school-based eating disorder prevention program: Building physical self-esteem and personal competencies. In N. Piran, M. Levine, C. Steiner-Adair (Eds.), *Preventing Eating Disorders: A Handbook of Interventions and Special Challenges.* Philadelphia: Brunner/Mazel.

Piran, N. (1999). On the move from tertiary to secondary and primary prevention: Working with an elite dance school. In N. Piran, M. Levine, C. Steiner-Adair (Eds.), *Preventing Eating Disorders: A Handbook of Interventions and Special Challenges.* Philadelphia: Brunner/Mazel.

Piran, N., (1999). The reduction of preoccupation with body weight and shape in schools: A feminist approach. In N. Piran, M. Levine, C. Steiner-Adair (Eds.), *Preventing Eating Disorders: A Handbook of Interventions and Special Challenges.* Philadelphia: Brunner/Mazel.

Piran, N., Levine, M., Steiner-Adair, C. (1999). *Preventing Eating Disorders, A Handbook of Special Challenges.* New York: Taylor & Francis.

Piran, N. (1995). Prevention: Can early lessons lead to a delineation of an alternative model? A critical look at prevention with schoolchildren. *Eating Disorders: The Journal of Treatment and Prevention, 3(1),* 28-36.

Piran, N. (1995, January-March). What it takes for eating disorder prevention to make a difference. *Newsletter of the National Eating Disorders Organization, 18,* 1-2, 4-5, 10.

Reijonen et al. (2003). Eating Disorders in the Adolescent Population: An Overview. *Journal of Adolescent Research, 18,* 209-222.

Rutter, M. (1985). Resilience in the face of adversity: Protective factors and resistance to psychiatric disorder. *British Journal of psychiatry, 147,* 598-611.

Rutter, M. (1990). Psychosocial resilience and protective mechanisms. In J. Rolf, A. S. Masten, D. Cicchetti, K. H. Nuechterlein, & S. Weintraub (Eds.), *Risk and Protective Factors in the Development of Psychopathology* (pp. 181-214). New York: Cambridge University Press.

Shisslak, C. M., & Crago, M.. (1994). Toward a new model for the prevention of eating disorders. In P. Fallon, M. A. Katzman, & S. C. Wooley (eds.), *Feminist Perspective on Eating Disorders* (419-437). New York: Guilford.

Shisslak, C., Crago, M., Estes, L. S. & Gray, G. (1996). Content and method of developmentally appropriate prevention programs. In L. Smolak, M. Levine, & R. Striegel-Moore (Eds.), *The Developmental Psychopathology of Eating Disorders: Implications for Research, Prevention, and Treatment* (pp. 341-364). Mahwah, NJ: Lawrence Erlbaum Associates.

Smolak, B., Harris, B., Levine, M. P. & Shisslak, C. (2001). Teachers: The forgotten influence on the success of prevention programs. *Eating Disorders: The Journal of Treatment and Prevention, 9(3),* 261-65.

Smolak, L. (1999). Elementary school curricula for the primary prevention of eating problems. In N. Piran, M. Levine, C. Steiner-Adair (Eds.), *Preventing Eating Disorders: A Handbook of Interventions and Special Challenges.* Philadelphia: Brunner/Mazel.

Smolak, L. (2004). Body image in children and adolescents: Where do we go from here? *Body Image, 1,* 15-28.

Smolak, L., & Levine, M. . (1994A, July-September). The role of parents in the prevention of disordered eating. *National Eating Disorders Organization Newsletter,* 1-9.

Smolak, L., & Levine, M. (1994B). Toward an empirical basis for primary prevention of eating problems with elementary school children. *Eating Disorders: The Journal of Treatment & Prevention, 2,* 293-307.

Steiner-Adair, C., and Vorenberg, A. (1999). Resisting weightism: Media literacy for elementary school children. In N. Piran, M. Levine, C. Steiner-Adair (Eds.), *Preventing Eating Disorders: A Handbook of Interventions and Special Challenges.* Philadelphia: Brunner/Mazel.

Striegel-Moore, R. H. (1992). Prevention of bulimia nervosa: Questions and challenges. In J. H. Crowther, D. L. Tennebaum, S. E. Hobfoll, & Stephens (Eds.), *The Etiology of Bulimia Nervosa: The Individual and Familial Context* (pp. 203-223). Washington, DC: Hemisphere.

8) Biological determinants of weight, health risks attributed to weight, trends and developments regarding health and weight.

Andres, R., Muller, D. C., Sorkin, J. D. (1993). Long-term effects of change in body weight on all-cause mortality: A review. *Annals of Internal Medicine, 119,* 737-743.

Beaumont, P. J. V. (1998). Neurobiology of eating behavior and weight control. In H. W. Hoek, J. L. Treasure, & Katzman, M. A. (Eds.), *Neurobiology in the Treatment of Eating Disorders.* Chichester, UK: Wiley and Sons.

Bennett, W. I. (1995). Beyond overeating. *New England Journal of Medicine, 332,* 673-674.

Berg, F. (1995). Customers want bigger meals. *Healthy Weight Journal, 9(1),* 26

Berg, F. (1997). *Afraid To Eat: Children and Teens in Weight Crisis.* Hettinger, ND: Healthy Weight Publishing Network.

Berg, F. (1999). Health risks associated with weight loss and obesity treatment programs. *Journal of Social Issues, 55,* 277-297.

Berg, F., (2003). *Underage and Overweight.* New York: Hatherleye Press.

Blair, S. N., Shaten, J., Brownell, K., Colling, G., Lissner, L. (1993). Body weight change, all--cause mortality, and cause-specific mortality in the Multiple Risk Factor Intervention Trial. *Annals of Internal Medicine, 119,* 749-757.

Bouchard, C., Despres, C. P, and Mauriege, P. (1993). Genetic and nongenetic determinants of regional fat distribution. *Endocrine Review, 14,* 72-93.

Bouchard, C., Pérusse, L., Rice, T., and Rao, D. C. (1998). The genetics of human obesity. In G. Bray, C. Bouchard, & P. James (Eds). *Handbook of Obesity* (pp. 157-190). New York: Dekker.

Bouchard, C., Despres, C. P, and Mauriege, P. (1993). Genetic and nongenetic determinants of regional fat distribution. *Endocrine Review, 14,* 72-93.

Coulston, A. (1998). Obesity as an epidemic: Facing the challenge. *Journal of the American Dietetic Association, 98,* 10(S2):16-22.

Di Domenico, P. (1994). Portion size: How much is too much? *Restaurants USA, 14,* 6:18-21.

Dyer, A.R., Stamler, J., & Greenland, P. (2000). Associations of weight change and weight variability with cardiovascular and all-cause mortality in the Chicago Western Electric Company Study. *American Journal of Epidemiology, 15,*: 324-333.

Dahlkoetter, J., Callahan, E., & Linton, J. (1979). Obesity and the unbalanced energy equation: Exercise versus eating habit change. *Journal of Consulting and Clinical Psychology, 47(5,* 898-905.

Ernsberger, P. & Haskew, P. (1987). *Rethinking Obesity: An Alternative View of its Health Implications.* New York: Human Sciences Press.

Feldman, W., Feldman, E., & Goodman, J. T. (1988). Culture versus biology: Children's attitudes toward thinness and fatness. *Pediatrics, 81(2,* 190-194.

Fields, A., Austin, S., Taylor, C., (2003). Relation between dieting and weight change among preadolescents and adolescents. *Pediatrics, 112(4).*

Fitzgerald, F. (1981). The problem of obesity. *American Annual Review of Medicine, 32,* 221-231.

Fitzgerald, F. T. (1994). The tyranny of health. *New England Journal of Medicine, 331,* 196-198.

Frazao, E. (1999). America's eating habits: Changes and consequences. *Agriculture Information Bulletin No. 750.* Washington, DC: USDA.

Gasser, G. .A. (1996). *Big Fat Les: The Truth about Your Weight and Your Health.* New York: Fawcett Columbine.

Goodrick, G. K., Poston, W. S., Kimball, K. T., Reeves, R. S., & Foreyt, J. P. (1998). Nondieting versus dieting treatments for overweight binge-eating women. *Journal of Consulting and Clinical Psychology, 66,* 363-368.

Guo, S., Roche, A., Chumlea, W., Gardner, J., & Siervogel, R. (1994). The predictive value of childhood body mass index values for overweight at age 35. *American Journal of Clinical Nutrition, 59,* 810-819.

Kassirer, J. P., Angell, M. (1998, January). Losing weight: An ill-fated new year's resolution. *New England Journal of Medicine,* 52-54.

Keys, A. (1980). Overweight, obesity, coronary heart disease and mortality. *Nutrition Review, 38,* 297-307.

Knapp, T. R. (1983). A methodological critique of the "ideal weight" concept. *Journal of the American Medical Association, 250,* 506-510.

Lee, C., Blair, S. N., Jackson, A. (1999). Cardiorespiratory fitness, body composition, and all-cause and cardiovascular disease mortality in men. *American Journal of Clinical Nutrition, 69(3),* 373-80.

Madaras, L. (1988). *The What's Happening to My Body Book for Girls.* New York: Newmarket Press.

Madaras, L. (1988) *The What's Happening to My Body Book for Boys.* New York: Newmarket Press.

McGinnis, J. M., & Foege, W. (1993). Actual causes of death in the United States. *Journal of the American Medical Association, 270,* 2207-2212.

McGinnis, J. M., & Foege, W. (1998). The obesity problem (letter). *New England Journal of Medicine, 338,* 1157.

Mokdad, A. H., Serdula, M. K., Dietz, W. H., Bowman, B. A., Marks, J. S., Koplan, J. P. (1999). The spread of the obesity epidemic in the United States, 1991-1998. *Journal of the American Medical Association, 282(16),*: 1519-1522.

Meyer, J., & Stunkard, A. (1993). Genetics and human obesity. In A. Atunkard & T. Wadden (Eds.), *Obesity:*

Theory and Therapy (2nd ed.) (pp. 137-150). New York: Raven.

Miller WC, Jacob AV. (2001). The health at any size paradigm for obesity treatment: the scientific evidence. *Obes Rev*;2:37–45 [review].

Obesity: preventing and managing the global epidemic. (2000). Report of a WHO consultation. Geneva, *World Health Organization (WHO Technical Report Series,* No. 894).

Ozer, E. M., Brindis, C. D., Millstein, S. G., et al. (1998). America's adolescents: Are they healthy? San Francisco: University of California, School of Medicine.

Richards, M., Abell, S., & Petersen, A. (1993). Biological development. In P. Tolan & B. Cohler (Eds.), *Handbook of Clinical Research and Practice with Adolescents* (pp. 21-44). New York: Wiley.

Robinson, J. (1997). Weight management: Shifting the paradigm. *Journal of Health Education, 28 (1)*, 28-34.

Rosenbaum, M., Leibel, R. L., Hirsch, J. (1997). Obesity. *New England Journal of Medicine, 337*, 396-407.

Sallis, J. (1993). Epidemiology of physical activity and fitness and children and adolescents. *Critical Review in Food Science and Nutrition, 33(4/5),* 403-408.

Schools Health Education Unit. (2003). Trends in young people's food choices; Attitudes about healthy eating and weight control 1983–2001.. Exeter, UK: SHEA.

Shapiro, L. (l997, April 21). Is fat that bad? *Newsweek,* 59-64.

Stice, E., Cameron, R., Killen, J. D., Hayward, C., & Taylor, C. B. (1999). Naturalistic weight reduction efforts prospectively predict growth in relative weight and onset of obesity among female adolescents. *Journal of Consulting and Clinical Psychology*, *67*, 967-974.

Stunkard, A. J. (1993). Introduction and overview. In A. J. Stunkard & T. A. Wadden (Eds.), *Obesity: Theory and Therapy* (2nd ed.) (pp. 1-10). New York: Raven Press.

Stunkard, A. J., Sorenson, T., Hanis, C., Teasdale, T., Chakraborty, R., Schull, W., & Schulsinger, F. (1986). An adoption study: Human obesity. *The New England Journal of Medicine, 314(4),* 193-198.

Stunkard, A. J., Foch, T., & Zdenek, H. (1986). A twin study of human obesity. *Journal of the American Medical Association, 256,* 51-54.

Troiano, R. P., Flegal, K. M., Kuczmarski, R. J., Campbell, S. M., & Johnson, C. L. (1995). Overweight prevalence and trends for children and adolescents: the National Health and Nutrition Examination Surveys 1963 to 1991. *Archives of Pediatric Adolescent Medicine,* 149, 1085–1091.

Tufts University. (1996). Sedentary living. *Obesity Research, 4,* 1S:8S.

Warren, M. P., & Peterson, A. (1983). Physical and biological aspects of puberty. In J. Brooks-Gunn (Ed.), *Girls at Puberty: Biological and Psychosocial Perspectives* (pp. 3-28). New York: Plenum.

Warviek, P., Toft, R., & Garrow, J. (l978). Individual differences in energy expenditure. In G. A. Gray (ed.), *Recent Advances in Obesity Research, Vol. 2.* London: Newman.

Wing, R. R., Mathews, K. A., Kuller, L. H., Meilahn, E. N., & Plantinga, P. (1991). Waist to hip ratio in middle-aged women: Associations with behavioral and psychosocial factors and with changes in cardiovascular risk factors. *Arteriosclerosis Thrombosis,* 11, 1250-1257.

Wooly, S. C., & Garner, D. M. (1991). Obesity treatment: the high cost of false hope. Journal of American Dietetic Association, 91, 1248 – 1251.

9) Nutritional and health

Acheson, J. (1993). Do carbohydrates make you fat? *Nutrition*, 9, 185.

American Dietetic Association Fact Sheet(s) for Dietetics Professionals. Chicago: ADA.

Bennett, W. I. (1995). Beyond overeating. *New England Journal of Medicine,* 332, 673-674.

Berg, F. (May/June). Nutritionists call for new approach. *Healthy Weight Journal/Obesity & Health, 5,* 3-6.

Center for Disease Control and Prevention: Guidelines for School Health Programs to PromoteLifelong Healthy Eating. (l997, March). USDHHS.

Developing Positive Eating Habits, Wisconsin Dept of Health and Social Services.

Guidelines for Adolescent Preventive Services (GAPS). (l995). Department of Adolescent Health, AMA. 515 North State Street, Chicago, Il 60610.

Ikeda J. If my child is too fat, what should I do about it? (1990). Berkeley, CA: Nutrition Education, Cooperative Extension, Dept of Nutritional Sciences, University of California.

Jequier, E. (1993). Body weight regulation in humans: The importance of nutrient balance. *NIPS*, 8, 273-276.

Kennedy, E., Bowman, S., Spence, J., Freedman, & King, J. (2001). Popular diets: Correlation to health, nutrition, and obesity. *Journal of the American Dietetic Association, 101*, 411-420.

Lytle & Achterberg. (1995). Changing the diet of America's children: What works and why? *Journal of Nutrition Education, 27,* 250-260.

Omilchinski, L. (1995). *Teens & Diets:: No Weigh*, HUGS International, Inc., Box 102A, RR#3, Portage la Prairie, Manitoba, RIN 313, Canada.

Prewitt, S., Keoh, G., Prentice, A., et al. (1991). Changes in body weight, body composition, and energy intake in women fed high and low-fat diets. *American Journal of Clinical Nutrition, 54*, 304-310.

Reaching Consumers with Meaningful Health Messages: Putting the Dietary Guidelines into Action. (1996). Dietary Guidelines Alliance.

Satter, E. (1995, November/December). The new paradigm of trust. *Healthy Weight Journal, 9(6)*, 107-108.

Satter, E. (1987). *How To Get Your Kids To Eat—But Not Too Much*. Palo Alto, CA: Bull Publications.

United States Department of Agriculture (2005). *Dietary Guidelines for Americans*, USDA, USDHHS.

Vitality Leader's Kit. (1994). Health Services and Promotion, Health and Welfare Canada. Ottawa, Ontario, Canada KiA 1B4.

Wolk, A., Manson, J., Sampfer, et al. (1999). Long term intake of dietary fiber and decreased risk of coronary heart disease among women. *Journal of the American Medical Association, 281*, 1998-2004.

10) Physical activity and health

ACSM position stand on the recommended quantity and quality of exercise for developing and maintaining cardiorespiratory and muscular fitness and flexibility in healthy adults. (1998). *Medicine and Science in Sports Exercise, 30*, 975-991.

R.J. & Wen S.J. (1994). Exercise and diet in the prevention and control of the metabolic syndrome. *Sports Medicine, 18,* 218-228. Fitness in Youth. *Medicine and Science in Sports and Exercise: 24*, 237-247.

Blair, S., Cheng, Y., & Holder, J. (2001). Is physical activity or physical fitness more important in defining health benefits? *Medicine and Science in Sports and Exercise*, 33, (Supplement) S379-399.

Blair, S., Dunn, A., Marcus, B., Cooper, K., & Jaret, P. (2001B). *Active Living Every Day: 20 Weeks To Lifelong Vitality.* Champaign, IL: Human Kinetics.

Blair, S. N., Kohl, H. W., Paffenbarger, R. S., Clark, D. G., Cooper, K. H., & Gibbons, L. W. (1980). Physical fitness and all-cause mortality: A prospective study of healthy men and women. *Journal of the American Medical Association, 262*, 2395-2401.

Berg, F. (1993, January/February). Why teenage girls drop out of sports. *Healthy Weight Journal, 8(1),* 13.

Center for disease control and prevention: Guidelines for school health programs to promote lifelong physical activity, (1997, March)., U.S. Department of Health and Human Services.

Flatt, J. P. (1987). Dietary fat, carbohydrate balance, and weight maintenance: Effects of exercise. *American Journal of Clinical Nutrition, 45,* 296-306.

Lutter, J., & Jaffe, L.,(1996). *Bodywise Woman.* Champaign, IL: Human Kinetics.

Jaffee, L. (1996, Summer). After school activities and self-esteem in adolescent girls. *Melpomene J, 15(2),* 18-25.

Jaffee, L., and Ricker, S. (1993). Physical activity and self-esteem in girls: The teen years. *Melpomene J. 12(3)*, 19-28.

Johnston, G. (1992, November/December). New vision for exercise. *Healthy Weight Journal, 6(6),* 108.

Lee, C., Blair, S., & Jackson, A. (1999). U.S. weight guidelines: Is it also important to consider cardiorespiratory fitness? *International Journal of Obesity, 22,* (Supplement 2): S2-S7.

McGinnis, J. J. (1992). The public health burden of a sedentary lifestyle. *Medicine and Science in Sports and Exercise, 24,* 196-200.

Mensink, G., Ziese, T., & Kok, F. (2000). Benefits of leisure-time physical activity on the cardiovascular risk profile at older age. *International Journal of Epidemiology, 28,* 659-666.

Pate, R., et al. (1995). Physical activity and public health: A recommendation from the CDC and the American College of Sports Medicine. *Journal of the American Medical Association, 273*, 402-407.

Schlicker, S. A., et al. (1994). The weight and fitness status of U.S. children. *Nutrition Reviews, 52(1)*, 11-16.

Stucky-Ropp, R., & DiLorenzo, T. (1993). Determinants of exercise in children, *Preventive Medicine, 22,* 880-889.

U.S. Department of Health and Human Services, Center for Disease Control. (1995, March). *Youth Risk Behavior Surveillance--U.S. Morbidity and Mortality Weekly Report, 44,* (SS-1).

Zelasko, C. (1995). Human performance laboratory recommendations. *Journal of American Dietetic Association, 95,* 1414-1417.

LESSON HANDOUTS AND OVERHEADS TO REMOVE FOR PHOTOCOPYING

HOME EDUCATION SLIPS

The following slips may be used to encourage the interest and involvement of adults at home in these *Healthy Body Image* lessons. Send the relevant slip along with the handouts from each corresponding lesson for parents or caregivers to read and sign, indicating they discussed the handouts with their student.

HOME EDUCATION

Building a Healthy Body and a Healthy Body Image

We recently began a new Unit to promote health and a healthy body image. In the Unit Introduction, we discussed the following *Body Image Building Block:*

The way we look will change as we grow up.

Please read and let your child tell you about the handouts from this unit that he or she is bringing home today. Your signature below will let us know that you received these materials.

Thank you!

Child's name ____

Your signature____

HOME EDUCATION

Building a Healthy Body and a Healthy Body Image

In Lesson 1 of this Unit we discussed this *Body Image Building Block:*

People become unhappy trying to control something that is not in their power to control. As for looks, it's best to make the most of who we were born to be.

Please read and let your child tell you about the worksheets and handouts that he or she has brought home. Your signature below will let us know you have done this.

Thank you!

Child's name ____________________________________

Your signature____________________________________

HOME EDUCATION

Building a Healthy Body and a Healthy Body Image

In Lesson 2 of this Unit we discussed this *Body Image Building Block:*

The way we look is only one part of us. We need to pay attention to all of who we are.

Please read and let your child tell you about the worksheets and handouts that he or she has brought home. Your signature below will let us know you have done this.

Thank you!

Child's name ____________________________________

Your signature____________________________________

HOME EDUCATION

Building a Healthy Body and a Healthy Body Image

In Lesson 3 of this Unit we discussed this *Body Image Building Block:*

There are many different normal ways for looks to change in puberty. Sooner or later, most girls and boys gain weight and fill out.

Please read and let your child tell you about the worksheets and handouts that he or she has brought home. Your signature below will let us know you have done this.

Thank you!

Child's name ____

Your signature____

HOME EDUCATION

Building a Healthy Body and a Healthy Body Image

In Lesson 4 of this Unit we discussed this *Body Image Building Block:*

Most of the way we look is determined before we are even born: taller, shorter, fatter, thin —all are normal, all built in.

Please read and let your child tell you about the worksheets and handouts that he or she has brought home. Your signature below will let us know you have done this.

Thank you!

Child's name ____

Your signature____

HOME EDUCATION

Building a Healthy Body and a Healthy Body Image

In Lesson 5 of this Unit we discussed this *Body Image Building Block:*

Each person's body works to grow and maintain a weight that is right for him or her.

Please read and let your child tell you about the work-sheets and hand-outs that he or she has brought home. Your signature below will let us know you have done this.

Thank you!

Child's name ____

Your signature____

HOME EDUCATION

Building a Healthy Body and a Healthy Body Image

In Lesson 6 of this Unit we discussed this *Body Image Building Block:*

Hardly anyone looks as perfect as the models in advertisements. I will be careful not to compare myself or others to them.

Please read and let your child tell you about the worksheets and handouts that he or she has brought home. Your signature below will let us know you have done this.

Thank you!

Child's name ____

Your signature____

HOME EDUCATION

Building a Healthy Body and a Healthy Body Image

In Lesson 7 of this Unit we discussed this *Body Image Building Block:*

Weight-loss diets are not a good idea. We can hold back hunger at first but will eat more to make up for it later.

Please read and let your child tell you about the worksheets and handouts that he or she has brought home. Your signature below will let us know you have done this.

Thank you!

Child's name ____

Your signature____

HOME EDUCATION

Building a Healthy Body and a Healthy Body Image

In Lesson 8 of this Unit we discussed this *Body Image Building Block:*

Satisfy hunger completely with enough wholesome food at regular meals and snacks.

Please read and let your child tell you about the worksheets and handouts that he or she has brought home. Your signature below will let us know you have done this.

Thank you!

Child's name ____

Your signature____

HOME EDUCATION

Building a Healthy Body and a Healthy Body Image

In Lesson 9 of this Unit we discussed this *Body Image Building Block:*

It is important not to sit around too much in our free time. Being active is one of the best things we can do for our health and self confidence.

Please read and let your child tell you about the worksheets and handouts that he or she has brought home. Your signature below will let us know you have done this.

Thank you!

Child's name ____

Your signature____

HOME EDUCATION

Building a Healthy Body and a Healthy Body Image

In Lesson 10 of this Unit we discussed this *Body Image Building Block:*

Choose role models you admire for things deep inside and who make you feel good about who you are.

Please read and let your child tell you about the worksheets and handouts that he or she has brought home. Your signature below will let us know you have done this.

Thank you!

Child's name ____

Your signature____

HOME EDUCATION

Building a Healthy Body and a Healthy Body Image

Throughout this Unit we discussed this *Body Image Building Block:*

It helps to support each other in having a healthy body image, in eating well, and in being active.

Please read and let your child tell you about the worksheets and handouts that he or she has brought home. Your signature below will let us know you have done this.

Thank you!

Child's name ____

Your signature____

I-A TERRY THE TADPOLE LEARNS TOOLS FOR CHANGE

Terry was a tadpole.
She lived in Silver Pool.
Every day she went to swim
With pals from her own school.

But one day Terry woke up,
Felt a pang of awful horror.
A leg was growing out of her
Where none had grown before!

Terry thought this must be bad,
She felt she was a freak.
She didn't know the facts, and so
Her fear just made her weak.

She tried to hide her leg,
But she was sure it had to show.
She felt like staying home.
She didn't want her friends to know.

The next day in the classroom
Teacher jumped into the pool
And said, "Today's the day you'll learn
You'll all be hopping soon."

"The facts are not uncertain.
For a while you may feel odd.
You're not quite tadpoles anymore,
But neither grown-up frogs."

Ms. Frog taught what would happen,
While not for everyone the same.
A few brave tadpoles raised their hands
And said they'd noticed change.

Some had legs that grew on bellies.
Some were growing fatter butts.
Some were getting bigger muscles.
Some felt awkward, like a klutz.

Some even wondered right out loud
What was wrong with them?
They hadn't noticed anything
From head to tail-end fin!

The teacher had the answers —
Terry knew she could feel great!
They had a lot in common.
It was *normal*—a tadpole's fate!

When Terry told her family
How she'd woken feeling strange,
How the teacher said it right OUT LOUD,
It wasn't strange, but CHANGE!

Her family told their stories
Of how they'd felt anxious, too.
How they had wondered, "What's the deal?"
When their body change was new.

They said at first they'd worried, too,
When friends grew more or less.
Taller, shorter, fatter, thin,
Each different than the rest.

Terry was glad to have the facts
And glad that she had talked.
The answers helped to calm her —
Now she knew that soon *she'd* hop.

Her body sure was changing,
Her friends would soon change, too.
It would take some time to get there,
But she knew now what to do.

She had to wait and watch and wonder
How her looks would be.
Meanwhile, just play and learn and grow
And keep herself HEALTHY.

I-B TOOLS FOR COPING WITH CHANGE

When your body starts to grow
from a child into a teen,
you will want to know the facts about
what will be happening.
You will want to get good answers
from the grown-ups you can trust;
those who have your health at heart
will give you answers you can trust!

It will help to hear from classmates
who are growing now with you.
You'll see you're not alone,
but just one of the group.
These body image lessons
will help you day by day
as you watch your body grow
in a healthy, "just right" way!

HEALTHY BODY IMAGE LESSONS WILL HELP ME IN THESE WAYS:

1) I will feel comfortable knowing my body is growing in a

n _ _ _ _ _ and **h** _ _ _ _ _ _ way .

2) I will understand my growth is pre-determined. This means

it is **s** _ _ - _ _ ahead of time to **b** _ a certain way.

3) I will understand what makes one person's body look

d _ _ _ _ _ _ _ _ from another's.

4) I will understand it is important not to **j** _ _ _ _

appearances during puberty or any other time.

5) I will understand what I **c** _ _ and **c** _ _ _ _ _

c _ _ _ _ _ _ about my body's size and shape.

6) I will understand how to have a good **b** _ _ _

i _ _ _ _ (feel good about my body).

I-D BODY IMAGE BUILDING BLOCKS

UNIT INTRODUCTION: The way we look will change as we grow up

LESSON 1: People become unhappy trying to control something that is not in their power to control. As for looks, it's best to make the most of who we were born to be.

LESSON 2: The way we look is only one part of us. We need to pay attention to *all* of who we are.

LESSON 3: There are many different normal ways for looks to change in puberty. Sooner or later, most girls and boys will gain weight and fill out.

LESSON 4: Most of the way we look is determined before we are even born: taller, shorter, fatter, thin—all are normal, all built in!

LESSON 5: Each person's body works to grow and maintain a weight that is natural for him or her.

LESSON 6: Hardly anyone looks as perfect as the models in advertisements. I will be careful not to compare myself or others to them.

LESSON 7: Weight-loss diets are not a good idea. We can hold back hunger for a while but will eat more to make up for it later.

LESSON 8: Satisfy hunger completely with enough wholesome food at regular at regular meals and snacks.

LESSON 9: It's important not to sit too much in our free time. Being active is one of the best things we can do for our health and self-confidence.

LESSON 10: Choose role models you admire for things deep inside and who make you feel good about who you are.

ALL LESSONS: Support each other in having a healthy body image, in eating well, and in being active.

The Body Image Building Blocks

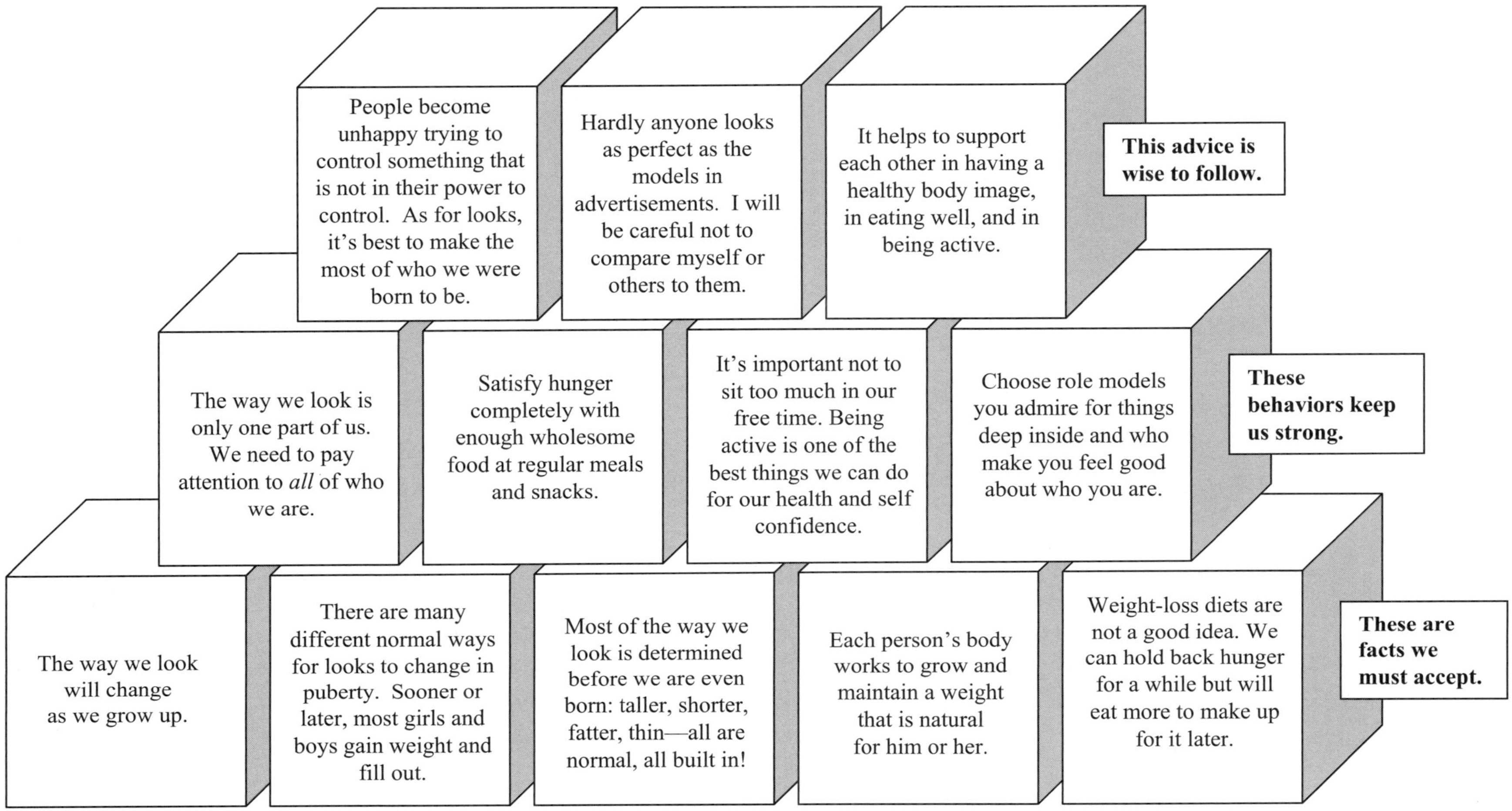

1-A

The Namuh were beings who hung many portraits on their walls. Draw a portrait of two or more people of different sizes and shapes who are important to you.

Portrait

YOUR IDENTITY: MANY PARTS MAKE YOU STRONG

Check or circle all of the items below that are part of who you are.

This may include:

- All of the things you enjoy doing, whether or not you do them well.
- All of the things you do well, even if you do not do them often.
- All of the things you have never tried but dream of doing in the future.

I AM PHYSICALLY ACTIVE

I can:

____ Run ____ Jump
____ Throw ____ Climb
____ Catch ____ Lift heavy things
____ Have energy to be active for a long time
____ Dance

I enjoy: ____ Playing outside

____ Skiing ____ Skating
____ Swimming ____ Bicycling
____ Gymnastics ____ Wrestling
____ Basketball ____ Tennis
____ Football ____ Soccer
____ Horseback riding ____ Volleyball
____ Track ____ Hockey
____ Walking ____ Dancing

List other physical activities or specific sports that are part of who you are:

____

____

____

I HAVE INTELLIGENCE. I CAN DO:

____Math ____Spelling
____Foreign language ____Science
____Reading ____Writing
____Creative Problem Solving ____ History
____Other______________________________

____

I TAKE PRIDE IN MY APPEARANCE

____ I take care of my health, eat well, stay fit, rest
____ I comb or brush my hair
____ I keep clean my hands and face
____ I like to wear my favorite colors
____ I like clothes that say something about me
____ I wear hats, jewelry, or other "decorations"
____ I like to appear friendly

Color of my hair______________________________

Eyes________________ Skin______________

My hair is: Short Medium Long
Curly Straight

Overall size (for my age): Big Small Average

Another thing about my looks is:___________

____

I AM CREATIVE OR ARTISTIC

_____ I like to draw, paint, or color

_____ I write poetry or stories _____ I dance

_____ I am in theater _____ I sew

_____ I build things or do crafts (What kind?)

_____ I am musical (In what way?)

List other creative or artistic abilities:

____

____

____

I AM OPEN TO LEARNING

_____I try new things
_____I learn from mistakes
_____I like to solve problems
_____If something is hard, I keep at it
_____I finish projects or assignments

I AM A CITIZEN (part of my community)

_____I am respectful
_____I pitch in to help
_____I am responsible
_____I work up to my ability
_____I participate (do my part)
_____I take care of the environment
_____I think about others as well as myself.

I HAVE RELATIONSHIPS

_____ I am friendly
_____ I am caring
_____ I am reliable
_____ I am loving
_____ I am kind
_____ I Communicate well
_____ I include people who are not my best friends
_____ I have fun ideas

_____ I have interests to share
_____ I am a team player—do what I'm asked for the sake of the team
_____ I can be a leader, take charge
_____ I can laugh at myself and at my mistakes
_____ I care about how people feel
_____ I can resolve conflicts

_____ I am fun to be with
_____ I enjoy humor
_____ I like to learn new things
_____ I am polite
_____ I can be serious
_____ I am a good listener
_____ I share

I MANAGE MY PHYSICAL AND EMOTIONAL HEALTH

_____I shower or bathe regularly
_____I eat healthy food
_____I am physically active
_____I play safe
_____I play smart
_____I think about healthy choices
_____I know what I need and ask for it

_____I take time to relax
_____I have realistic expectations of myself
_____I can accept it when things don't work out
_____I organize and manage my time
_____I organize and manage my belongings
_____I am able to make decisions
_____I can say no and disagree if I need to

I have many feelings:
_____happy
_____sad
_____afraid
_____hurt
_____angry
_____excited
_____anxious
_____grateful

I HAVE MANY INTERESTS (Add as many as you like!)

_____I collect things (list things that you collect):
____
____
_____I have a pet (what kind(s)?________________

List other hobbies and interests:
____
____
____

I enjoy:
_____ Cards or other indoor games
_____Miniature golf
_____Magic
_____Scuba diving
_____Cooking
_____Computers
_____Have a pen pal
_____Building things
_____Reading
____
____
____

I HAVE VALUES AND/OR BELIEFS ABOUT LIFE

Do you have a religious faith? What is it called?

____

Do you have strong cultural or ethnic ties? What are they?

____

List a few of the values you think are most important in life: ______________________________

____

MY PREFERENCES OR FAVORITES: (You may list one or more than one)

Color
Food
Drink
Quiet activity
Busy activity
Person
Teacher
Animal
Way to dress
Memory
Hobby
Sport
Fruit
Vegetable
Subject in school
Song
Game
TV show
Movie
Book
Hero

ATTRIBUTES OF MY IDENTITY

Choose two or more attributes from each category of your identity survey (2-A) that are most important to you. Write your choices in the appropriate rectangles below. You may write attributes on both sides of each card if you wish. Glue this page to a sheet of construction paper to make it stronger. Cut the rectangles into cards. Use the supplies provided by your teacher to make an Identity Mobile. Use your Identity Mobile to remember there are many parts to who you are—even more than are included here.

I am PHYSICALLY ACTIVE.	**I am CREATIVE OR ARTISTIC.**
I take PRIDE IN MY APPEARANCE.	**I have INTELLIGENCE. I do:**
I LEARN NEW THINGS.	**I am a CITIZEN (part of my community). I am:**
I have OTHER INTERESTS.	**I have RELATIONSHIPS.**
I manage my HEALTH and well being.	**I have VALUES AND/OR RELIGIOUS BELIEFS.**

3-A

HOW APPEARANCE CHANGES IN PUBERTY

By

____

Age ________

HOW APPEARANCE CHANGES IN PUBERTY

Dear Puberty Expert,
There is a lot to learn about how kids' bodies grow during puberty. I have some ideas, but I don't know if they are correct or true for everybody. Some kids in my class are already growing in new ways. I heard you had a class on this, and you might have the answers to my questions.

1. ***Does everybody go through puberty sometime?*** **Yes No**
2. ***Will growth be more than just getting taller?*** **Yes No**

   As you develop you will also be ______________________ ______________.

3. ***Is everybody supposed to change at the same time?***

   Everyone changes at ____________________________ times, according to their own inner "body ____________________________," or pre-determined ____________________________.

4. ***Do boys and girls change at the same time?*** **Yes No**

Compared to each other: (Circle. Fill in the ages)				Average age	As early as	As late as
GIRLS change:	sooner	same	later	_______	_______	_______
BOYS change:	sooner	same	later	_______	_______	_______

5. ***So it's normal for many girls to be taller than most boys at our age?*** **Yes No**
6. ***I heard someone say my friend was having a "growth spurt." What is that?***

   Growth spurts are when you grow ______________________ than ever before. During puberty, instead of growing about __________ ______________________ per year, you may grow __________ ______________________. You may hear your family say, "You are growing out of your clothes too fast." But, you can't help it!

7. ***Is it better to start puberty sooner or better to start later?* (circle)**

Better sooner **Better later** **Not better either way**

8. ***Why doesn't everybody start puberty at the same time?***

How and when we grow (circle) **is** **is not** something anyone has control over. The timing for this is ________________ - ____________________________ before birth. Whether you start your growth spurt earlier or later (circle) **will** **will not** affect how big or small you will be in the end.

9. ***What if I'm really early or late in starting puberty?*** *I don't want to be different.*

Differences in body changes: (circle) **are** **are not** something that can be judged as________________________ or __________________. No one has control over when or how changes occur. It is like the color of your eyes, or how fast your hair grows. It is not something anyone should ever have to feel bad about. Even if it would be easier to change at the same time or in the same ways as your friends, differences are a ______________________________and a ______________________________ part of life.

10. ***What if someone teases me?***

It may mean they do not understand the facts about ____________________________ or once in a while a person may intend to be mean.

You could try ____________________________________ or even ____ them. Or you could try telling a ________________________and getting his or her ________________________.

If that doesn't help, you should ask a trusted ____________________________ to stop the teasing.

11. ***Please tell me all the details about puberty changes. Will I grow everywhere all at once?***

Some parts of your body will grow ______________________________, while other parts will grow ______________________________. It is different for everyone, but here is the usual order: First ____________________________. Feet can be full-size long before you are! Then________________________________ and

____________________________________. Then________________________________

____________________________ and other bones.

12. ***What exactly will make me "fill out?" What should I expect?***

It is ____________________________________ to ________________________

____________________________________ from adding ______________________

______________________________ and ____

_________________________________ during puberty. In later teen years, you will also gain some ______________________________________.

13. ***Isn't fat bad?***

Sometimes fatness is talked about as if it were just plain "bad." There are at least three reasons why this idea is not accurate. Many people need to learn the A B Cs of body fat:

A) The body ___________________________ ______________________ without fat. It is critical for health. Fat lubricates our joints, and protects our vital organs. Body fat is also needed to help the body absorb vitamins needed for health. In addition, 60% of the solid part of the brain is made of fat. Last but not least, fat is the body's storage container for energy. We will learn more about this later.

B) ____________ people are naturally pre-disposed (set-up before they are even born) to be ___________________________, ______________________________, or in-between. When something in nature is pre-disposed, there is a *very strong* tendency for it to be a certain way. If a fatter person is ____________________ _______________, _____________________, and _______________, then his or her fatness is probably just right. No matter what people say or think, a naturally thin pre-disposition is not better than a fit and healthy fatter one; just different. The important thing is to be fit at any size.

C) When something is not in a person's control, then it is ignorant to judge it as "bad." It is also not fair. When we state that someone is "fatter" or "thinner," this should only be a way to _________________________________ that person, never a way to _______________________________ them as "good" or "bad"—as if size could be "right" or "wrong." This would be the same as judging someone because of their eye or skin color, or because they were good at music, but not at sports. Because so many people have learned incorrect information about body size and weight, we will be talking more about this in later lessons.

14. ***Besides developing earlier than boys, are there other differences for girls?***

    Yes **No**

LET'S TALK ABOUT CHANGES FOR GIRLS:

1. ***While everyone is different, it is normal for girls to gain body fat rapidly in puberty.***

   Girls may gain __________________ ___________________________ or more in one year. This does not mean they are getting fat.

2. ***Why do girls gain more body fat than boys?***

   This is the beginning of the normal, healthy rounding out of a girl's body as she grows into a young woman. Nature ___________________________ adult women to carry more body fat than most boys and men. This is part of a woman's special design for bearing children, and should not be confused with becoming unhealthily fat. It is perfectly ______________________________ for a woman to have a more ______________________________ figure than a man. Puberty is when this rounding-out begins.

3. ***What does a girl's body do with the added fat?***

   At first a girl may develop a layer of fat _____________ ______________________, like an extra layer under the skin. Then it will begin to be more obvious in certain parts: ___________________________________, ______________________________, and ____________________________.

4. ***Do girls get taller before they add fat, or rounder first?***

   Either way. Everyone is different. Some may get rounder first, and only later gain height. Others may get quite tall and thin first, later adding curves or roundness. A ________________________ girls will remain very thin and not very rounded all their lives, whether they are taller or shorter. But, despite what people think, a very thin body (circle)

   is **is not** the most common or natural body shape for a woman.

5. ***Are there any other changes for girls that boys don't share?***

Girls' pelvic bones (just above her hips) very gradually begin to ______________________________. This is essential for a woman to be capable of having a ____________________________________ when she is an adult. For example, this occurred to allow your ______________________________ to have you. Wider pelvic bones are the _______________________________________ reason why women normally have bigger hips than men. Overall, girls do develop different shapes than boys. Following are some ways girls may grow early in puberty. *(Draw the figures according to scale.)*

IN PUBERTY, GIRLS MAY GROW

Taller first	Rounder first	Not much taller or rounder	Taller and rounder	The most common adult female shape: narrower at the shoulders, wider at the hip.

LET'S TALK ABOUT CHANGES FOR BOYS

1. ***Aren't men usually bigger than women? How can boys begin their development later than girls?***

   Once outward growth begins, boys quickly catch-up. Most, but not all boys eventually become ______________________________ and more ________________________________ than most girls.

2. ***Is it normal for boys to gain body fat during puberty too?*** (circle)

Often **Sometimes** **Rarely**

Some boys become fatter before they get taller. However, as boys grow taller, many stretch out their fatness into a taller, slimmer body. While there are natural differences, most adult males carry (circle) **more** **less** body fat overall than most females.

3. ***What other changes occur for boys?***

Later in puberty, ___________________________________ can become wider, and eventually more muscular. However, boys usually do not ___________________ ___________________ their bodies until later teen years. Then, they will begin to look less like boys and more like adult males. (Draw the figures according to scale.)

IN PUBERTY, BOYS MAY GROW				
Taller first	Rounder first	Not much taller or fatter	Taller and always slim	The most common adult male shape: broader at the shoulders than at the hips.

4. ***Anything else?***

More than half of all boys will have some___________________ _________________________ in puberty. This is normal and does not mean he is developing breasts. The swelling will go away in 1 to 2 years. Boys do not need to worry about this.

5. ***What happens to a boy's voice during puberty?***

   When a boy's voice box has grown larger, usually by age 14 or 15, his voice becomes ______________________________. This may happen somewhat suddenly, or in a gradual and less noticeable way. Some boys may experience a ___________________________________ of their voices as they're going through this change. Their voices may become high-pitched or squeaky unexpectedly.

6. ***Isn't that embarrassing? What if a boy gets teased?***

   There is no reason to be embarrassed, because voice changes are simply part of growing up. But teasing is always wrong unless the person being teased is genuinely having fun.

7. ***Aren't there some other outward changes for both boys and girls in puberty?*** (circle)

   Yes **No**

LET'S TALK ABOUT CHANGES BOYS AND GIRLS HAVE IN COMMON

1. ***What are some changes boys and girls have in common?***

   Boys and girls grow hair in new places. First ______________________________ and underarm hair, then on ________________________________ and ________________________________, and for boys only, eventually _________________________ and _______________________ hair. Also, two glands become more active: __________________ and ______________________.

2. ***What about the glands?***

   When oil glands are more active, you may notice your hair gets __________________ faster. Also, many kids have some pimples or skin acne when they are further along in puberty. (More about this in later grades.) When sweat glands are more active we perspire more. Also, perspiration may have a more __________________________ _____________ odor. When oil and sweat glands become more active, kids usually need to bathe or shower and wash hair more often. You may want to ask a parent or guardian for deodorant.

3. ***It sounds like this puberty business goes on for a while. I guess it doesn't happen overnight.***

   That's: (circle) **true** **not true.**

4. ***It also sounds like different parts of the body grow earlier or later than others. If some bones grow faster than others, if I add body fat before I get taller, or if I'm getting taller before I fill out—won't I look kind of out of proportion?*** (circle)

   Yes **No** **Maybe**

   It may take several ______________________________ before you see how you will end up looking.

It is important to understand that the way you grow in puberty may not be even.

For example, your arms and legs may grow long, while your backbone is still short. Your feet may be as big as an adult's feet, even 2 or 3 years before the rest of you grows taller. Your ears and chin may grow before the rest of your face.

For a while the way you look may be very different than how you will end up. One day you may look in a mirror and enjoy seeing the changes. Another day, you may not be so crazy about them.

It may help to know many kids feel this way at one time or another. Most kids feel a little awkward or clumsy when some parts of their body are growing faster than other parts. Remember, you are not a finished product yet! That is why teasing about body changes is especially unfair and hurtful.

Remember Terry the Tadpole and picture him as half tadpole and half frog. This is not a time to judge or worry about looks. It is a time to be amazed at the many wonderful changes your body is going through as you are growing up.

THINK ABOUT IT THIS WAY:

It probably took from ________________ to ________________ years for you to gain your first fifty pounds, and longer yet to get to be four feet tall. When you start your growth spurt you may very well gain another ______________ pounds in only two or three years, and more than another foot or two of height in that same amount of time. That's a *BIG* change in a short amount of time.

My advice is:

A) ______________________ B) __________________ ________________________,

and C) give your body ________________________ to show you how it's going to end up.

If you A) ______________________ ______________________, B) stay) ______________________________, ____________________________________, and ______________________ as well as C)____________________________, you will see your body develop naturally, into the size and shape it was born to be!

Remember the *Tools for Change* from our first body image lesson:

When your body starts to grow from a child into a teen You will want to know the facts about what will be happening. You will want to get good answers from the grown-ups that you trust; those who have your health at heart will give you answers you can trust!	It will help to hear from classmates who are growing now with you. Then you'll see you're not alone, but just one of the group. These body image lessons will help you day by day As you watch your body grow in a healthy, "just right" way!

DRAW A PICTURE OF YOURSELF AS A BABY, At 5 YEARS OLD, AND NOW.

Think about all the things your body can do now
that it could not do when you were younger!

Me as a baby	Me at 5 years old
Me NOW!	

Regardless of eating behavior or activity, *genes* will determine the following:

1. How ***l—o—n—g***, **short**, narrow, or **wide** your bones will be.

   This will affect your height but also how long your arms and backbone are, how wide your shoulders and hips are, how big your feet will grow, the shape of your nose, the rest of your skull, and MORE.

2. **Whether you will be more, medium, or** less fat.

   This could be overall thinner or fatter, or thinner in some parts and fatter in other parts.

WHAT DETERMINES THE SIZE AND SHAPE OF BODIES?

- Many things may influence weight and shape. But most of the way we look is determined before we are born: taller, shorter, fatter, thin—all are normal, all built in!
- The internal "programming" for our body's size and shape is genetic. This means a natural weight range and overall body shape is *built into* our bodies before we are born.

REGARDLESS OF EATING BEHAVIOR OR ACTIVITY, *GENES* WILL DETERMINE THE FOLLOWING:

1. How *l—o—n—g*, **short,** narrow, or **wide** your **bones** will be.

This will affect your height but also how long your arms and backbone are, how wide your shoulders and hips are, how big your feet will grow, the shape of your nose, the rest of your skull, and MORE.

2. Whether you will be **more,** medium, or less fat.

This could be overall thinner or fatter,
or thinner in some parts and fatter in other parts.

PEOPLE BECOME UNHAPPY TRYING TO CONTROL SOMETHING THAT IS NOT WITHIN THEIR POWER TO CONTROL. AS FOR LOOKS, TAKE CARE OF YOUR HEALTH, AND MAKE THE MOST OF WHO YOU WERE BORN TO BE.

DO YOU KNOW WHO MAY HAVE PASSED THESE CHARACTERISTICS TO YOU?

CHARACTERISTIC	WHAT IS YOURS?	WHO IN YOUR FAMILY HAS THIS CHARACTERISTIC?
HAIR COLOR		
HAIR TYPE (straight, curly, etc.)		
EYE COLOR		
SHAPE OF NOSE		
SHAPE OF MOUTH		
SKIN COLOR		
Other Abilities or Talents: ATHLETIC		
MATHEMATIC		
ARTISTIC		
MUSICAL		
OTHER *(name other abilities you think may be inherited.)*		

YOUR GENETIC FAMILY TREE

I. Use the following plan to draw your own *Genetic Family Tree* on a *larger paper.*

A. FOR CHILDREN WHO KNOW THEIR BIOLOGICAL FAMILY:

Draw a *rough* picture of your blood relatives. Include brothers and sisters, parents and grandparents. If possible, also add aunts and uncles and great-grandparents. Get help from adults at home who may be able to describe relatives you do not know well. Show as many of the following as possible:

- hair color
- hair type (straight or curly)
- eye color
- skin color
- height (taller, medium, shorter)
- body type or overall shape (thinner, medium, or fatter)

It is not important that your drawings be artistic. What is important is that your pictures help you think about all the genes you have inherited that will determine how you will look.

B. FOR CHILDREN WHO DO NOT KNOW THEIR BIOLOGICAL RELATIVES:

If you or the adults you live with do not know your blood relatives, or know only a few, this activity is still a great one for you. Your genetic heritage is important. All you have to do is look at yourself. Then imagine and draw a Family Tree that includes characteristics your blood relatives MUST have had—because *you* have those characteristics! Let an adult or your teacher help you.

II. If you have special abilities or talents, you may have inherited these as well. Write them next to any people who also have those talents.

SAMPLE: (make yours large enough so you can sketch and color the characteristics.)

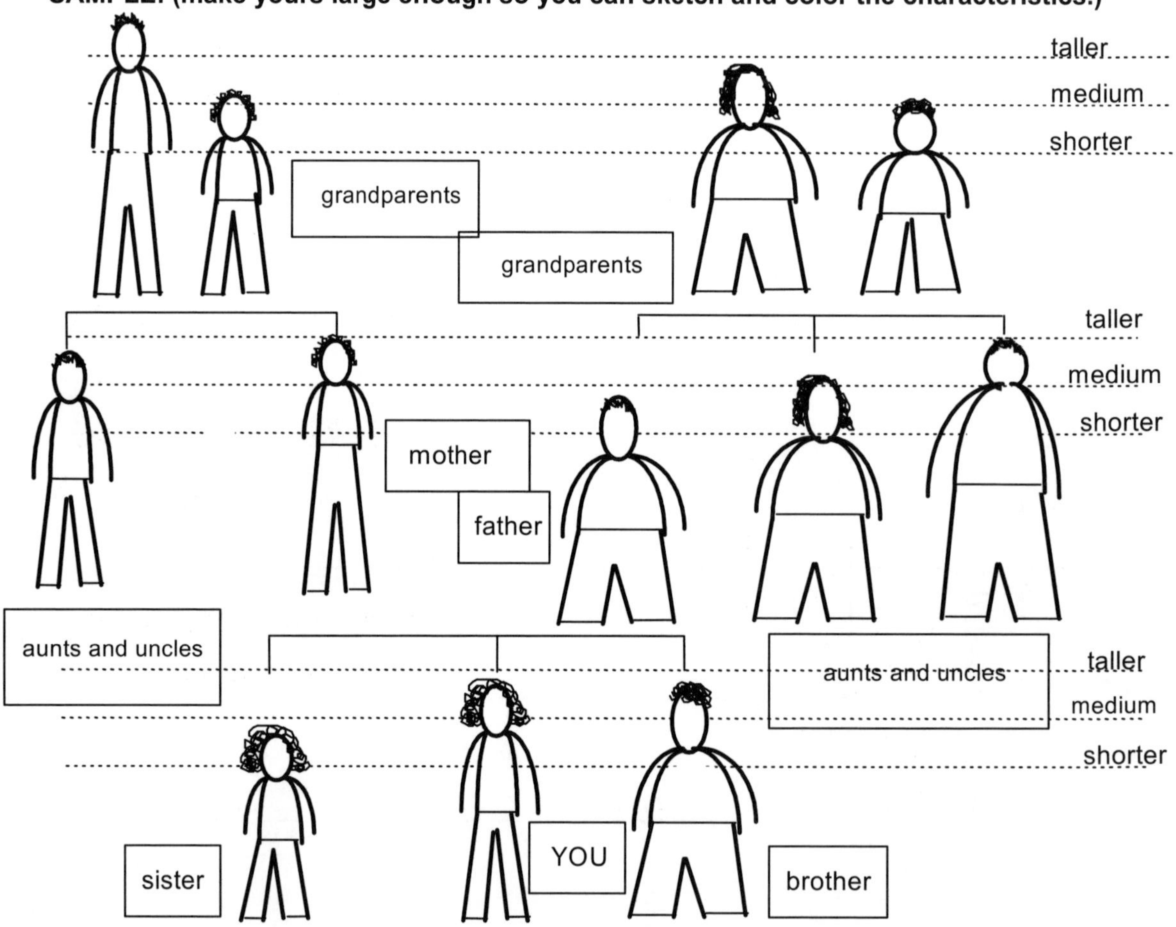

5-A **WHAT IS THE MAIN INFLUENCE FOR FATNESS OR THINNESS?**

Understanding the Internal Weight Regulatory System

If you forget to put gas in your car, it will stall—unless you have a "reserve" tank of gas.

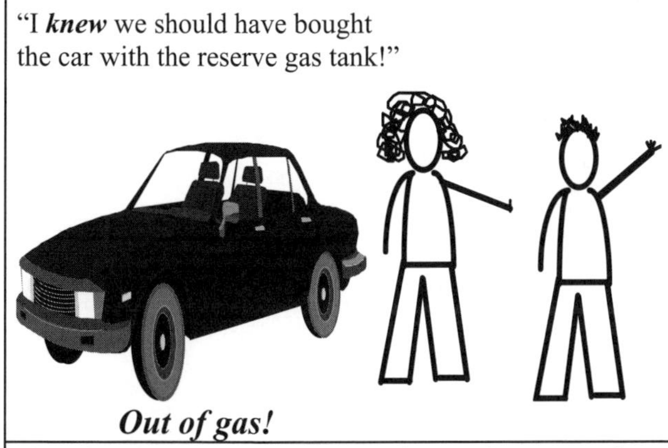

Fortunately, nature built in a way for bodies not to "stall" when there is not enough to eat. Fat is fuel that is stored "in reserve." Why do some people store more of it than others?

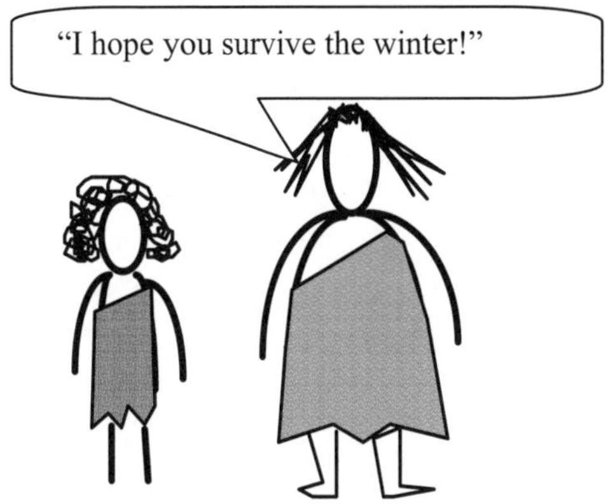

People often assume that people are fatter or thinner entirely because of how they eat or how active they are. But this is a myth.

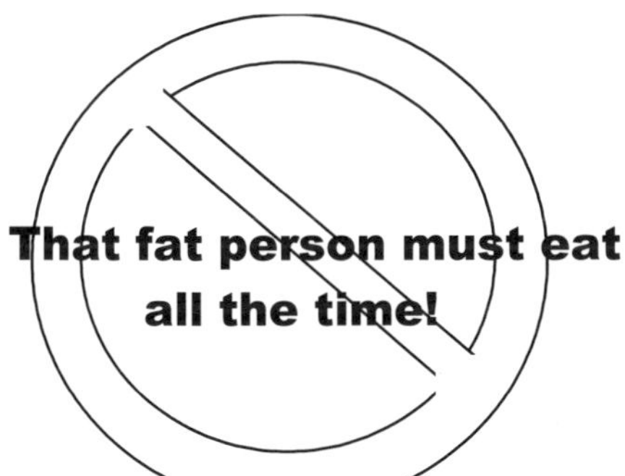

Bodies work from the inside to grow and to maintain a weight that is natural for each one. For this to work, we must listen to the messages our bodies send.

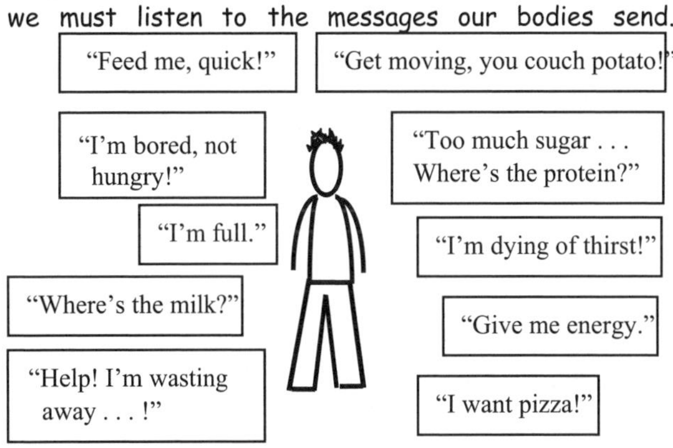

If everyone ate exactly the same food and was active in exactly the same ways all the time, they would still be many different shapes and sizes.

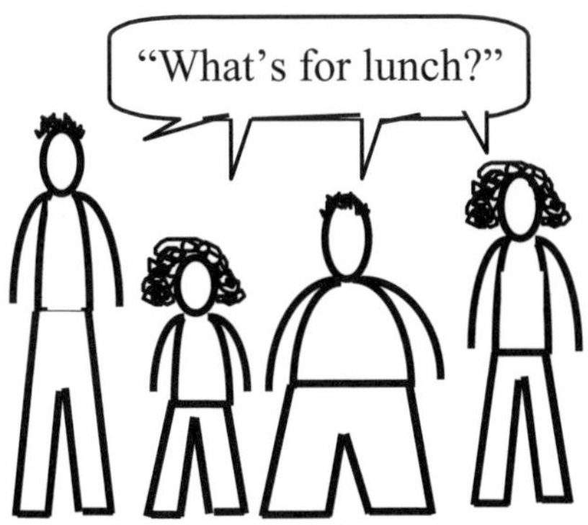

Same-age friends

Eat well and be active for nutrition, energy, satisfaction of hunger, and enjoyment.

Trust your body to find a healthy weight for you.

LUNCH

1) Cut out the foods below for your lunch.
2) Cut up the foods into "bites" along the dotted lines. You should have 16 portions, or "bites," of lunch when you are finished.

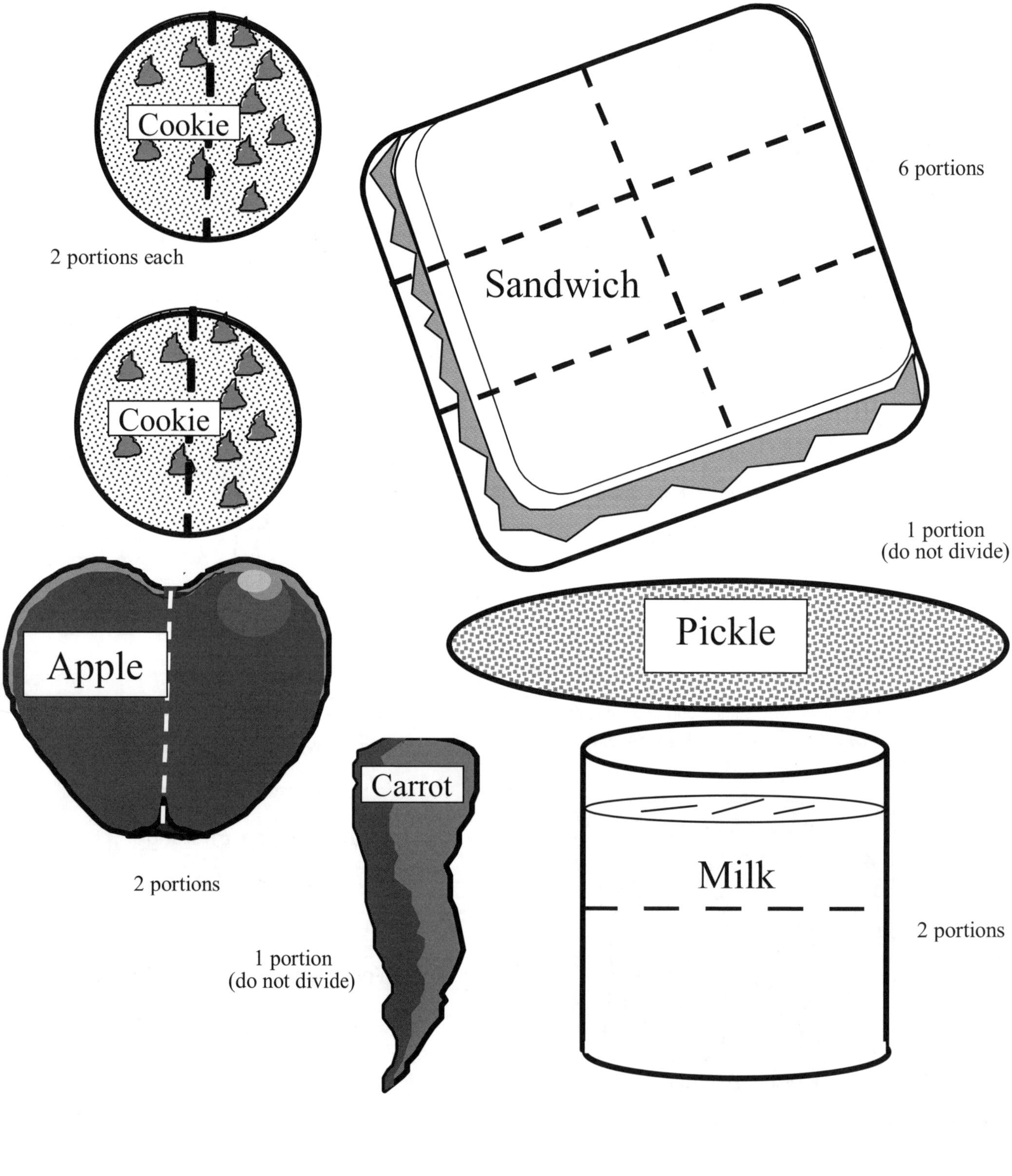

5-C

METABOLISM RATE HANDOUT

(Copy and cut the number needed according to a normal distribution, as directed.)

METABOLISM RATE DIRECTIONS 1

Your body will metabolize your food at this rate:
ONE BITE EVERY OTHER "15 MINUTES"

You will put one bite of your lunch into your body's Metabolism Energy Converter *every other* time your teacher signals.

METABOLISM RATE DIRECTIONS 2

Your body will metabolize your food at this rate:
ONE BITE EVERY "15 MINUTES" — except YOU WILL SKIP EVERY 4TH "FUELING"

You will put one bite of your lunch into your body's Metabolism Energy Converter every time your teacher signals— *except* you will skip every 4th signal.

METABOLISM RATE DIRECTIONS 3

Your body will metabolize your food at this rate:
ONE BITE EVERY "15 MINUTES"

You will put one bite of your lunch into your body's Metabolism Energy Converter every time your teacher signals.

METABOLISM RATE DIRECTIONS 4

Your body will metabolize your food at this rate:
ONE BITE EVERY "15 MINUTES" — except for EVERY 4TH "FUELING," when you will "burn up" 2 bites.

Every time your teacher signals, you will put one bite of your lunch into your body's Metabolism Energy Converter— *except* you will put 2 bites into the converter every 4th signal.

METABOLISM RATE DIRECTIONS 5

Your body will metabolize your food at a rate of
TWO BITES EVERY "15 MINUTES"

Every time your teacher signals, you will put two bites of your lunch into your body's Metabolism Energy Converter.

HOW STORIES ARE TOLD BY PICTURES IN ADVERTISING

Our Product is for YOU:	
	moms, dads, teens, animal lovers, old people, tough guys, cool girls, teachers, dancers, athletes, gardeners, swimmers, cooks, etc.
You are a person who is or could be:	
	happy, safe, loved, popular, adventurous, cool, healthy, gorgeous, successful, etc., or lonely, stressed out, in pain, worried, etc.
You believe in:	
	family life, getting ahead, being good, taking care of yourself, winning, looking good, working hard, having fun, a religious faith, etc.
You want:	
Beauty:	**great hair, white teeth, beautiful eyes, to lose weight, thin thighs, big muscles, smooth hands, clear skin, long fingernails, young skin, the "right" look, etc.**
Popularity:	**attractiveness, pizzazz, what it takes, etc.**
Power:	**control, to be "in charge," money, wisdom, fame, prestige, the "right" image, etc.**
Interest:	**a cause, fun, laughs, color, excitement, speed, quiet, energy, the meaning of life, etc.**
Balance:	**time, health, comfort, peace of mind, etc.**
You need: **OUR PRODUCT!**	

READ AND DISCUSS AT HOME

How stories are told by pictures in advertising

OUR PRODUCT IS FOR YOU: moms, dads, teens, animal lovers, old people, tough guys, cool girls, teachers, dancers, athletes, gardeners, swimmers, cooks, etc.

YOU ARE A PERSON WHO IS OR COULD BE: happy, safe, loved, popular, adventurous, cool, healthy, gorgeous, successful, etc., or lonely, stressed out, in pain, worried, etc.

YOU BELIEVE IN: family life, getting ahead, being good, taking care of yourself, winning, looking good, working hard, having fun, a religious faith, etc.

YOU WANT:

Beauty: great hair, white teeth, beautiful eyes, to lose weight, thin thighs, big muscles, smooth hands, clear skin, long fingernails, young skin, the "right" look, etc.

Popularity: attractiveness, sparkle, pizzazz, what it takes, etc.

Power: control, to be "in charge," money, wisdom, fame, prestige, the "right" image, etc.

Interest: a cause, fun, laughs, color, excitement, speed, quiet, energy, the meaning of life, etc.

Balance: time, health, comfort, peace of mind, etc.

YOU NEED: OUR PRODUCT!

EXAMPLES: Product, Words, and Picture	Unspoken Story
Car: *"The only mini-van to earn five stars in the crash test."* Beautiful, smiling, slim mother dressed in the latest style, standing by a van with five smiling, good-looking kids.	You value your family and want to be a top-notch mom. You also want to be a fun, trendy, attractive lady. You can have the good looks that lead to happiness and a happy, attractive family if you buy our product!
Hair conditioner: *"No more tug of war!"* (*Before*: Ungroomed, mad mom with comb and tearful girl with messy hair and clothing. *After*: Well-groomed, attractive, hugging, happy pair.)	Relationships are important to you. You feel bad and guilty when you fight with your daughter. To help you daughter achieve the good looks that will make her love and admire you, just buy our product!
Antacids: *"How do you spell RELIEF?"* (Miserable, pudgy, balding man in a sweat-suit at football game. Next to him are two slim, handsome, well-dressed happy men with two very pretty women.)	You could be a fun, eye-catching guy. Why let indigestion make you unattractive? To enjoy life, be the good looking guy you were meant to be, and *attract a pretty date*, you *need* our product!
Toy: Two very attractive, bright-eyed, laughing girls with shiny hair and stylish clothes are playing together with a *brand-name toy*. They are surrounded by other happy, attractive children who are eagerly watching.	No need to be left out or worry that you might not have friends and be popular. Without a doubt you will be one of the attractive, happy, popular kids when you buy our product!
Weight-loss plan: *"Diet magic! Lose 30 pounds in 30 days with No Hunger!"* Two photos: One is a black/white, grainy photo of a fat, sad-looking, woman with uncombed hair and unstylish clothing. The other is a color photo of the same woman, now slim, wearing a swimsuit and walking with a handsome man.	Hasn't your fatness kept you alone and unhappy long enough? No need for you to be shunned. Lose weight quickly and get the relationships you've been waiting for. To be slim and find happiness by next summer, just buy our product!

READ AND DISCUSS ADVERTISING STRATEGY AT HOME

Advertisements featuring models with "ideal" looks contain this common story:
"You need something. In fact, if you compare yourself and your life to what you see in this picture, you will know there is a *lot* you could improve upon. See how these models are completely happy, healthy, and appear in control? See how attractive they are? Without a doubt, they are having better lives than you. *You can tell this because of how good they look.* If you compare yourself and your life to what you see in these models, you will quickly know that you are missing something. The models and their products *go together*. If you buy the products, you and your life will be *more like theirs."*

Advertisers want you to believe you need improvement and that their products will correct what you are lacking. Be careful before you "buy" this idea!

Advertisements suggest there is a "right way" for men to look. Is it realistic?
Male models look strikingly handsome. Their bodies have broad shoulders balanced over narrow hips. Often they have intense eyes that look cool, detached, and far away, or they seem to look right through you. The "take-charge" eyes above strong chins and straight noses suggest these men are tough, on top of things, and clearly have no insecurities or worries. Some even look a little mean. Do most men look like this?

Advertisements suggest there is a "right way" for women to look. Is it realistic?
Most female models look extraordinarily beautiful, sophisticated, sleek, and very, very slim. They have only smooth lines and no fat. Their clothes hang perfectly, without a lump or bulge. Their skin is completely clear, without a wrinkle or blemish; their mouths are perfectly drawn and colored; and their eyes are bright and even, with long, divided lashes. Every hair shines. Do most women look like this?

Think about it.
Do you think you should try to copy the look of beautiful models in photo ads? Should you look for a girlfriend or boyfriend who looks like a model? Why or why not?

Fewer than three in 100 women naturally have the "ideal" body type of models shown in most advertisements. More than 97% of women do not. This strategy is very successful in convincing the majority of women that, by comparison, they are "too fat" or otherwise inadequate. After creating this insecurity, advertisers claim that buying their product will help. What do you think?

Neither male nor female models look as "good" as their pictures. Media images are "enhanced." Special lighting, make-up, and computer imaging make models look better than anyone could look in real life. It is normal to want to feel special. Advertisers hope to "wake up" your natural wish for this when you look at images of "beautiful" people. Think twice before you are "sold" on the idea that a certain look will make you special.

When basic needs for life are not fully met, you can expect the following:

1. You will be constantly thinking about what is missing: sleep, water, air, food, warmth.

2. It will be hard to concentrate or think about anything else.

3. There will be a powerful craving (drive) to satisfy the need (tiredness, thirst, hunger, etc.)

4. Until satisfied, the craving will be very uncomfortable. You may become crabby and self-centered. It will be hard to think about anyone else's needs.

5. When the need is finally met, more than a normal amount will be needed in order to feel satisfied.

CONSEQUENCES OF DIETING

1. A dieter is almost constantly thinking about <u>FOOD</u>.
2. When dieting, it is hard to <u>CONCENTRATE</u> on or think about anything else.
3. There is a <u>POWERFUL</u> craving for <u>FOOD</u>, especially fast-energy foods like sweets and high-fat foods.
4. Not satisfying hunger is very <u>UNCOMFORTABLE</u>. It is not surprising that dieters may feel <u>CRABBY</u> and may think most about <u>THEIR</u> <u>OWN</u> needs.
5. A <u>HUGE</u> hunger is felt when a dieter stops dieting. This makes a dieter feel he or she cannot get enough food. It is normal to expect to rapidly eat a <u>LARGE</u> amount of food when going off a diet—far <u>MORE</u> than a normal amount. Dieters may not know they are full until they feel "<u>STUFFED</u>."
6. The longer and more often a dieter diets, the <u>MORE</u> overeating occurs. <u>DIETING</u> is one of the most common causes of overeating.
7. After losing weight on a diet, most people <u>REGAIN</u> the weight plus <u>ADDED</u> pounds.
8. The more people diet, the harder it is to tell when they are full and when they are still <u>HUNGRY</u>. They may always <u>FEEL</u> <u>HUNGRY</u> even if they are not. If they stop dieting long enough, they may get back their normal hunger sensor.

7-C DIETING FOR WEIGHT LOSS CAN CAUSE BIG PROBLEMS

Many believe that eating less than they are hungry for is good for losing weight. But food is a *basic need*. When basic needs are not fully satisfied, here's what you can expect:

1. You will be constantly thinking about what is missing (sleep, water, air, warmth, food).
2. It will be hard to concentrate or think about anything else.
3. There will be a powerful craving to satisfy the need.
4. Until satisfied, the craving will be very uncomfortable. You may become crabby or self-centered. It will be hard to think about others' needs.
5. When you can finally satisfy the need, *more* than a normal amount will be needed for complete satisfaction.

Water, air, food, sleep, and warmth satisfy basic needs.

You can expect these consequences if you restrict your hunger to lose weight:

1) A dieter is almost constantly thinking about ________________.

2) When dieting, it is hard to ________________ on or think about anything else.

3) There is a________________ craving for ________________, especially fast-energy foods like sweets and high-fat foods.

4) Not satisfying hunger is very ________________. It is not surprising dieters may have ________________ patience, feel ________________, and may be thinking most about________________ ________________ needs.

5) A ________________hunger is felt when a dieter stops dieting. This makes a dieter feel he or she cannot get enough food. It is normal to expect to rapidly eat a very ________________ amount of food when going off a diet—far ________________ than a normal amount. Dieters may not know they are full until they feel "________________."

6) The longer and more often a dieter diets, the ________________ overeating, or "stuffing," occurs. ________________ is one of the most common causes of overeating.

7) After losing weight on a diet, most people ________________ the weight plus ________________ pounds.

8) The more people diet, the harder it is to tell when they are full and when they are still hungry. They may always ________________ ________________ even if they are not. If they stop dieting long enough, they may get back their normal ________________ sensor.

When you need a drink, it's hard to think! Can you concentrate when your lunch is late?	***Dieting to lose weight is not a good idea. To find the natural weight that's best for you, eat well and be active for fun and fitness.***

My Pyramid

STEPS TO A HEALTHIER YOU

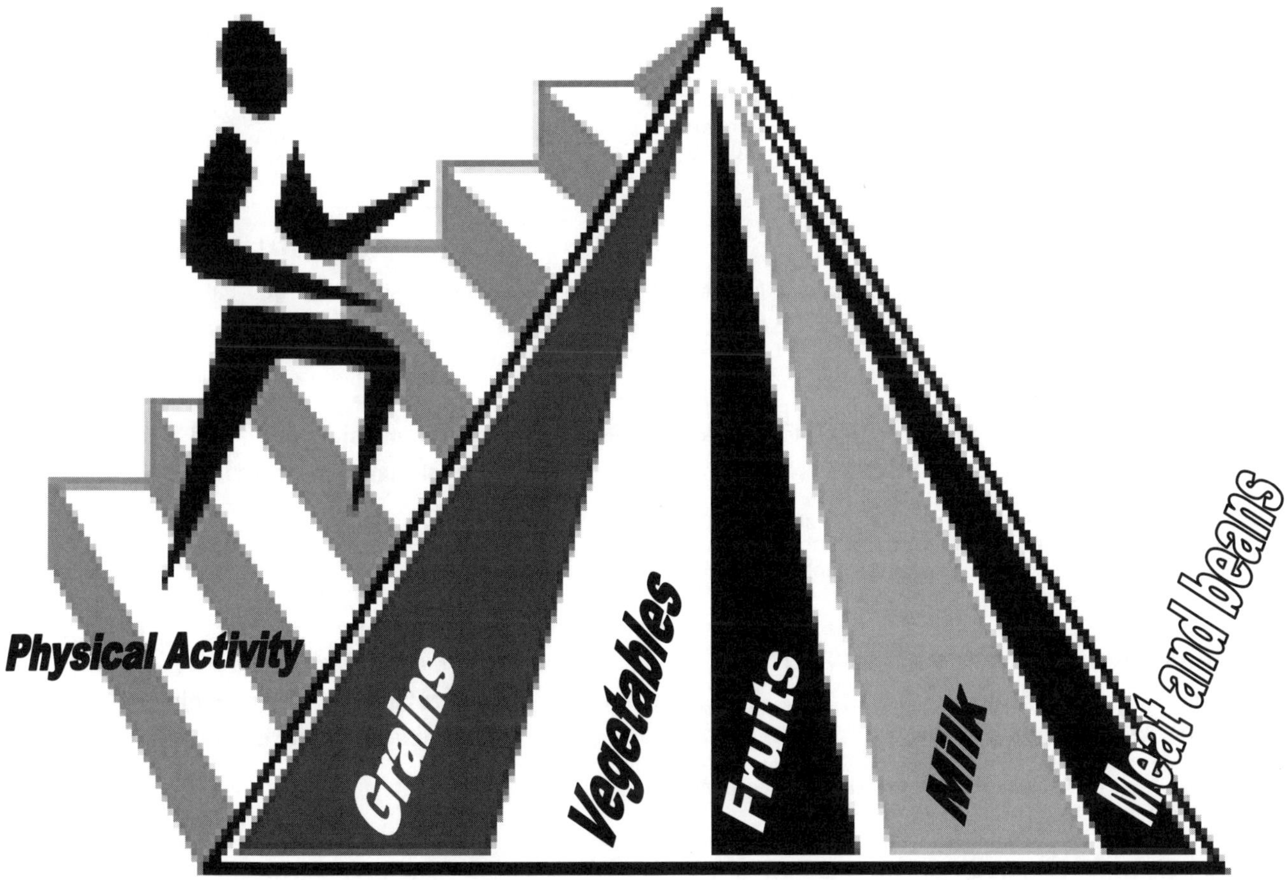

Food Guidelines—DO YOU EAT ENOUGH?

FOOD GROUP	DO YOU EAT ENOUGH FOR HEALTH?
GREAT GRAINS Build your body with great grains from the earth. Make at least half of your choices *whole* grains, like *whole wheat* bread, pasta, and cereal, and brown and wild rice. Don't be fooled by caramel-colored "wheat" bread or cereal. Whole oats, barley, buckwheat, bulgur, corn, wheat, and rye are all examples of whole grains.	**EAT at least 5-6 servings of grain a day. Make half or more of these *whole* grains.** A serving is 1 average slice of bread, 1/2 bagel, 1 cup of flaked cereal, or ½ cup of pasta or rice. Most people need more than one serving of grain in a meal to satisfy hunger and to get in enough grain in a day.
VERY VARIED VEGETABLES Eat veggies raw or cooked, fresh or frozen, canned or any other way you like to get a variety of types and colors every day. Dark green, orange, brown, red, white, or yellow—choose a variety of colors to get all the different nutrients these provide.	**EAT at least 4 servings of vegetables a day.** A serving is about the size of ½ cup. Eat 2 or more cups of different vegetables each day.
FRUIT FOR FUN Eat fruit fresh, whole or cut up, canned or cooked. Mix it into yoghurt, put it on your cereal, make a smoothie, or freeze it into popsicles. Choose 2-3 different fruits every day just for the health of it.	**EAT at least 3 servings of fruit a day.** A serving is about the size of ½ cup. Eat 1½ or more cups of different fruits each day.
MILK, YOGURT AND CHEESE, AND OTHER CALCIUM-RICH FOODS Your bones need a lot of calcium to grow strong. Choose low-fat milk, yogurt, cheese, and ice cream. If you cannot drink dairy products, choose calcium-fortified foods, soy-based foods, and some fish.	**DRINK 3 glasses of skimmed or 1% milk a day, or an equal amount of other calcium-rich foods.**
MEAT AND BEANS FOR LEAN PROTEIN Eat protein to build strong muscles. Choose chicken, turkey, lean beef, pork, or lamb without visible fat. Choose more low-fat lunch meats than those with a greasy feel, like salami. Peanut butter and eggs are also rich in protein.	**EAT low-fat meat, brown beans, peanut butter, eggs, tofu, or other high-protein foods at least once or twice a day.**
FATS FROM PLANTS AND FISH Fats are essential for health. However, we now know that fats that come from animals, like butter and fat that is hidden in cheese, meat, and cream, can contribute to heart problems. Fats that come from vegetables, nuts, or fish do not cause the same health concerns.	Many foods have fat built into them. Therefore, *added* fats are not required for most people. However, fats carry the flavor in foods and make them very satisfying. Use butter, mayonnaise, salad dressings, or oils used for cooking with some restraint for the taste, hunger satisfaction, and enjoyment they provide. Eat deep-fried foods occasionally rather than as a rule.
SUGAR Sugar is a fun food. Almost everyone enjoys its sweetness. But sugar contains calories without nutrients. Satisfy hunger with nutritious food before too much is spent on sweet treats.	No added sugar is needed for health.

8-C

Do You Eat Enough? Daily Food Record ©

DIRECTIONS: Use a new copy of this page for each day that you record what you eat. At the end of each day, count the number of servings that you have eaten from each food group and write that number in the "count" column. When you have records for up to 5 days, record your results on 8-D—the *Do You Eat Enough?* graph. The graph will show you whether you are giving your body enough of the nutrients it needs.

MEAL ⇨ **FOOD GROUP** ⇩	**BREAKFAST**	**LUNCH**	**DINNER**	**SNACKS:** Morning Afternoon Evening	**COUNT**
GRAIN (note which are whole grains Cereal, rice, pasta, breads, wild rice, grits, tortillas, cous cous, popcorn, pancakes, waffles, etc.					
VEGETABLES Corn, peas, beans, potatoes, carrots, broccoli, beets, parsnips, lettuce, tomatoes, peppers, avocados, mushrooms, sprouts, etc.					
FRUIT Apples, bananas, oranges, melons, grapes, pineapple, peaches, pears, berries, mangos, etc.					
MILK/CALCIUM Low-fat milk, cheese, ice cream, yogurt (if these are made with cream and sugar, count also as fat/sugar), other calcium-rich foods.					
MEAT AND BEANS Fish, meats, eggs, tofu, nuts, peanut butter, brown beans, and other legumes.					
ADDED FAT/ SUGAR Butter, oil, margarine, mayonnaise, cream, cheese, cream, sugar, all foods combined with fats & sugars so most of their energy comes from the fat and/or sugar.					
WATER (Count the number of times you take a drink.)					

8-D

Do You Eat Enough? Graph Daily Food Intake

- **Mark the number of servings you ate each day from each food group.**
- **Reach to touch the gray for the minimum each day!**

GRAINS—At least 5-6 servings per day. Try to make more than half of your choices *whole* grains.

Servings	1	2	3	4	5	6	7	8	9
Day 1									
Day 2									
Day 3									
Day 4									
Day 5									

1. Do you eat enough from each food group?

VEGETABLES—4 or more servings per day

Servings	1	2	3	4	5	6	7	8	9
Day 1									
Day 2									
Day 3									
Day 4									
Day 5									

2. If not, how can you make room for what you need?

FRUITS—3 or more servings per day

Servings	1	2	3	4	5	6	7	8	9
Day 1									
Day 2									
Day 3									
Day 4									
Day 5									

MILK, OR CALCIUM-RICH FOODS—3 glasses per day or the equivalent

Servings	1	2	3	4	5	6	7	8	9
Day 1									
Day 2									
Day 3									
Day 4									
Day 5									

MEAT AND BROWN BEANS OR LEGUMES—Once or twice per day

Servings	1	2	3	4	5	6	7	8	9
Day 1									
Day 2									
Day 3									
Day 4									
Day 5									

ADDED FATS AND SUGAR—No portions needed; enjoy in limited amounts.

Servings	1	2	3	4	5	6	7	8	9
Day 1									
Day 2									
Day 3									
Day 4									
Day 5									

Water fulfills a basic need. On average, how many drinks did you have each day? ______

8-E

In my neighborhood, stores that sell treats are everywhere.
When I see the signs, I always think, "Let's stop and get some!" (Second-grade student)

Draw an advertisement urging people to eat a variety of wholesome foods. What "story" will your advertisement tell?

Does advertising affect what you choose to eat?

CATEGORIES OF MOVEMENT

1. **Passive sitting**—Awake but sitting with both upper and lower body still. EX: Watching a video, reading, thinking, writing a letter, talking quietly, playing a hand-held game, or using a computer.

2. **Active sitting**—Sitting but with the upper body busy. EX: Doing artwork, playing cards, eating, enjoying lively conversation, or playing a more active game in which your upper body is moving.

3. **Normal movement**—Everyday movement on your feet. EX: Walking normally, doing chores, playing on your feet, going shopping, walking to school or the corner store, rehearsing a play.

4. **Vigorous movement**—On the go at a faster pace. EX: Walking fast, playing a start-stop running game, climbing trees, playing in the water, or riding a bike. This kind of movement includes a rise in heartbeat and breathing but either for short bursts of time or for sa moderate rise that is sustained for a longer time.

5. **Aerobic movement**—Working large muscles so the heart is beating rapidly for an extended time (15 to 30 minutes or more). EX: Dancing fast, swimming hard, aerobic walking, soccer or another running sport, skiing, rollerblading, or biking at a fast pace.

Sample Activity Diary

	Sedentary	Active sitting	Movement	Vigorous	Aerobic
Before school		**Played with cat: 15 min.** **Ate breakfast: 15 min.** **Rode bus: 15 min.**	**Showered: 15 min.** **Got dressed: 15 min.**	**Played & did handstands at bus stop: 15 min.**	
School-day morning	**Read and listened: 1/2 hr.**	**Worked at desk: 1 hr.**	**Library: 30 min.** **Walking: 15 min.**	**Phys. ed. warm-up: 15 min.**	**Phys. ed. running games: 15 min.**
Lunch period		**Ate lunch and talked with friends: 30 min.**	**Talked on playground: 15 min.**	**Played keep-away: 15 min.**	
School-day after-noon	**Read and listened, saw video: 1-1/4 hr.**	**Wrote a test: 30 min.** **Worked in small group: 30 min.**	**Choir practice: (standing) 30 min.** **Walked: 15 min.**	**Spelling "bee"— (standing & nervous): 15 min.**	
After school until dinner	**TV: 1 hr.**	**Rode bus: 15 min.** **Homework: 30 min.**	**Walked dog: 15 min.**	**Warmed up for soccer and on sidelines: 30 min.**	**Played soccer: 35 min.**
Dinner and until bed	**Computer game: 30 min.** **Read: 15 min.**	**Dinner: 30 min.** **Played cards: 15 min.** **Talked on phone: 15 min.** **Piano: 30 min.**	**Walked dog: 15 min.** **Did dishes: 15 min.** **Played with sister: 30 min.**		
TOTALS:	***2 hours, 30 min.***	***5 hours, 30 min.***	***3 hours, 15 min.***	***1 hour, 30 min.***	***35 min.***

9-C

HOW MUCH ARE YOU ACTIVE? HOW MUCH DO YOU SIT?

Directions: Record your activity for at least two days using the following key. Use a separate Activity Diary for each day. "Guestimate" the time to the nearest 15 minutes.

Sedentary activity: Sitting very still, absorbed and focused: TV, computer games, reading, etc.
Active sitting: Sitting but busy: writing, artwork, playing cards, eating, etc.
Normal movement: Up and moving: normal walking, building an indoor fort, doing dishes, shopping
Vigorous movement: On the go: swinging, climbing, hide & seek, playing catch, heavy chores, etc.
Aerobic activity: Any activity that makes your heart race for several minutes or more without stopping.

	Sedentary	**Active sitting**	**Movement**	**Vigorous**	**Aerobic**
Before school					
School-day morning					
Lunch period					
School-day afternoon					
After school until dinner					
Dinner and until bed					
TOTALS:					

9-D ACTIVITY PYRAMID

How will you use your free time?

Sedentary: **Sitting with little movement.**

Limit when possible

Active sitting: **Sitting but with upper body movement.**

Do a little less

Vigorous movement: **Examples: Fast walking, playing in water, swinging, hide & seek, playing catch, heavy chores, karate, riding bike, etc.**

Do a lot or regularly

Heart-pumping movement: **Examples: Fast dancing, long-distance running or swimming, aerobic walking, playing soccer, jumping rope, tag with the dog, skiing, skating, or biking fast, etc.**

Do more. Do 30 minutes every day in 10 minute or longer intervals.

Everyday chores and activities on your feet: **Walking to school, building a fort, shopping, taking the stairs, playing outside, walking the dog, making the bed, helping a neighbor, rehearsing a play, painting a wall, giving a speech, sweeping the floor, baby-sitting, etc.**

Do plenty every day.

9-E ACTIVITY PYRAMID

How will you use your free time?

Sedentary:

Limit when possible

Active sitting:

Do a little less

Vigorous movement:

Do a lot or regularly

Heart-pumping movement:

Do more. Do 30 minutes every day in 10 minute or longer intervals.

Everyday chores and activities on your feet:

Do plenty every day.

10-A Overhead

WHAT DO YOU THINK?

A. What if the swan had stayed with the ducks?

B. If one choice is "*good*," are other choices "*bad*"?

C. We all like things that are "cool." Are there times when what is considered to be cool isn't right for everyone?

D. Does it matter to what or to whom we compare ourselves?

- If apples compared themselves to oranges, how would they feel about being apples?
- The Namuh compared themselves to tall, thin, unusually beautiful models. How did this affect them?

E. How can the experience of the *Ugly Duckling* help you in your life?

10-B WHO WILL YOU CHOOSE FOR YOUR ROLE MODELS?

1. People we admire often become our role models. Think of two people you admire and might choose as role models. At least one should be someone you know personally. The other may be someone you do not know but have read or heard a lot about.
   - *You should know more than one quality about your role model. For example, you may admire a famous athlete, but if you only know he or she is a great athlete, and nothing more, that would not be enough.*

2. List at least five qualities about each of these people that you admire and would like to develop in yourself. If you cannot think of five, choose a different person for your role model.
   - *Consider deeper qualities in your role model, not merely what you see on the surface. For example, what type of person he or she is, what does he or she believe in and how does he or she act?*
   - *If you were to try to be like the role models you have chosen, would you feel healthy and stronger, or would you feel mismatched, like the Ugly Duckling?*

Name of your role model:	**Name of your role model**
______________________________	______________________________
Five qualities you admire in this person:	**Five qualities you admire in this person:**
______________________________	______________________________
______________________________	______________________________
______________________________	______________________________
______________________________	______________________________
______________________________	______________________________
______________________________	______________________________
______________________________	______________________________
______________________________	______________________________
______________________________	______________________________
______________________________	______________________________
______________________________	______________________________
______________________________	______________________________
______________________________	______________________________
______________________________	______________________________
______________________________	______________________________
______________________________	______________________________
______________________________	______________________________
______________________________	______________________________
______________________________	______________________________

10-C **Adults may also answer the following question and share their responses with students.**

Draw a picture or write about a time when you or someone you know felt like the Ugly Duckling

Just about everyone has felt like the *Ugly Duckling* sometime. Think of a real-life example of this from your own or someone else's life. Then draw a picture or write about this. How did you or the person cope with this? What ideas do you have now about what might have helped?

Remember what helped the Ugly Duckling? The same things could help you:

- He did not keep trying to be something he was not meant to be.
- He did not keep trying with those who would not appreciate him.
- He did not give up. He knew he needed to belong somewhere.
- He let caring companions help him along the way.
- When he met those who did not have his best interests at heart, he moved on.
- He paid attention to what had touched him in a good way *deep inside.*
- He found others with whom he naturally shared things in common and saw their beauty in himself.
- He recognized he could not change the ducks, but he knew they were wrong about him.
- He realized he could feel good about himself.

SUPPLEMENTAL HANDOUTS AND OVERHEADS
TO REMOVE FOR PHOTOCOPYING

The Model for Healthy Body Image

<table>
<tr><th>Conceptual Building Blocks</th><th>Foundation</th><th>Desired Outcome</th><th>Goal</th></tr>
<tr><td>Developmental change is inevitable.

Normal changes of puberty include weight gain and temporary out-of-proportion growth; fat does not by itself define "overweight."

Genetics and other internal weight regulators strictly limit the degree to which shape, weight & Body Mass Index (BMI) can be manipulated through healthy means.

Restricted or restrained hunger (dieting) results in predictable consequences that are counterproductive to weight loss and interfere with normal hunger regulation.</td><td>Recognize and respect basic biology; understand what is not in our control regarding size, shape, weight, and hunger.</td><td>Accept the innate body: "This is the body I was born to have."</td><td rowspan="3">Healthy Body Image

Prevention of Unhealthy and Disordered Eating</td></tr>
<tr><td>Balance attention to many aspects of identity. Looks are only one part.

Consistently satisfy hunger with enough varied, wholesome food in a stable, predictable manner.

Limit sedentary choices to promote a physically active lifestyle at all ages.

Choose role models who reflect a realistic standard.</td><td>Emphasize what can be influenced or chosen.</td><td>Enjoy eating for health, energy, and hunger satisfaction. Create a physically active lifestyle for fitness, endurance, fun, relaxation and stress relief.</td></tr>
<tr><td>Promote historical perspective on today's cultural attitudes related to body image.

Teach critical thinking about media messages that influence body image.

Support each other in resisting unhealthy norms about weight, dieting, low nutrient food choices, eating for entertainment, and sedentary entertainment.</td><td>Develop social and cultural resiliency.</td><td>Develop autonomy, self esteem, confidence, and the ability for critical thinking.</td></tr>
</table>

The Body Image Building Blocks

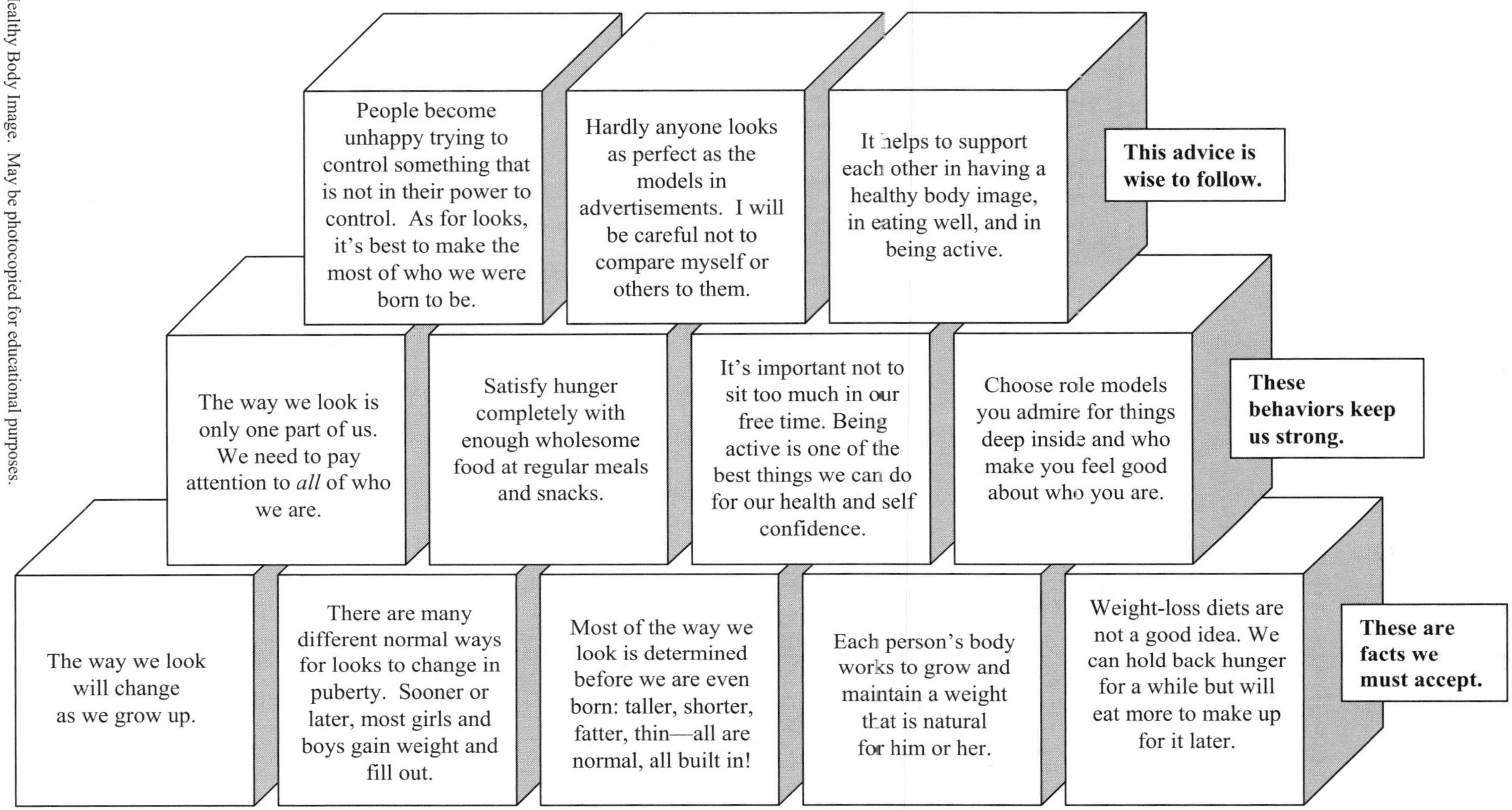

Toxic Cultural Myths Underlying Body Image, Eating, Fitness, Nutrition, and Weight Problems

IMAGE IS VALUED OVER SUBSTANCE: ***"How I look" is more important than "who I am." An essential criterion for the "right" look is a thin/lean body.***

DENIAL OF BIOLOGICAL DIVERSITY: ***Anyone can be slim if he or she works at it. Fatter people eat too much or are inactive. Fat is bad/wrong.***

DENIAL OF THE EFFECTS OF EXTERNALLY PRESCRIBED HUNGER REGULATION: ***Dieting is an effective weight-loss strategy.***

DISCOUNTING THE VALUE OF HEALTH; complacency about choices that do not result in the desired look: ***Eat, drink, & be merry… Healthy choices for health's sake are too much work!***

WHAT CAUSES DISORDERED EATING?

Five known factors contribute to body image and disordered-eating problems.

The first four of these depend on individual circumstances. Prevention or intervention is therefore required on an individual basis or with small groups of people who have been identified as experiencing that risk factor in common.

1) Psychological Stress:	A person who feels emotionally overwhelmed or out of control due to a stressful situation may channel difficult emotions into excessive pre-occupation with controlling body size, eating, and/or exercise.
2) Personality Traits:	People who by nature tend toward anxiety and perfectionism are more are more likely than others to fixate on rigid and unrealistic standards regarding weight, eating behaviors, and/or exercise.
3) Biochemical Imbalances:	Persons with biochemical imbalances may develop depression, anxiety, or compulsive tendencies. Since eating behaviors are known to have a soothing effect, certain people may develop a dependency on dysfunctional eating to temporarily relieve a difficult mood.
4) High-Risk Vocations:	The choice of a vocation or activity that emphasizes a thinner/leaner size as a predictor of success can contribute to disordered eating as people attempt to manipulate eating and/or exercise to control weight without regard to health and internal hunger.

While the above factors may contribute to disordered eating, experts agree that this result would almost never occur in the absence of the fifth factor, *socio-cultural pressures.*

5) Socio-Cultural Pressures:	The primary risk factors for body image problems and disordered eating are conveyed through cultural messages that encourage the drive to be thin, prejudices about diverse body sizes, the belief that calorie-restrictive "dieting" is an effective weight-loss method, and eating for entertainment versus energy and health. The U.S. has the highest incidence of disordered eating in the world, although other cultures that have embraced America's "thinness schema" are increasingly affected.

Since it is within our power to change or resist socio-cultural influences, these should be the focus of primary prevention efforts. Young people can and should be educated at an early age, preferably before puberty, about the unhealthy cultural myths that promote unhealthy body image, eating, and weight-related attitudes. Prevention and intervention should a part of mainstream child development.

Promoting Healthy Body Image, Eating, and Weight-Related Attitudes

To develop a healthy body image in today's social context, challenge toxic cultural myths that encourage body dissatisfaction, eating, fitness, and weight problems.

Challenge myths promoting image over substance: *"How I look" is more important than "who I am." An essential criterion for the "right" look is a thin/lean body.*

Teach students to understand and resist objectification:

- Acquire historical perspective on today's body image attitudes. Understand that an emphasis on superficial appearance is a formula for unhappiness.
- Become media-literate and recognize advertising strategies. Think critically about media messages that encourage unrealistic, unhealthy body image attitudes.
- Develop a strong sense of identity based on *inner* qualities, *not* on appearance.

Challenge myths that deny biological diversity: *Anyone can be slim if they work at it. Fatter people inevitably eat too much, and/or are not active. Fat is bad/wrong.*

Teach students the biological principals of size diversity:

- Understand the normal, expected addition of body fat that is common during puberty and other developmental stages of life.
- Respect and appreciate vast genetic diversity of body shapes and sizes.
- Understand how the internal weight regulatory system *limits* the extent of long-term control that is possible over weight. Many factors influence fatness/slimness. It is presumptuous and prejudicial to judge an individual's lifestyle behaviors by his or her appearance.

Challenge myths that deny the universal and negative effects of externally prescribed hunger regulation: *Dieting is an effective weight-loss strategy.*

Teach students the facts about dieting for weight loss:

- Recognize there are predictable, counterproductive results when hunger is not satisfied. Ninety percent of weight lost through dieting is regained, usually with added pounds.

Challenge myths that discount health as a value and that encourage complacency about choices that do not result in the desired look: *"Eat, drink, and be merry!" Healthy choices for health's sake are too much work.*

Teach children of every size to value health:

- Eat well. Satisfy hunger completely with a balanced variety of wholesome food that provides all the nutrients and energy your body needs. Enjoy "entertainment eating" in limited doses that do not interfere with nutritional needs or ignore hunger satiation.
- Make movement a priority. Spend enough time and energy engaged in physical activity to maintain your body's fitness level throughout the life cycle. Enjoy sedentary entertainment in limited doses that do not interfere with physical endurance, strength, and agility.
- Look for realistic role models that help you to feel good about who you are. Resist pressures, prescribed unrealistic weight standards, dieting, low-nutrient foods, and sedentary entertainment.

What Contributes to a Healthy Body and a Healthy Body Image?

- Integrity is valued over appearance.
- Innate size diversity is accepted and affirmed.
- Internal hunger regulation is trusted. Dieting is avoided.
- Hunger is routinely satisfied with food that balances wholesome nutrition, energy, enjoyment, and good taste.
- Physical activity is part of the daily routine and is maintained throughout life for fitness, self-confidence, and overall well-being.
- Role models reflect a realistic standard.

Ten Essential Lessons to Build Body Esteem

Start by accepting what is *not in your control*:

1) Accept your body's genetic predisposition. All bodies are wired to be fatter, thinner, or in between. This includes fatter in some places and thinner in others. Regardless of efforts to change it, over time your body will fight to maintain or resume the shape it was born to be. You may force your body into sizes and shapes that you prefer, but you can't beat Mother Nature without a tremendous cost.

2) Understand that all bodies change developmentally in ways that are simply not in your control through healthy means. You may positively influence changes of puberty, pregnancy and lactation, menopause, and aging by making healthy lifestyle choices, but you will not "control" these changes, no matter how much you try.

3) Never "diet." Hunger is an internally regulated drive and demands to be satisfied. If you restrict the food needed to satiate hunger, it will backfire, triggering preoccupation with food and ultimately an overeating or compulsive-eating response. You may lose weight in the short run, but 95% of weight that is lost through dieting is regained, plus added pounds. Dieters who go off their diets only to binge are not "weak willed." They are mammals whose built-in starvation response has kicked in—both physically and psychologically, going after what has been restricted. Scientific evidence has been available on this since the early 1950s, but most people remain unaware of the biologically predictable results of "dieting."

Then focus your attention and energy on what *is* possible to achieve:

4) Satisfy hunger completely with plenty of wholesome, nutrient-rich foods chosen from the core of the food pyramid: *eat well!* In today's world, surrounded by taste-stimulating, cheap, cleverly advertised, readily available, low-nutrient entertainment foods, learning to *feed* your body versus merely "eat" is an essential difference.

5) Limit sedentary entertainment. Move aerobically, if possible, on a regular basis. Everyone who is not medically inhibited, regardless of size, can and should develop a reasonable level of fitness and maintain it throughout the life cycle.

6) Understand that, if you eat well and maintain an active lifestyle over time, your best, natural weight will be revealed. Set a goal to eat well and be active. Don't be swayed by whether or not this makes you thin. Healthy, well-fed, active bodies are diverse in size and shape, from fat to thin and everything in between. Don't let anyone tell you otherwise, not even your doctor, who may be caught in unhealthy cultural myths about weight.

7) Choose role models who reflect a realistic standard against which you can feel good about yourself. If the Ugly Duckling had continued to compare herself to the ducks, she'd *still* be miserable, no matter how beautifully she developed.

8) Maintain your integrity as a human being. In spite of advertisements seducing you to believe that "image is everything," never forget that how you look is only one part of who you are. Develop a sense of identity based on all the many things you can do, the values you believe in, and the person that you are deep inside.

9) Become media savvy. Educate yourself about the hidden power of advertisements. Advertisers spend tons of money on strategies specifically designed to make you feel there is something wrong with you. Why? If they *first* advertise an unrealistic standard of beauty that leaves you feeling deficient by comparison, a product that promises to improve your condition is an easy sale. Don't be sold this bill of goods.

10) Encourage your friends and co-workers to join you in developing a healthy, realistic body image. Use the collective energy you might have spent criticizing your bodies to make the world a better place. Help the next generation to develop healthy body image attitudes and learn positive lifestyle habits.